GENRE IN ENGLISH MEDICAL WRITING, 1500–1820

Sociocultural Contexts of Production and Use

Written by an interdisciplinary team of scholars, this book offers novel perspectives on the history of medical writing and scientific thought styles by examining patterns of change and reception in genres, discourse, and lexis in the period 1500–1820. Each chapter demonstrates in detail how changing textual forms were closely tied to major multifaceted social developments: industrialisation, urbanisation, expanding trade, colonialisation, and changes in communication, all of which posed new demands on medical care. It then shows how these developments were reflected in a range of medical discourses, such as bills of mortality, medical advertisements, medical recipes, and medical rhetoric, and provides an extensive body of case studies to highlight how varieties of medical discourse have been targeted at different audiences over time. It draws on a wide range of methodological frameworks and is accompanied by numerous relevant illustrations, making it essential reading for academic researchers and students across the human sciences.

IRMA TAAVITSAINEN is Professor Emerita of English Philology at the University of Helsinki. Her research focuses on historical pragmatics, corpus linguistics, genre and register variation, and the evolution of scientific thought styles in medical writing.

TURO HILTUNEN is University Lecturer in English at the University of Helsinki. He has authored several studies on corpus pragmatics, corpus compilation, phraseology, and the language of science and medicine.

JEREMY J. SMITH is Professor Emeritus of English Philology at Glasgow University, and a Fellow of the Royal Society of Edinburgh. His interests include English historical linguistics, the history of Scots, and book history. Recent publications include *Transforming Early English* (2020).

CARLA SUHR is University Lecturer in English at the University of Helsinki. Her research focuses on early modern English medical writing and early news discourse, which she examines with methods adopted from historical (corpus) pragmatics, genre studies, and book history.

STUDIES IN ENGLISH LANGUAGE

The aim of this series is to provide a framework for original studies of English, both present-day and past. All books are based securely on empirical research, and represent theoretical and descriptive contributions to our knowledge of national and international varieties of English, both written and spoken. The series covers a broad range of topics and approaches, including syntax, phonology, grammar, vocabulary, discourse, pragmatics and sociolinguistics, and is aimed at an international readership.

Already published in this series:

Haruko Momma: *From Philology to English Studies: Language and Culture in the Nineteenth Century*
Raymond Hickey (ed.): *Standards of English: Codified Varieties around the World*
Benedikt Szmrecsanyi: *Grammatical Variation in British English Dialects: A Study in Corpus-Based Dialectometry*
Daniel Schreier and Marianne Hundt (eds.): *English as a Contact Language*
Bas Aarts, Joanne Close, Geoffrey Leech and Sean Wallis (eds.): *The Verb Phrase in English: Investigating Recent Language Change with Corpora*
Martin Hilpert: *Constructional Change in English: Developments in Allomorphy, Word Formation, and Syntax*
Jakob R. E. Leimgruber: *Singapore English: Structure, Variation, and Usage*
Christoph Rühlemann: *Narrative in English Conversation: A Corpus Analysis of Storytelling*
Dagmar Deuber: *English in the Caribbean: Variation, Style and Standards in Jamaica and Trinidad*
Eva Berlage: *Noun Phrase Complexity in English*
Nicole Dehé: *Parentheticals in Spoken English: The Syntax-Prosody Relation*
Jock O. Wong: *The Culture of Singapore English*
Marianne Hundt (ed.): *Late Modern English Syntax*
Irma Taavitsainen, Merja Kytö, Claudia Claridge and Jeremy Smith (eds.): *Developments in English: Expanding Electronic Evidence*
Arne Lohmann: *English Coordinate Constructions: A Processing Perspective on Constituent Order*

Nuria Yáñez-Bouza: *Grammar, Rhetoric and Usage in English: Preposition Placement 1500-1900*
Anita Auer, Daniel Schreier and Richard J. Watts (eds.): *Letter Writing and Language Change*
John Flowerdew and Richard W. Forest: *Signalling Nouns in English: A Corpus-Based Discourse Approach*
Jeffrey P. Williams, Edgar W. Schneider, Peter Trudgill and Daniel Schreier (eds.): *Further Studies in the Lesser-Known Varieties of English*
Jack Grieve: *Regional Variation in Written American English*
Douglas Biber and Bethany Gray: *Grammatical Complexity in Academic English: Linguistics Change in Writing*
Gjertrud Flermoen Stenbrenden: *Long-Vowel Shifts in English, c. 1050-1700: Evidence from Spelling*
Zoya G. Proshina and Anna A. Eddy (eds.): *Russian English: History, Functions, and Features*
Raymond Hickey (ed.): *Listening to the Past: Audio Records of Accents of English*
Phillip Wallage: *Negation in Early English: Grammatical and Functional Change*
Marianne Hundt, Sandra Mollin and Simone E. Pfenninger (eds.): *The Changing English Language: Psycholinguistic Perspectives*
Joanna Kopaczyk and Hans Sauer (eds.): *Binomials in the History of English: Fixed and Flexible*
Alexander Haselow: *Spontaneous Spoken English: An Integrated Approach to the Emergent Grammar of Speech*
Christina Sanchez-Stockhammer: *English Compounds and Their Spelling*
David West Brown: *English and Empire: Language History, Dialect, and the Digital Archive*
Paula Rodríguez-Puente: *The English Phrasal Verb, 1650-present: History, Stylistic Drifts, and Lexicalisation*
Erik. R. Thomas (ed.): *Mexican American English: Substrate Influence and the Birth of an Ethnolect*
Thomas Hoffmann: *English Comparative Correlatives: Diachronic and Synchronic Variation at the Lexicon-Syntax Interface*
Nuria Yáñez-Bouza, Emma Moore, Linda van Bergen and Willem B. Hollmann (eds.): *Categories, Constructions, and Change in English Syntax*
Raymond Hickey (ed.): *English in the German-speaking World*
Axel Bohmann: *Variation in English World-wide: Registers and Global Varieties*
Raymond Hickey (ed.): *English in Multilingual South Africa: The Linguistics of Contact and Change*
Jeremy J. Smith: *Transforming Early English: The Reinvention of Early English and Older Scots*
Tobias Bernaisch: *Gender in World Englishes*
Lorena Pérez-Hernández: *Speech Acts in English: From Research to Instruction and Textbook Development*
Elisabeth Reber: *Quoting in Parliamentary Question Time: Exploring Recent Change*
Marco Condorelli: *Standardising English Spelling: The Role of Printing in Sixteenth and Seventeenth-century Graphemic Developments*

Earlier titles not listed are also available

GENRE IN ENGLISH MEDICAL WRITING, 1500–1820

Sociocultural Contexts of Production and Use

EDITED BY

IRMA TAAVITSAINEN

University of Helsinki

TURO HILTUNEN

University of Helsinki

JEREMY J. SMITH

University of Glasgow

CARLA SUHR

University of Helsinki

CAMBRIDGE
UNIVERSITY PRESS

CAMBRIDGE
UNIVERSITY PRESS

Shaftesbury Road, Cambridge CB2 8EA, United Kingdom

One Liberty Plaza, 20th Floor, New York, NY 10006, USA

477 Williamstown Road, Port Melbourne, VIC 3207, Australia

314–321, 3rd Floor, Plot 3, Splendor Forum, Jasola District Centre, New Delhi – 110025, India

103 Penang Road, #05–06/07, Visioncrest Commercial, Singapore 238467

Cambridge University Press is part of Cambridge University Press & Assessment, a department of the University of Cambridge.

We share the University's mission to contribute to society through the pursuit of education, learning and research at the highest international levels of excellence.

www.cambridge.org
Information on this title: www.cambridge.org/9781009100090

DOI: 10.1017/9781009105347

First published 2022

A catalogue record for this publication is available from the British Library.

Library of Congress Cataloging-in-Publication Data
NAMES: Taavitsainen, Irma, editor. | Hiltunen, Turo, editor. | Smith, J. J. (Jeremy J.), editor. | Suhr, Carla, editor.
TITLE: Genre in English medical writing, 1500–1820 : sociocultural contexts of production and use / edited by Irma Taavitsainen, Turo Hiltunen, Jeremy J. Smith, Carla Suhr.
DESCRIPTION: Cambridge; New York, NY: Cambridge University Press, 2022. | Series: Studies in English language | Includes bibliographical references and index.
IDENTIFIERS: LCCN 2022023392 (print) | LCCN 2022023393 (ebook) | ISBN 9781009100090 (hardback) | ISBN 9781009108683 (paperback) | ISBN 9781009105347 (epub)
SUBJECTS: LCSH: Medical literature–Great Britain–History. | Medical literature–Europe–History. | English language–Medical English. | English language–Discourse analysis. | Sociolinguistics. | BISAC: LANGUAGE ARTS & DISCIPLINES / Linguistics / Historical & Comparative
CLASSIFICATION: LCC R118.6 .G455 2022 (print) | LCC R118.6 (ebook) | DDC 610.1/4–dc23/eng/20220615
LC record available at https://lccn.loc.gov/2022023392
LC ebook record available at https://lccn.loc.gov/2022023393

ISBN 978-1-009-10009-0 Hardback

Contents

Figures

Image Gallery

Tables

Notes on Contributors

CHIARA BENATI is Professor of Germanic Philology at the University of Genoa, Italy. Her research interests include Middle High German literature, Middle Low German-Scandinavian language contact, Faroese language and literature, Germanic charms and blessings, the earliest (Low) German surgical treatises, and their specialised terminology.

ISABEL DE LA CRUZ-CABANILLAS is Full Professor of English Philology at the University of Alcalá, Spain. Her interests include medical manuscript studies, and lexicology and semantics in the history of the English language. She has published widely in these fields.

TURO HILTUNEN works as University Lecturer in English at the University of Helsinki, Finland. He has authored several studies on corpus pragmatics, corpus compilation, phraseology, and the language of science and medicine.

ALPO HONKAPOHJA is based at the University of Oslo, Norway, working on an EU MSCA IF project on the Cotton manuscript group. His research interests include historical linguistics, codicology, lexicology, digital humanities, and medieval medicine. The research in this volume is based on the British Academy–funded project Tracing John of Burgundy.

LORI JONES is a medical historian at Carleton University and the University of Ottawa, Canada. Her research focuses primarily on plague texts and images. A monograph version of her dissertation and two edited volumes on disease in the medieval and early modern worlds are appearing in 2022.

PETER MURRAY JONES is Fellow at King's College, Cambridge, UK, and a medical historian affiliated to the Department of History and

Philosophy of Science at the University of Cambridge. His publications focus on medicine from the Middle Ages to the eighteenth century. He has a particular interest in relations between knowledge and practice as expressed in texts and images.

ÁGNES KUNA is Assistant Professor at the Department of Applied Linguistics and Phonetics, Eötvös Loránd University of Budapest, Hungary. Her main research interest is the linguistic study of doctor–patient interaction and medical language in historical and modern contexts.

MARTTI MÄKINEN works as University Lecturer of English at Hanken School of Economics, Helsinki, Finland. His research interests are genre studies, early and current scientific writing, learner academic writing, and manuscript studies. He has published several articles on these themes.

RODERICK MCCONCHIE, formerly of the University of Helsinki, Finland, is now an independent researcher working on the history of medical dictionaries and the history of lexicography more generally. He is currently writing a biography of Dr Robert James (1703–76).

ANNA ILONA RAJALA has a multidisciplinary background in philosophy, politics, and health sciences. She has clinical experience in physiotherapy, and her research focuses on critical physiotherapy studies, critical theory, and ethics with a special interest in dementia, disability, and representations of health and illness in literature.

MAURA RATIA has been working as University Lecturer in English at the University of Helsinki, Finland. Many of her publications are on medical writing, especially that of the early modern period. At the moment, her main research interests include genre analysis, historical pragmatics, and the London plague epidemics.

JEREMY J. SMITH is Professor Emeritus of English Philology at Glasgow University, and a Fellow of the Royal Society of Edinburgh, Scotland. His interests include English historical linguistics, the history of Scots, and book history. Recent publications include *Transforming Early English* (Cambridge University Press, 2020).

CARLA SUHR is University Lecturer in English at the University of Helsinki, Finland. Her research focuses on early modern English medical writing and early news discourse, which she examines with methods adopted from historical (corpus) pragmatics, genre studies, and book history.

IRMA TAAVITSAINEN is Professor Emerita of English Philology at the University of Helsinki, Finland. Her research focuses on historical pragmatics, corpus linguistics, genre and register variation, and the evolution of scientific thought styles in medical writing. She has published widely in these fields.

ALBERTO TANTURRI is Associate Professor of Early Modern History at the Catholic University of the Sacred Heart, Milan, Italy. His main research interests are concentrated within the fields of social history of medicine, history of medical thought, and history of welfare institutions.

TIMO UOTINEN specialises in English literature and philosophy, especially in the intersections between Shakespeare and early modern and modern philosophy. His research focuses on Shakespearean tragedies and the philosophy of Sir Francis Bacon, and he is also interested in Shakespearean influences on the Finnish novelist Aleksis Kivi.

Preface

In recent years, medical writings from the past have attracted a great deal of attention from scholars in a variety of related disciplines, and research on these materials, as in medical humanities more generally, has become increasingly multidisciplinary. This diversity of approach was reflected in the papers presented at the Second International Conference on Historical Medical Discourse (CHIMED-2) organised at the University of Helsinki in June 2019. Presentations at the conference drew upon a wide variety of cognate disciplines, including the history of medicine, linguistic and literary studies, and book history. Several themes emerged during CHIMED-2, and several underpin this collection of papers, all contributing to the current recuperation of philology within the wider frame of interdisciplinary research. The current volume contains not only revised versions of these papers, but several invited contributions, reflecting the richness of this field of research. All offer new insights into the ways in which medical discourse was deployed, both within and beyond explicitly medical situations.

With the advent of digital corpora and large digital archives capturing linguistic 'big data', empirical methods have become mainstream in historical linguistics. But while these resources improve the objectivity, reliability, and generalisability of research results, they also place additional requirements on selecting relevant data for analysis and appropriate conceptual classification. It is clear that textual research needs categories such as genres, text types, and registers that can serve as structural guides for corpus compilation. They are discussed in this volume together with textual traditions and changing conventions, pertinent to the creation of genres in the diachronic perspective. The richness of the medical register is what inspired this collection, and specifically the contexts of production and use of medical genres. In other words, context matters, and this concern has driven the current collection of papers.

Acknowledgements

The richness of the medical register with its recent discoveries of long-forgotten materials and new digital databases offers ample opportunities for original research. The contributors of this volume have been inspired by this state of affairs, and we are very happy to see this collective volume come true without overdue delay, in spite of the challenges posed by the pandemic. Several contributors faced problems from COVID-19, as some countries were particularly hard hit, libraries were shut down for longer periods and their role in supporting research activities suffered. Nevertheless, the difficulties were overcome, and we would like to thank these institutions for their collaboration and permission to use images from their collections.

The point of departure for this book, the CHIMED-2 Conference in 2019, received funding from the Federation of Finnish Learned Societies and the University of Helsinki. We would like to thank these institutions for their support. Our thanks are also due to the devoted and efficient conference secretary Noora Kumpulainen, who worked tirelessly behind the scenes to make sure the event became friendly and inspiring. As editorial secretary, Noora's contribution to preparing the book for publication was also invaluable.

We would like to thank the CUP team – Helen Barton, Isabel Collins and Stephanie Taylor – for their support, advice and collaboration. The series editor Merja Kytö deserves our special word of thanks for her constructive and helpful comments during the editorial process, and for accepting our volume into the series.

We are also grateful to the anonymous reviewers of the book proposal and the individual chapters for their insightful comments and constructive criticism that improved the volume as a whole a great deal.

CHAPTER 1

Medical Discourse and Sociocultural Contexts 1500–1820

Irma Taavitsainen, Jeremy J. Smith, Turo Hiltunen, and Carla Suhr

This volume illustrates the wide-ranging forms and functions of medical discourse, expressed through a variety of genres across several centuries from the early modern period to the long eighteenth century. In the background are dynamic and complex societal developments such as increasing trade and sea travel, and colonialisation leading to intercultural encounters of greater and lesser aggression and – as a result – pandemic outbreaks. The authors of the chapters in the collection come from many different disciplinary backgrounds: linguistic, philological, codicological, historical, and literary. Nevertheless, despite this variety of approaches, there are clear cross-cutting themes – organising principles – that run through the whole book, most importantly genre and tradition, and multimodality and interdisciplinarity. These themes are conceptual pillars supporting the volume's architecture, pointing to future directions for research.

1.1 Research Questions

All chapters in this book engage with the register of medical discourse, but take a broad view of what is meant by the notion. We aim to show how medical texts were modified to new uses and forms across several centuries, and how medical discourse was deployed in different cultural contexts. Central research questions addressed in this collection include how medical discourse was created and deployed by authors, how medical texts were used by different readers for different purposes, and how medical ideas were transmitted across time and space.

In answering these research questions the importance of *genres* has proved key to understanding the history of medical discourse. Thus, genre theories and qualitative analyses of instantiations of individual genres receive special attention, bringing together the analysis of text traditions with cultural, textual, contextual, and sociohistorical perspectives.

We hold, uncontroversially, that sociocultural contexts are crucial for identifying particular shades of meaning and cultural signification in medical discourse, whether expressed linguistically or visually. And we are fully aware of the importance of breaking down the traditional boundaries imposed by periodisation, illustrating in our discussions how profound and dynamic societal changes have informed the materials under review. We consider that our focused discussions on the evolution and life cycle of medical texts provide potential models for the advancement of future textually oriented historical genre studies.

1.2 Definitions of Key Terms

The term *genre* and its relatives *register*, *text type*, and *style* are slippery notions used in different ways by various researchers. According to Biber and Conrad (2009), *register* combines linguistic characteristics with situational use, and researchers often rely on text extracts in digital corpora to pinpoint typical characteristics. Following this definition, medical discourse includes both written and spoken registers of situational language use.[1]

By contrast, the *genre* perspective focuses on conventions, employing linguistic analysis to take into account different contexts. Genre has proved a particularly useful analytical concept in highlighting different aspects of the production, structure, and reception of medical discourse. Pertinent examples include Atkinson's (1992) overview of the diachronic development of genres, in particular the case report; Salager-Meyer, Alcaraz Ariza, and Pabón Berbesí's (2007) analysis of medical book reviews; and Taavitsainen's (2016) study of changing genre dynamics drawing upon literary studies on genre (see Fowler 1982).[2] Other related terms include *text type* (Werlich 1982), typically categorised into five subtypes according to linguistic features,[3] and *style*, which, despite being commonly associated with literary analysis, can usefully be applied to non-literary texts as well (Crystal & Davy 1969; Leech & Short 1981; Fowler 1986; see also Locher & Jucker 2021). In addition to these concepts, this collection

[1] The two terms are widely used and well established, though otherwise the uses of *register* and *genre* are not as streamlined. More recently, the distinction launched by Biber and Conrad (2009) has gained wide acceptance, see e.g. Claridge (2017 [2012]).

[2] See also Atkinson (1999) and Gross, Harmon, and Reidy (2002) on the evolution of scientific genres beyond medicine.

[3] The five text types are narrative, argumentative, descriptive, expository, and instructive.

provides insights into *textual traditions* involving diachronic sequences of intertextually linked texts (Taavitsainen 2001: 150).

From early on, register and genre studies have employed corpus-linguistic methods in stylistic applications,[4] but the availability of digital corpora has enabled the raising of novel research questions on register variation and opened up new ways of dealing with language variability.[5] Biber's (1988) influential study of registers belongs to *variational genre analysis* and demonstrates how a synthesis of corpus-linguistic and statistical methods (in this case factor analysis) can be used to map language variation along several dimensions.[6] These and other studies have contributed to increased precision, objectivity, and replicability in language research. Historical genres vary and change through time in relation to each other and with respect to the oral-literate dimension. Biber and Finegan (1989) observed a 'drift' towards orality across different genres and have inspired further diachronic studies on popularisation and democratisation (e.g. Farrelly & Seoane 2012; Hiltunen & Loureiro-Porto 2020).

Genre studies have moreover long been a staple in Applied Linguistics, where the emphasis has been on the communicative function of genres, mostly in present-day writings (Swales 1990, 2004). Central to these studies is the question of how the results of genre analysis can be applied in the context of teaching English for specific purposes, but otherwise the approach is essentially the same as in variational genre analysis: to identify and describe conventional text structures and genre conventions. In all cases it is, however, clear that a full understanding of historical genres necessitates a careful contextualisation of textual evidence and an appraisal of contemporaneous communicative contexts. Another source of complexities in historical genre analysis is the notion of *hybridity* that pertains to genre dynamics: changes in existing genres, formations of new ones, and the interlinkage between them. Such hybridity in the context of the long traditions of medical writing often goes unnoticed in studies focusing on modern genres.[7]

[4] Some articles in Sebeok (1960) use statistical methods for defining stylistic characteristics of the assessed texts.

[5] The CHIMED-2 conference yielded material for another collected volume, *Corpus Pragmatic Studies on the History of Medical Discourse*, edited by Hiltunen and Taavitsainen (in press a).

[6] The most important ones from the diachronic perspective are Informational vs Involved Production, Narrative vs Non-Narrative Concerns, Explicit vs Situation-Dependent Reference, and Overt Expression of Persuasion.

[7] For example, a study of narrativity in blogs, medical case reports, and medical case presentations in recent writing (Dorgeloh 2016) ignores the earlier phases where the doctors' and the patients' narratives are closely interwoven. See in particular Taavitsainen (2011) and Lehto and Taavitsainen (2019).

1.3 Genre and Tradition

The distinction between the terms suits the present collection, as variability of language related to conventions and traditions of writing is a leading theme in several chapters and surfaces in various contexts in other chapters as well. The major contribution of the book in the area of discourse and genre analysis is placing texts into a larger frame of traditions, where both the social and cultural contexts of production and use as well as the meaning-making processes of written texts as communicative events receive attention. All contributions emphasise the notion of context in its variable forms in textual production and use.

Traditionally, philological scholarship on textual transmission focused on geographical dialect variation or the comparison between different versions to establish 'original' readings. This goal has increasingly given way to more sociopragmatic and sociolinguistic concerns, the successful integration of which into philological studies, together with corpus linguistics, has given new vitality to this ancient discipline – especially as the 'digital turn' has rendered manuscript resources and early printed data more accessible (see Fulk 2016; Hiltunen & Taavitsainen in press b). Philology has thus undergone a renewal in both goals and methods. Philologists commonly seek to show how texts, seen as cultural products, reached their audiences and were used by their readers, a research goal that aligns well with the exciting and more recent theoretical paradigm known as historical pragmatics (e.g. Jucker 2008; Taavitsainen 2015; Włodarczyk & Taavitsainen 2017), which emphasises how meaning-making processes exist within multilayered contexts. Textual forms, in sum, are intimately linked to their sociocultural functions. This shift in philological orientation applies as much to the analysis of scientific and medical registers as to literary interpretation.

Research in this conceptual and contextual frame is necessarily wide in scope, ranging from attention to minute detail to engagement with overarching 'worldviews' and humanity's place within them. For instance, in medical discourse before the 'new science', humoral medicine and medical astrology saw celestial influences as projected on all worldly affairs, not only health and disease (a view still current in some popular discourse), and this 'holistic' view of medicine was reflected in the terminology deployed by contemporary writers. Chapters in this collection thus range from delicate analysis of detail to wider textual surveys engaged with the cultural construction of diseases such as the plague (see Figures 1 and 2 in the Image Gallery). New methodologies have been developed to meet the new challenges. Cues to interpretation are provided by material characteristics of textual witnesses, including hands, illustrations, layout and quality of paper, and other aspects that aid in pragmatic meaning-making assessments (see Pahta & Jucker 2011; Smith 2020). Comparisons between various versions show how texts were modified, transcribed, translated, revised, and published in new formats, and shared across wider geographical areas within Europe. In addition to comparisons between text realisations with possible modifications revealing what the people involved considered important, the chapters in this volume draw on this kind of discourse variation, largely ignored in previous studies.

Another feature of the chapters in this book is their emphasis on variation in discourse forms in texts that were repurposed for new readerships removed in time from the original compositions, often by decades or centuries, and thus within new sociocultural settings. All highlight the common European core to be found in medical writing. Text traditions in Western medical writing go back to classical antiquity. Several genres were created in Greek and Latin science and, modified by Arab scientists, mediated to later periods, and finally to several European languages (Pahta & Taavitsainen 2010). The vernacularisation boom in medical texts started in the late medieval period and went on for several centuries (see Voigts 1989; Siraisi 1990; Crossgrove 1998). In the early modern period, medical texts were produced by a wide variety of practitioners with different levels of medical training, and the readership expanded as well. University-educated physicians such as William Bullein (see Figure 3 in the Image Gallery) were joined by authors with careers as apothecaries, quacks, or man-midwives, for example (see Figures 4–6 in the Image Gallery). Several chapters in the volume trace the transmission of key texts and their text conventions, first developed in late medieval times but 'reinvented' in the early modern period. The analyses describe various modifications as the texts moved through time and space, being adapted to different target audiences in both contents and material features, showing once more how textual forms and sociocultural functions are closely intertwined. For instance, a stable genre like recipes, drawing on more than two thousand years of 'wisdom', demonstrates how exceptionally strong and binding traditions of writing can be (see below and e.g. Görlach 2008; Alonso-Almeida 2013). Recipes were repeatedly translated and copied, and became more complicated and hybridised over time when mixed with other emerging genres. Individual recipes were compiled into collections – produced in manuscript and print – but they could also be embedded into other established genres of medical discourse such as treatises and health guides. But while the prototypical form of recipes remained constant through the medieval period into the early modern period and beyond, their language and style were influenced by historical, cultural, and societal changes.

1.4 Multimodality, Interdisciplinarity, and 'Normal Science'

A notable feature of this collection is its deployment of interdisciplinary and cross-disciplinary approaches, as researchers borrow methodologies from different areas, contributing to the reimagining of the philological enterprise and new empirical approaches. A pertinent example is provided by multimodal analysis, which analyses not only the linguistic characteristics of texts but also the physical aspects of manuscripts, printed books, and visual images, in order to discern more implicit meanings that were perhaps explicit at their time but are lost to modern readers.

Multimodality with regard to physical aspects of the page also receives attention with a meaning-making potential that may pass unnoticed without careful analysis (see Peikola et al. 2017). Material forms of books with wear and tear, whether in manuscript or in print, are susceptible to various interpretations, but it is not straightforward to determine how these texts were used by their readers, or how we can gain access to past reception. Methods of dealing with possible appropriations are in need of further elaboration, as the answers to pertinent questions tend to be elusive and hard to come by (Chartier 1992: viii–ix). However, steps in this direction have already been taken.

Several chapters illustrate the ways in which dominant paradigms of thinking underpin what Thomas Kuhn calls 'normal science' at particular points in time, bearing out his dictum that 'there is no standard higher than the assent of the relevant community' (1970: 94). As Kuhn (1970) and others have regularly insisted, all scientific discourses – and medical discourse is not an exception – are culturally situated; thus (for instance) 'Enlightenment' or 'Romantic' medical discourses are inflected with 'Enlightened' or 'Romantic' ideological assumptions and concerns, both within the community of medical practitioners and more widely in society.

Medical discourses, reflecting these ideological assumptions, have a broad currency, and again chapters in this collection demonstrate their pan-European reach. The focus of the volume is on Britain, but of course medical issues were discussed in contemporaneous German and Hungarian medical literature as well as Italian historical texts. Spain and Portugal are also involved, since they played an important role as an intermediary between the Old World and the Americas, introducing unknown medical ingredients and new ways of looking at nature by direct observation instead of relying on inherited wisdom. Many chapters display different forms of engagement with new developments in medical science stemming from the pan-European Enlightenment.

Contributions to this volume show that regardless of the considerable geographical distances, medical discourses exhibit similar patterns as texts travelled across Europe both at the time of vernacularisation and in the post-medieval period, and English writers shared profoundly in this pan-European medical culture. This culture forms an additional major theme in this volume and is particularly prominent in relation to the cultural construction of disease. On the one hand, we can assume that the diseases under a label like *pestilence* or *fever* remained much the same, although viruses also mutate, as we know so well from the COVID-19 pandemic. On the other hand, as has already been emphasised, diagnoses and treatment of diseases are always culturally constructed and vary in time.

1.5 Organisation of the Volume

Although all the contributions in this book can be read as independent pieces of research, they nevertheless fall into distinct groups. The four chapters at the beginning, by Peter Murray Jones, Lori Jones, Chiara Benati, and Alpo Honkapohja, are firmly anchored in late medieval texts, but consider what the transition from medieval to early modern and beyond involved. Chapter 2 by Peter Jones describes how a treatise by the fourteenth-century master surgeon John Arderne continued to be in common use into the seventeenth century, but in manuscript form; Jones argues that studying the afterlives of this work 'overturns assumptions made about periodisation and the coming of print culture to Europe'. Similarly focused on textual afterlives are Chapter 3 by Lori Jones, which traces how the late fourteenth-century *Gouernayl of Helþe* by John Mirfield was reworked in the sixteenth century to reflect changes in medical practice, and Benati's Chapter 4, which describes the way in which two early German translations of medical works negotiated the transition from script to print. Honkapohja's Chapter 5 describes the textual afterlives, during the early modern period, of *John of Burgundy's Treatise*, a plague tract from the medieval period. Through detailed examination of the language, contents, and material contexts of later reworkings of this text, Honkapohja demonstrates the *Treatise*'s continuing societal impact, as a link between medieval and early modern medicine.

The following four chapters by Alberto Tanturri, Roderick McConchie, Jeremy J. Smith, and Isabel de la Cruz-Cabanillas focus on the terminology of medical science, including its transition into wider culture. Tanturri's description of medical responses to the Noja plague of 1815–1816 in Chapter 6 shows how the 'Brunonian' system of thought skewed treatment practices in the face of an appalling pandemic; Chapter 7, a short supplementary commentary to Tanturri's paper by Smith, offers a bridge to the remaining papers in the set. McConchie's study of eighteenth-century medical dictionaries and encyclopaedias in Chapter 8 demonstrates the systematisation of knowledge associated with Enlightened thinking, represented on a larger scale by the great French encyclopaedists. Next, in Chapter 9 Smith shows, through an analysis of vocabulary, how literary responses to medical debates in the early nineteenth century drew not only on the Enlightened inheritance – including Brunonianism – but also new transformative, Romantic developments in what has been called 'imaginative intensity'. Smith's chapter introduces a literary theme that is picked up again in the last contribution to the volume (Rajala and Uotinen's Chapter 16). Finally in this part, Chapter 10 by de la Cruz-Cabanillas traces the adoption of a wide range of new substances into the lexis of medical recipes from the sixteenth, seventeenth, and eighteenth centuries. The origins of these substances are located in the Americas and in Asia, as well as in continental Europe.

The next three chapters, by Irma Taavitsainen, Maura Ratia, and Carla Suhr, address the process of change and how it takes place in specific genres: how does an existing template, which is familiar to both medical authors and readers and as such guides the production and reception of discourse, adopt new components and lose others? In what ways are these changes linked to social, ideological, and disciplinary changes? Taavitsainen's Chapter 11 focuses on one prominent medical writer's use of genres, which constructs a unique discourse type that responds to the rhetorical needs of the communicative situation at the crossroads of old and new medical science. She shows how Walter Bailey skilfully draws on long-standing genres like *commentaries* and *recipes* and mixes them with discourse forms characteristic of the emerging empiricist repertoire. Ratia in Chapter 12 investigates *Bills of Mortality*, a hybrid genre that despite its linkage with core medical genres has received relatively little attention in previous philological scholarship. Bills of mortality operate at the intersection of several discourses – for instance religious discourse, medical discourses of aetiology and advice-giving, as well as the emerging commercialisation of medicine – whose prominence in individual texts varies diachronically. Finally in this group the themes of genre hybridity and the commercialisation of medicine are at the core of Suhr's Chapter 13 on pamphlet advertisements. Applying move analysis to the material, Suhr traces the changing repertoire of genre components from which pamphlet advertisements were derived. Some of these components can be traced back to medieval medical writing and beyond, while others were contemporary innovations.

The chapters by Ágnes Kuna and Martti Mäkinen take a different approach, focusing on early modern medical recipes and the communicative function of persuasion. In Chapter 15, Mäkinen approaches persuasion in English texts through the lens of metadiscourse by mapping metadiscourse items onto the three rhetorical concepts of *ethos*, *pathos*, and *logos*, while Kuna identifies and examines the conceptual categories used for persuasion in Hungarian medical recipes in Chapter 14. Kuna applies reliability testing of semantic categories in analysing her historical data, drawing on methods of qualitative analysis widely adopted in psychology, for instance, but rarely adopted in linguistics (but see Jucker 2008). The methodologies chosen for these two complementary studies illustrate the complexity of the concept of persuasion as a textual strategy. Both studies stress the necessity of factoring in contextual information about contemporary society and culture in the classification of linguistic features.

The final chapter in this volume makes use of the results from multiple disciplines, including literary analysis, disability studies, and medical archaeology, thus underlining the interdisciplinary nature of the collection's scope. In Chapter 16, Anna Ilona Rajala and Timo Uotinen describe the deployment of medical tropes in depictions of the body of Richard III, the last Plantagenet king. In doing so, they focus on the role of myth and interpretation in descriptions of Richard's physical and social disability in early modern English historiography, Shakespeare's plays, and modern scientific reports written after the discovery of Richard's bones in 2012. This chapter shows us that medical topics are not restricted to medical discourses, but play a role in the history of representation, the politics of narrative, and the subjectivity of interpretation, regardless of time and place.

The Image Gallery at the end of the volume gives illustrations of textual features and highlights some of the above themes with concrete examples. References to pertinent plates are inserted in the chapters.

It will be clear from these short summaries that the collection ranges widely, illustrating the richness of the field. We hope to have offered in this volume a kaleidoscopic, 'cubist,' and – we believe – novel angle on the history of medical discourses, in which significant new insights are achieved by approaching the materials under review from a variety of perspectives.

REFERENCES

Alonso-Almeida, Francisco. 2013. Genre conventions in English recipes, 1600–1800. In Michelle DiMeo & Sara Pennell (eds.), *Reading and writing recipe books, 1550–1800*, 68–90. Manchester: Manchester University Press.

Atkinson, Dwight. 1992. The evolution of medical research writing from 1735 to 1985: The case of the *Edinburgh Medical Journal*. *Applied Linguistics* 13: 337–74.

Atkinson, Dwight. 1999. Scientific discourse in sociohistorical context: The *Philosophical Transactions of the Royal Society of London*, 1675–1975. Mahwah, NJ: Erlbaum.

Biber, Douglas. 1988. *Variation across speech and writing*. Cambridge: Cambridge University Press.

Biber, Douglas, & Susan Conrad. 2009. *Register, genre and style*. Cambridge: Cambridge University Press.

Biber, Douglas, & Edward Finegan. 1989. Drift and the evolution of English style: A history of three genres. *Language* 65(3): 487–517.

Chartier, Roger. 1992. *The order of books*. Cambridge: Polity Press.

Claridge, Claudia. 2017 [2012]. Styles, registers, genres and text types. In Alex Bergs & Laurel Brinton (eds.), *Historical outlines from sound to text: Reprint articles from English historical linguistics: An international handbook*, 218–37. Berlin: Walter de Gruyter.

Crossgrove, William. 1998. Introduction. In William Crossgrove, Margaret Schleissner, & Linda Ehrsam Voigts (eds.), *Early Science and Medicine* 3 (2): 81–7. Special issue.

Crystal, David, & Derek Davy. 1969. *Investigating English style*. London: Longmans.

Dorgeloh, Heidrun. 2016. The interrelationship of register and genre in medical discourse. In Christoph Schubert & Christina Sanchez-Stockhammer (eds.), *Variational text linguistics: Revisiting register in English*, 43–65. Berlin: de Gruyter.

Farrelly, Michael, & Elena Seoane. 2012. Democratization. In Terttu Nevalainen & Elizabeth Closs Traugott (eds.), *The Oxford handbook of the history of English*, 392–401. New York: Oxford University Press.

Fowler, Alistair. 1982. *Kinds of literature*. Oxford: Oxford University Press.

Fowler, Roger. 1986. *Linguistic criticism*. Oxford: Oxford University Press.

Fulk, Robert D. 2016. Philological methods. In Merja Kytö & Päivi Pahta (eds.), *English historical linguistics*, 95–107. Cambridge: Cambridge University Press.

Görlach, Manfred. 2008. *Text types and the history of English*. Berlin: De Gruyter Mouton.

Gross, Alan G., Joseph E. Harmon, & Michael Reidy. 2002. *Communicating science: The scientific article from the 17th century to the present*. Oxford: Oxford University Press.

Hiltunen, Turo, & Lucía Loureiro-Porto. 2020. Democratization of Englishes: Synchronic and diachronic approaches. *Language Sciences* 79: 101275.

Hiltunen, Turo, & Irma Taavitsainen (eds.). In press a. *Corpus pragmatic studies on the history of medical discourse*. Pragmatics and Beyond New Series, vol. 330. Amsterdam: Benjamins.

Hiltunen, Turo, & Taavitsainen, Irma. In press b. Corpora, pragmatics, and historical medical discourse. In Turo Hiltunen & Irma Taavitsainen (eds.), *Corpus Pragmatic Studies on the History of Medical Discourse*, 1–19. Pragmatics and Beyond New Series, vol. 330. Amsterdam: Benjamins.

Jucker, Andreas H. 2008. Historical pragmatics. *Language and Linguistic Compass* 2(5): 894–906.

Kuhn, Thomas. 1970. *The structure of scientific revolutions*, 2nd ed. Chicago: University of Chicago Press.

Leech, Geoffrey N., & Mick Short. 1981. *Style in fiction: A linguistic introduction to English fictional prose*. Milton: Routledge.

Lehto, Anu, & Irma Taavitsainen. 2019. Medical case reports in Late Modern English. In Irma Taavitsainen & Turo Hiltunen (eds.), *Late Modern English medical texts: Writing medicine in the eighteenth century*, 89–111. Amsterdam: John Benjamins.

Locher, Miriam A., & Andreas H. Jucker. 2021. *The pragmatics of fiction: Literature, stage and screen discourse*. Edinburgh: Edinburgh University Press.

Pahta, Päivi, & Andreas H. Jucker. 2011. *Communicating Early English manuscripts*. Cambridge: Cambridge University Press.

Pahta, Päivi, & Irma Taavitsainen. 2010. Scientific discourse. In Andreas H. Jucker & Irma Taavitsainen (eds.), *Historical pragmatics*, 549–86. Vol. VIII of Wolfram Bubliz, Andreas H. Jucker, & Klaus P. Schneider (eds.), *Handbook of pragmatics*, vols. I–X. Berlin: Mouton de Gruyter.

Peikola, Matti, Aleksi Mäkilahde, Hanna Salmi, Mari-Liisa Varila, & Janne Skaffari (eds.). 2017. *Verbal and visual communication in Early English texts*. Turnhout: Brepols.

Salager-Meyer, Francoise, María Ángeles Alcaraz Ariza, & Maryelis Pabón Berbesí. 2007. Collegiality, critique and the construction of scientific argumentation in medical book reviews: A diachronic approach. *Journal of Pragmatics* 39, 1758–74.

Sebeok, Thomas (ed.). 1960. *Style in language*. New York: Massachusetts Institute of Technology.

Siraisi, Nancy G. 1990. *Medieval and early Renaissance medicine: An introduction to knowledge and practice.* Chicago: University of Chicago Press.

Smith, Jeremy. 2020. *Transforming Early English: The reinvention of Early English and Older Scots.* Cambridge: Cambridge University Press.

Swales, John M. 1990. *Genre analysis: English in academic and research settings.* Cambridge: Cambridge University Press.

Swales, John M. 2004. *Research genres: Explorations and applications.* Cambridge: Cambridge University Press.

Taavitsainen, Irma. 2001. Changing conventions of writing: The dynamics of genres, text types, and text traditions. *European Journal of English Studies* 5 (2): 139–50.

Taavitsainen, Irma. 2011. Medical case reports and scientific thought-styles. *Revista de Lenguas para Fines Específicos* 17, Special issue, Francisco Alonso Almeida (ed.), 75–98.

Taavitsainen, Irma. 2015. Historical pragmatics. In Douglas Biber & Randy Reppen (eds.), *The Cambridge handbook of English corpus linguistics*, 252–68. Cambridge: Cambridge University Press.

Taavitsainen, Irma. 2016. Genre dynamics in the history of English. In Merja Kytö & Päivi Pahta (eds.), *English historical linguistics*, 271–85. Cambridge: Cambridge University Press.

Voigts, Linda E. 1989. Scientific and medical books. In Jeremy Griffiths & Derek Pearsall (eds.), *Book production and publishing in Britain 1375–1475*, 345–402. Cambridge: Cambridge University Press.

Werlich, Egon. 1982. *A text grammar of English.* Heidelberg: Quelle & Meyer.

Włodarczyk, Matylda, & Taavitsainen, Irma. 2017. Historical (socio)pragmatics at present. *Journal of Historical Pragmatics* 18(2): 159–74.

CHAPTER 2

John Arderne's Afterlife in Manuscript and Print

Peter Murray Jones

This chapter will explore the fortunes of one particular fourteenth-century English surgical text, written by the master surgeon John Arderne (1307–c. 1380), which remained in active use (that is to say it continued to act as a guide to practice) until late into the seventeenth century. It will argue that the long life of this text, particularly in its manuscript form, overturns assumptions made about periodisation and the coming of print culture to Europe. The first of these assumptions is ingrained in modern scholarly disciplines. The year 1500 is often taken by historians and literary specialists to be the point at which 'medieval' turns into 'early modern'. Scholars in these fields define their individual specialisms by identifying with one side or another of the divide at 1500. They will typically write books and articles that use this date as a boundary beyond which they do not trespass. To take one pertinent example, *The Cambridge History of Science*, Volume 2 (Lindberg & Shank 2013) deals with *Medieval Science*, Volume 3 with *Early Modern Science* (Park & Daston 2006), with 1500 as an implicit dividing line, and they employ different sets of contributors. A second similar assumption is paradigmatic for book history, in which the incunabular era (pre-1501) is distinguished from later printing, and which treats manuscript books as co-existent with incunables, but as having more or less lost the battle for media supremacy by 1500. Admittedly this assumption has been questioned vigorously over the last twenty-five years, but here again specialists in manuscripts and specialists in printed books still tend to retain career identities predicated on this division of manuscript and print eras. *The Cambridge History of the Book in Britain* divided its Volume 3 (Hellinga 1999) from Volume 4 (Barnard 2002) at 1557, taking the royal charter given to the Stationers' Company in that year as marking a more significant boundary for books than the year 1500. But the theme of Volume 3 is the transition from manuscript to print, thus perpetuating the idea of modernity attaching to print first stated so compellingly by Sir Francis Bacon in his *Instauratio Magna* of 1620.

2.1 Arderne's Writings

The publishing history of the *Practica* on fistula in ano written by the English surgeon John Arderne (Jones 2004) in 1376 will be the subject of this chapter, and will be used to test the assumptions described in the paragraph above. John Arderne's writings on surgery for fistula in ano and his book of medical recipes or *Experimenta*[1] both enjoyed a wide circulation in England in the century afterwards (Power 1910; Jones 1994; Sharpe 1997: 202–4). There are more surviving manuscript copies of Arderne's texts than of any other English surgical writing. He wrote in Latin, but at least four separate Middle English translations of his works were also made (Jones 1989).[2] Deviating from the organising conventions of scholastic surgeries written by his university-trained competitors, Arderne visualised and described his surgical operations in temporal sequence from beginning to end. He could be said to provide a 'how-to' descriptive manual for an apprentice surgeon, rather as if demonstrating how to assemble flat-pack furniture or repair a car. The crucial accompanying pictures were called for in the text. Thus manuscripts of Arderne's writings were heavily illustrated within and alongside the text-block on the page, reinforcing the bias of the text towards visualisation and personal witness (Jones 1987, 2002). All but one of the manuscripts are codices, some produced by highly proficient 'professional' scribes and illuminators; others were copied by the owner in their own hand with crude illustrations. In one spectacular exception Arderne's *Experimenta* are sampled in a text written and illuminated on a roll (London, c. 1420) made up of six parchment membranes sewed together. The illustrations on the roll include a sequence of fistula in ano operations, but not the text that describes the operations. It is almost certain that this manuscript was commissioned by a very high-status individual whose interest was not in carrying out surgery but in enjoying the anecdotal flavour of Arderne's text and a collection of spectacular medical images (Svenberg & Jones 2014).[3]

2.2 Arderne Manuscripts after 1500

After 1500 John Arderne's writings on surgery and his *Experimenta* continued to be copied by hand in England, in both Latin and English. This is

[1] I will use the title *Experimenta* for the work also known as the *Liber medicinarum sive receptorum*. This is simply for the sake of brevity.

[2] More than forty Latin manuscripts of the *Practica* survive, another ten of the four Middle English translations.

[3] www.wdl.org/en/item/11631/view/1/1 (accessed 14 July 2020).

not such a surprise given that the essential techniques of fistula in ano surgery have not changed radically up to the present day, and the condition itself is still encountered by surgeons in modern hospitals. The need for guidance on how to perform Arderne's operations thus remained a constant, we may suppose. But it is less obvious why Arderne's text was not replaced or updated in the sixteenth and seventeenth centuries. In its original Latin version the text of the *Practica* on fistula in ano is not a very polished work and, despite its focus on describing the fistula in ano operations in time sequence, there are interpolations of a puzzling kind that suggest a jumbling of several different texts. One at least of the Middle English translations attempted to reorder and give the *Practica* text a more coherent organisation; the translator was also in effect an editor. This was the translation that had the longest textual tradition, the only one represented after 1532 (Power 1910). Even so, the Middle English Arderne text of the early fifteenth century must have seemed increasingly difficult for sixteenth- and seventeenth-century readers, with regard to both its grammar and lexis (Jones 2015). Examination of manuscripts of Arderne's text written in the sixteenth century may help us to understand the dynamics of this textual transmission.

One feature shared by these later manuscripts of Arderne copied in the sixteenth century is significant. They were commissioned or owned by practising surgeons and medics, rather than by university teachers, scholars, or lay patients. This is not so clearly the case with most of the earlier manuscripts. The Stockholm roll of Arderne is exceptional in its format and the liberties that it took with text and illustrations, but it is like most other Arderne codices from the fifteenth century in that it cannot plausibly be claimed to have been made for surgical practitioners to follow as a guide. Very few of the other late medieval manuscripts have any clear evidence as to commissioning, ownership, or use. One that does, Cambridge, Gonville & Caius MS 190/223, seems to have been put together for the Premonstratensian abbey of Hagnaby, Lincolnshire. It is not very likely that one of the canons practised surgery given the prohibitions in canon law against shedding blood (McCall 2016; Jones 2019).[4] We do know, however, that one manuscript of Arderne was bequeathed in the will of the London surgeon Henry Assheborne in 1442 (Talbot & Hammond 1965: 75).

[4] The contents are analysed in the Appendix to Jones (2019): Arderne's *Experimenta* are found on fols. 7–43v, the *Practica* on fols. 50–91v of the manuscript.

There are three extant sixteenth-century manuscripts of Arderne. Two contain distinct Middle English translations of the *Practica*, while the other is in Latin. British Library, Sloane MS 776, can be dated to 1532, and was written for Charles White or Whyte, a London barber-surgeon, by one Nicholas Browne (Watson 1979: no. 926).[5] An inscription in the manuscript calls Charles Whyte the compiler of the book, but on the basis of the text his role seems to have been that of a commissioner, rather than someone who selected, combined, or edited different texts as might be expected of a compiler. In Whyte's will of 1545 this manuscript ('namyd John of Ardren') is bequeathed to the surgeon Nicholas Archepolle.[6] Another medical book compiled by Charles Whyte and supposedly written by Nicholas Browne was quite possibly one of those books left by Whyte to his apprentice John Colmay, and was sold at Christie's in 2016.[7] Sloane MS 776 contains the longest Middle English translation of Arderne, containing both the *Practica* and the *Experimenta*; this translation is otherwise known only through the early fifteenth-century manuscript Cambridge, Emmanuel College MS 69 (Power 1913). Sloane MS 776 is profusely illustrated in ink and colour wash, and the images are related in appearance to the programme in the Cambridge manuscript (Jones 2002: 211–13). While we cannot know for certain if Charles Whyte used his Arderne manuscript as a guide to performing fistula operations, he evidently thought of it as a useful handbook of practical information for himself and surgeons like Archepolle who belonged to the guild of barber-surgeons.

Glasgow University Library, Hunter MS 403, was written in the distinctive hand of Robert Green or Greene of Welby (Rampling 2020), and dated by Greene himself to 1544 (Young & Aitken 1908: 321–2). This is the last known reference to Greene, who wrote or owned a number of other manuscripts containing alchemical and medical texts (Watson 1985; Thomson 2011). In one of these (Oxford, Bodleian MS Ashmole 1415),

5 It has the inscription 'compylyd by me Charles Whytte Cittezen and Barboure Cirurgyon of london And Wrytton by the hande of Nycholas Browne the vj daye of Januarij in the yeare of oure lorde god M.v.c.xxxij ti and in the xxxiiij th yere of the Reygne of Kynge Henrye the viii th [. . .]'(fol. 271v). See www.bl.uk/catalogues/illuminatedmanuscripts/record.asp?MSID=1188&CollID=9&NStart=776 (accessed 14 July 2020).

6 The will is in The National Archives, PROB 11-30-337.

7 www.christies.com/lotfinder/Lot/a-tudor-barber-and-surgeons-handbook-in-6012437-details.aspx (accessed 14 July 2020). The handwriting however is not identical with that of Sloane MS 776.

Greene tells us that he was seventy-one years old in 1538, so was born c. 1467. Greene seems to have been both a medical practitioner and an experimental alchemist, to judge from the contents of his manuscripts. Alongside Greene's copy of the Latin *Practica* and *Experimenta* of John Arderne, the manuscript also contains the gynaecological treatise known as *The book of Rota* (on pp. 347–63), a late medieval translation of the *Trotula* corpus very much presented as if made for a male practitioner of women's medicine (Green 2008: 190, 285, 340). The manuscript also contains Robert Greene's own compilation of plasters and ointments ('Compilacio emplastrorum et unguentorum'). It is possible that Greene was still practising surgery in his seventies, though it would have unusual to have undertaken the complexities of the fistula operation at such an age. But it is clear in any case that he was very interested in the practice of surgery.

London, Wellcome MS 7117, is a compendium of medicine in English compiled for use by an unknown Elizabethan practitioner around the year 1575.[8] It contains an incomplete English translation of John Arderne's treatise on fistula, hundreds of medical recipes, notes on medical astrology, and lists and classifications of diseases and medicaments. There is also an illustrated guide to urine diagnosis. There are two distinct hands, a fine, cursive secretary hand, with headings in italic, for the treatise on fistula and the uroscopy section (fols. 5r–39v, 119r–22r), and a more stolid Tudor hand for the rest. Both, however, are probably the work of the same scribe. Arderne's treatise on fistula in ano in this manuscript is based on the most commonly met of the four Middle English translations, and is organised in twenty-five numbered chapters. The other contents of the manuscript (not the Arderne treatise) align closely with those of Cambridge, Trinity College MS R.14.52, copied by a single scribe (the 'Hammond' scribe) in the third quarter of the fifteenth century (Tavormina 2006, vol. I: 7–13, 40–6). The Trinity manuscript has many sixteenth- and seventeenth-century annotations, suggesting it was regarded as current and useful for long afterwards. One of the Trinity annotators, Henry Dyneley, twice dates his interventions to 1573, close to the date of writing of the Wellcome MS, though the Wellcome MS does not copy the Trinity MS directly.

[8] http://archives.wellcomelibrary.org/DServe/dserve.exe?dsqIni=Dserve.ini&dsqApp=Archive&dsqCmd=Show.tcl&dsqDb=Catalog&dsqPos=0&dsqSearch=%28AltRefNo%3D%277117%27%29 (accessed 14 July 2020).

2.3 Arderne in Print

The treatise on fistula in Wellcome MS 7117 corresponds quite closely to the first (and only) printed version of Arderne's *Practica* of fistula in ano dated to 1588. It is the same Middle English translation that forms the basis of both, and the chapter headings correspond. This printing formed a section of a compendium of various tracts on surgery edited by John Read, a surgeon. Its title was *A most excellent and compendious method of curing woundes in the head,* [...] *With a treatise of the fistulae in the fundament, and other places of the body, translated out of Iohannes Ardern. And also the description of the emplaister called dia chalciteos, with his vse and vertues. With an apt table for the better finding of the perticular matters, contayned in this present worke* (Read 1588). Read was practising in Gloucestershire in 1587, but must have arrived in London that same year, since he was licensed to practise surgery by the Archbishop of Canterbury in January 1588. In June 1588 he married the daughter of John Banister, lecturer in anatomy to the London Company of Barber-Surgeons. Read never joined the Company himself, but associated with some of its most prominent members, including Banister, William Clowes, and Thomas Gale, and like them sought in writing to associate himself with a tradition of learned surgery, and to disassociate himself from those he called 'quacks'. His one printed work appeared in 1588, but was evidently completed in the preceding year; it was entered in the Stationers' register on 10 November 1587 (Symons 2004). It is for the most part a translation of *De recta curandorum vulnerum ratione* by Franciscus Arcaeus, but also includes John Arderne's *Treatise* translated from the *Practica*, as well as an English version of the Hippocratic oath, various miscellaneous pieces, and substantial interpolations by Read. At the end of Arderne's *Treatise* there are two notes about practising on patients with fistula in ano by Read himself. The first begins:

(1) The true method of the fistulae practised and used of one Hall of Northfolke, to whom the people doth flocke as unto an Oracle, which thing came to my handes by chaunce, (by a Gentleman a patient of mine) and for that I would not have such a secret hidden [...]. (Read 1588: fol. 108r)

It is very clear here that Read's motive for publishing Arderne in translation was to make 'secrets' available to those who wanted to provide the most effective surgical treatment for fistula in ano.

What is remarkable about both Read's printed book and Wellcome MS 7117 is that neither contains any illustrations of the fistula in ano operations. There are illustrations of urine glasses in Wellcome MS 7117, probably scribal rather than the work of a professional, and there seems no good reason why the scribe should not have also copied the surgical images from their exemplar. Similarly amateur illustrations are found in fifteenth-century manuscripts of Arderne (for example London, British Library, Harley MS 5401). The Middle English translation copied by the scribe of Wellcome MS 7117 was usually accompanied in earlier manuscripts by a manageable number of line illustrations, not the full suite of two hundred or more images found in Sloane MS 776. For its part the failure of the Read printing to include illustrations of fistula in ano should be considered in the context of other printed works of surgery of the same generation. The works of William Clowes, Thomas Gale, and others were illustrated with a limited repertoire of woodcut images copied from earlier continental works of surgery (wound man, surgeon's chest, etc.), rather than using original images to convey surgical technique. The English barber-surgeons perhaps wanted, in any case, to identify themselves more closely with scholarly works of learned medicine and surgery than with artisanal handicraft (Chamberland 2010). John Banister, Read's father-in-law, did in fact make spectacular use of painted anatomical tables to teach anatomy to English surgeons, but did not carry this practice over as illustration into his printed output of writings on anatomy and surgery. Instead he borrowed the woodcuts of Andreas Vesalius's *De fabrica*, or rather the pirated versions of these first printed in England by Thomas Geminus (Banister 1578). It may be that the English surgical authors, or their printers (if they met the costs), were simply deterred from commissioning new woodcut illustrations because of the expense. The effect of such policies, however, was to limit significantly the effectiveness of the Arderne *Practica* in print as a practical tool, since the author explicitly points from the text to the illustrations found in manuscript copies of his work to convey essential information about the presentations of fistula, the instruments to be used, and the sequence of operation.

The only other appearance of Arderne in print was in the seventeenth century, when three of his remedies were credited to the fourteenth-century surgeon in the *Pharmacopoeia Londinensis* of 1632 (Royal College of Physicians of London 1632). This edition enlarged slightly on the original *Pharmacopoeia* issued by the College in 1618, and three entries under *Unguenta* (ointments) were taken from Arderne: *Valentia scabiosae*, *Tapsivalencia*, and *Tapsimel* were all drawn from the *Practica* on fistula in ano. The *Pharmacopoeia Londinensis* has a note about Arderne, remarking on his origin in Newark, and that he flourished around 1370. The note claims that the three remedies from Arderne were excerpted word for word from an ancient manuscript ('ipsissimis verbis ex antiquo manuscripto excerpta'). Many of Arderne's remedies indeed continued to circulate in manuscript, for instance those to be found in London, Wellcome MS 674, probably compiled in the late sixteenth century.[9] These particular three remedies remained in print in successive editions of the *Pharmacopoeia.* As late as 1733 James Alleyne's *A New Dispensatory in Four Parts* [. . .] was still recommending the three remedies from Arderne, quoting from the *Pharmacopoeia Londinensis* in English translation (Alleyne 1733: 336–7). John Freind in his *History of Physick* (1725) gave a favourable account of the English surgeon, and cited the same three remedies by Arderne as still current. Freind was aware of John Arderne manuscripts in circulation in his own time:

(2) he has left us a large volume of Physick and Surgery, but chiefly of the last; many Manuscripts of which we have among us; and one wou'd wonder that it has not yet been printed, since perhaps it may be as useful a work as any writ in that profession in these ages [. . .]. (Freind 1725, vol. 2: 325)

2.4 Walter Hamond, Chirurgian, and the Lentaigne Manuscript, 1645

Freind's surprise at Arderne's works not having been printed in his own time may be shared today. But the failure to print the *Practica* was not a matter of it having fallen out of surgical use. There is one valuable piece of evidence revealing a seventeenth-century English surgeon making use of a fifteenth-century manuscript of Arderne as a guide to the fistula in ano operation. This is a manuscript now in Dublin, in the Library of the Royal College of Surgeons in Ireland (RCSI), MS 97. It is also known as the Lentaigne Manuscript after its donor, Sir John Lentaigne, who gave it to the RCSI in 1851 (see Figure 7 in the Image Gallery). A former owner, Walter Hamond, 'Chirurgian', had the manuscript bound in leather in 1645 and interleaved the vellum leaves with paper pages for his own notes. It is not known how the manuscript came into Sir John Lentaigne's possession. The main texts of the manuscript are the *Practica* of fistula

[9] See Chapter 3 in this volume.

in ano and Arderne's *Experimenta* in Latin, written in an English hand of the early fifteenth century. Walter Hamond wrote the interleaved notes, which, though far from the complete commentary he may first have intended, provide evidence of his understanding of Arderne's text and of its importance to his own practice of the fistula in ano operation.[10]

Walter Hamond, whose date of birth and origins are unknown, was apprenticed to Arthur Doughton in the Barber-Surgeons' Company of London, and made free in 1616 (McConnell 2004). In 1617 he was responsible for the publication of *The method of curing vvounds made by gun-shot* [...] (Hamond 1617). This work was dedicated to Arthur Doughton, and described itself as intended for students and apprentices of the craft of surgery, more especially those who do their country service on the seas. Hamond was in the service of the East India Company. In 1630, as surgeon to the *Charles* and the *Jonas* (Captain Weddell), bound for the Far East, he spent four months on the island of Madagascar. This voyage gave Hamond the material for writing in 1639 a short pamphlet in favour of colonising the island for naval purposes (Hamond 1640). An expedition planned for 1639 never left port, but another opportunity arose in 1643, giving rise to Hamond's second advertisement (Hamond 1643). This expedition was much delayed but finally sailed in 1645. It is very unlikely that Hamond went himself. In any case, the colony soon failed. At Hamond's death in May or early June 1648, he left a wife, Marie, to execute his modest estate, but his will provided no clue as to his then residence or desired place of burial.

From the little we know of Walter Hamond, it seems then that he was for much of his life a sea surgeon. However, when in 1645 (the year the Madagascar expedition sailed) he assembled the interleaved volume of Arderne and had it bound, he was probably in his fifties, and was no longer practising his craft at sea. On the title page he wrote 'The Workes of Master John Arderne, Chirurgian, of Newark in Nottingham Shire written by his own hand in the yeeare of our Lord 1349 – with Some Observations collected in blank paper By Walter Hamond Chirurgian, 1645' (Widdess 1943: 80; O'Doherty 2013). On the first page of his 'Observations', opposite the first vellum leaf of Arderne's *Experimenta*, Hamond recorded a running title 'The Practice of M[aste]r John Arderne', and he began by

[10] Dublin, Royal College of Surgeons in Ireland Library, RCSI/MS/97: see http://heritage.rcsi.ie/CalmView/Record.aspx?src=CalmView.Catalog&id=RCSI%2fMS%2f97&pos=1 (accessed 14 July 2020).

translating Arderne's charm for staunching blood at the beginning of the text:

(3) Write in a paper the following letters and hang them about the arme or neck of the Hemorois [Humerus] and itt will stay itt [. . .] and if you will nott believe itt you may chuse otherwise Take a Hasell wand of one year's growth and slitt itt in the midell and so forth [. . .]. (RCSI 97, unpaginated)

So Hamond does not distinguish between the *Experimenta* and the *Practica*, all being subsumed as 'The Practice of M[aste]r John Arderne', and nor does he balk at what might be regarded as 'superstitious' or 'magical' experiments. Hamond's writing out of his 'Observations' soon become sporadic on the interleaved pages. He has nothing to say about the coloured illustrations in the *Experimenta* part of the Lentaigne Arderne manuscript.

This lack of interest in illustration changes dramatically when it comes to the section of the *Practica* where the instruments and the operative sequence for fistula in ano are described. In the Lentaigne *Practica* the images of the instruments to be used for the operation are found inserted within the text-block. On the blank page opposite Hamond drew his versions of the same instruments, with his own descriptions of the instruments in English. Neither the images nor the descriptions of them are straightforward copies of Arderne. On page 163 Hamond drew the probe, giving it the same title as Arderne, 'sequere me' ('follow me'). His description runs:

(4) This instrument named Sequere me ought to be made of lead that it may be pliant to bend every way, and it ought to have an eye to draw through the *frenum caesaris* [see below] (RCSI 97: 163)

He follows Arderne in emphasising pliability, but Arderne's version declares that the instrument should be like the pin that women use in their hair, and made of the same metal, and does not specify the need for an eye. In the medieval and early modern periods such pins were usually made of copper alloy (brass wire) or of iron – not lead as Hamond suggests. Hamond is specific about how to make the *frenum caesaris* where Arderne is not:

(5) Take 2 or 3 horse haires and ther will Twist a strong double silke called sticking silk of any collour save black, wax them well et reseruentur ad usum predictum [and keep for the use aforesaid]. (RCSI 97: 164)

For his drawing of the *Acus rostrata*, or pointed needle made of silver recommended by Arderne, Hamond writes: 'This Acus Rostratus [sic] semes onely to cut the orifices one unto another to passe the frenum cesaris.' For the *siringa* or clyster-pipe, Hamond draws what is evidently a seventeenth-century version of the instrument for administering enemas, with a circular fat pipe and plunger, and a narrower part for insertion. The drawing in the *Practica* does not have a plunger or the narrower part for insertion. Hamond calls his version 'The Siringue a Common Instrument needfull in this case' (see Figure 8 in the Image Gallery).

But the most significant departure from Arderne's model comes in relation to the *tendiculum*, an instrument Arderne claims to have invented himself. Hamond's *tendiculum* bears little resemblance to Arderne's, having a saw-toothed dial at the centre with which the *frenum caesaris* is progressively tightened once it is passed through the anus and comes out of the fistula hole. Hamond substitutes on page 163 of the manuscript his instrument for that of Arderne:

(6) A *tendiculum* devised by my selfe in the cure of Mr Richard Wild, and it ought to be made no greater than the patterne [i.e. this drawing] of silver [By] helpe of this instrument you may every day straine the frenum every day til you have fretted the part asunder. (RCSI 97: 163)

Arderne specifies that his *tendiculum* should be made of box wood. The Hamond instrument was devised for operating on a named patient, Richard Wild, presumably to the entire satisfaction of both. By naming the patient Hamond is following Arderne's example, for the earlier surgeon identified at the beginning of the *Practica* a series of patients he had successfully operated on for fistula in ano. But although the revised *tendiculum* performs the same function as that of Arderne, Hamond evidently wished to draw attention to his ability to strike out independently and to register his own improved design.

Hamond was interested in comparing the fees for the fistula in ano operation that Arderne claimed to charge with what he charged himself when operating on Richard Wild in 1630:

(7) the rates and rewards given to the author three hundred years since, were as he saith of a noble person for this cure was 40 lb a liverie gowne and 5lb a yeare during life of others 40lb or 40 marks with his cloak and he protesteth that never in his life did he take lesse of the poorest patient for his Cure than 100 shillings or 5lb wherby itt is evident that Mr Arderne was better paid in those dayes Considering

> that then the rate of silver , the price of victualls, and the rent of Houses was nott the twentieth part so much as itt is in these times. Yett I must with thankfullnes confesse that I rec[d?] from Mr Wild in anno 1630 the somme of 100 lb for effecting the same cure. (RCSI 97: 150)

Hamond was every bit as interested as Arderne in how much to charge for this difficult operation. It seems that Hamond recognised that Arderne's fees were very high for that period, but that in the case of Mr Wild, Hamond himself charged an amount quite outside his own usual fee structure. Perhaps Wild was the only patient he performed this operation on, or perhaps he charged others less in accordance with their ability to pay. But, like Arderne's statement at the beginning of the *Practica*, Hamond used his 'Observations' to show how much such outstanding skill might earn.

What is significant in the 'Observations' is the deep level of Hamond's engagement with this 'ancient' surgical text, and his ability not only to read Arderne's idiosyncratic Latin but also to grapple with the palaeography of a manuscript more than two hundred years old. The reward for his engagement was that he could compare his own practice of the tricky fistula in ano operation with that of Arderne. Hamond could also record for the use of others how to make improvements on the necessary surgical instruments Arderne described and illustrated, and what kind of fee to charge. Opposite the leaf on which Arderne depicted the successive stages of the fistula in ano operation, Hamond wrote:

> (8) My good and loving frend Mr Geofrey Guilbert died about the 1 September the news was brought me this day Sep 5 1645 of whome I had this booke. (RCSI 97: 164)

We learn two things here. First, that Hamond was writing on this page on 5 September 1645, making it likely that his 'Observations' on Arderne all date from that year. Second, that his friend Mr Geoffrey Guilbert gave Hamond this Arderne manuscript. We know nothing more of Guilbert, unfortunately. He does not appear to be recorded as a barber-surgeon under the name Guilbert or Gilbert. Guilbert must have known that Hamond would put the manuscript to good use. It is probable that Hamond interleaved the manuscript for his 'Observations' because he wanted to supplement Arderne's teaching with the fruits of his own experience. Within three years of Guilbert's death, however, Hamond himself was dead, and the Arderne manuscript does not feature in his will, nor is there any other sign of his giving it in turn to another surgeon.

Nevertheless, it is safe to assume that Hamond hoped that other surgeons would be able to profit from his 'Observations'.

2.5 Other Practical Users of Arderne in the Seventeenth Century

There is other significant evidence that the currency of Arderne's manuscripts in the seventeenth century was connected with their practical usefulness. Sir Theodore Turquet de Mayerne (1573–1655), the Huguenot court physician (Nance 2001: 8–9; Trevor-Roper 2006: ch. 22), copied in his own hand from a Latin manuscript containing both the *Practica* of fistula in ano and the *Experimenta*. He described his own transcript as 'collecta ex libro manuscripto' (collected from a manuscript book).[11] The other works excerpted in this volume in Mayerne's hand were by sixteenth- and seventeenth-century authors, English and continental. Mayerne dated the *Practica* accurately to 1376, but clearly felt that the considerable gap in time between Arderne's date of writing and his own did not reduce the usefulness of the earlier surgeon's work. Mayerne also cited a passage in Latin from the *Experimenta* concerning a charm against spasm and cramp in his commonplace book *De amuletis* (On amulets) (Skemer 2006: 145, n. 53). Another lengthy excerpt from the *Experimenta* is to be found in a fifteenth-century manuscript acquired by Sir Kenelm Digby (1603–1665), Bodleian Library, Digby MS 161. Digby is known to have been collecting medical recipes and experiments for his own use from 1625 onwards, and Digby MS 161, one of those he acquired after he inherited the library of Thomas Allen, reflects this interest clearly. Digby was a friend and collaborator of Mayerne (Foster 2004; Moshenka 2017). These men are not surgeons like Hamond, and belonged to a rather more courtly milieu (though Digby also was a sea voyager). But they were eager to learn from the unusual methods and practical bent of Arderne, the medieval surgeon, and to this purpose sought out his manuscripts and copied from them.

Another such practically minded user of an Arderne manuscript, but this time an ecclesiastic, was Samuel Knott (1613–1687). Knott obtained his BA at Trinity College in Oxford on 16 May 1632. He became vicar of Broadhembury in Devon in 1634, and in 1635 was nominated rector of Combe Raleigh, also in Devon. Ejected from the church in 1647, he was restored in 1660, only to be suspended again by the bishop in 1663 and definitely prohibited from preaching in 1664, as he did not conform to the

11 London, British Library, Sloane MS 1991, fol. 200v.

Act of Uniformity. Knott acquired a considerable collection of early manuscripts, most liturgical or theological, but twenty medical manuscripts now in the British Library Harley collection were also once Knott's. His very distinctive hand is found in all of these medical books. Relevant for our purposes is that Knott owned and annotated Harley MS 3371, a fifteenth-century Latin manuscript containing the *Practica* and *Experimenta* of Arderne, *inter alia*, and the exemplar for one of the Middle English translations (Jones 1990). It is clear from Knott's notes that he regarded these texts as important guides to medical practice. Knott's manuscripts later came into the hands of Robert Burscough (1650/1–1709), prebendary of Exeter in 1701, archdeacon of Barnstaple in 1703, and rector of Cheriton Bishop in 1705. The Arderne manuscript was no. 60 in his collection. In 1715 Robert Harley (1661–1724) acquired Burscough's manuscripts by purchase from the rector's widow, a purchase negotiated by Humfrey Wanley, which included all Knott's medical manuscripts (Nuvoloni 2008).

2.6 Collecting Arderne Manuscripts

The single most important gathering of Arderne's manuscripts was that of Sir Hans Sloane (1660–1753). No fewer than fifteen of the Sloane manuscripts now in the British Library contain Arderne texts, and one now in the Hunterian collection of Glasgow University Library (MS 339) formerly belonged to Sloane. This means that almost a third of the surviving Arderne manuscripts today were once in Sloane's collection. Although Sloane was a collector of collections on a scale unknown in his day or since, the concentration of Arderne manuscripts cannot be simply an accident caused by his absorbing so many smaller collections. His fortune was made as a medical practitioner (and through investments in land and slavery), and he was committed to collecting medical history. Arderne was arguably the most important English medical author before William Harvey, and so would have appealed to Sloane's patriotic instincts as well. No doubt the extraordinary illustrations were an attraction, for Sloane also collected illuminated manuscripts. Sloane's own medical practice would not have included treating fistula in ano surgically, as he defined himself as a physician and not a surgeon (Delbourgo 2017: 124), although he did certainly collect reports of successful remedies. Unlike Hamond, Mayerne, Digby, or Knott, Sloane did not collect these Arderne manuscripts primarily to improve his practice or to test Arderne's remedies. His interest was principally that of an antiquarian or connoisseur, whose specialist field of collecting was medical (Hunt 2012; Delbourgo 2017: 202–11, ch. 6).

Although Sloane's collections were not much used by scholars in his lifetime, Humfrey Wanley (1672–1726) did gain access to Sloane's manuscripts and took a particular interest in the Arderne texts held by Sloane (Heyworth 2004). Wanley's work on Edward Bernard's *Catalogi librorum manuscriptorum Angliae et Hiberniae* (1697) had already introduced him to Sloane's acquisitions (264 Sloane manuscripts were included), and when he moved from Oxford to London Wanley worked as Sloane's assistant while the latter was Secretary of the Royal Society (Blakeway 2011: 23–5). After 1708 he settled down as library-keeper to Robert Harley and to his son Edward Harley, building up the great Harleian collection of manuscripts (Jackson 2011). Wanley then was in a unique position to make a study of the Arderne manuscripts in both collections, and he took advantage of it. He was no doubt instrumental in the acquisition of several of these manuscripts and Wanley's hand is found in the margins of Arderne manuscripts owned by both Harley and Sloane. Wanley collated the various manuscripts and his notes in the margins are a result of this collation. We can see this impressive activity as the purest expression of the instincts of the textual scholar and librarian – while Sloane was Wanley's doctor, there is no hint that Wanley was interested in practising medicine himself. John Arderne and his *Practica* of fistula in ano were still very much relevant to the continuing practice of the surgical operation, but the manuscripts were no longer being quarried medically in the way that they had been in the sixteenth and seventeenth centuries.

2.7 Conclusion

On the basis of the evidence provided by the sixteenth- and seventeenth-century manuscripts of John Arderne's writings, it is clear that the work of the medieval surgeon was valued highly for its contemporary practical usefulness by surgeons, physicians, and apothecaries. He was of course far from being the only medieval medical author whose works enjoyed a long early modern afterlife.[12] Given that Arderne appeared late in print (1588) and that copying his work in manuscript remained attractive to

[12] See Chapter 5 (John of Burgundy) and Chapter 3 (John Mirfield) in this volume. Thomas Moulton, compiler of the medical bestseller *This is the myrrour or glasse of helth* [. . .] (London 1532 etc.), was in fact a fifteenth-century Dominican friar (Getz 1990: 10–11).

early modern medical practitioners, there is no question of the supposed distinction between manuscript and print eras acting as an obstacle to his continuing popularity. Nor did his 'barbarous' Latin or Middle English translations (Jones 2015) put off those who were used to reading and writing in early modern English. Only towards the end of the seventeenth century do we begin to find Arderne's manuscripts being treasured for their linguistic and editorial interest or for the light they throw on the historical past of English surgery, rather than their immediate practical usefulness.

REFERENCES

Alleyne, James. 1733. *A new English dispensatory, in four parts [. . .]*. London: Tho. Astley & S. Austen.

Banister, John. 1578. *The historie of man sucked from the sappe of the most approued anathomistes, in this present age, compiled in most compendious fourme, and now published in English, for the vtilitie of all godly chirurgians, within this realme, by Iohn Banister, Master in Chirurgerie, and practitioner in phisicke.* London: John Day.

Barnard, John (ed.). 2002. *The Cambridge history of the book in Britain*, vol. IV: 1557–1695. Cambridge: Cambridge University Press.

Blakeway, Amy. 2011. The library catalogues of Sir Hans Sloane: Their authors, organization, and functions. *Electronic British Library Journal*, 2011: article 16.

Chamberland, Celeste. 2010. Between the Hall and the market: William Clowes and surgical self-fashioning in Elizabethan London. *Sixteenth Century Journal* 41: 69–89.

Delbourgo, James. 2017. *Collecting the world: The life and curiosity of Hans Sloane.* London: Allen Lane.

Foster, Michael. 2004. Sir Kenelm Digby (1603–1665). *Oxford Dictionary of National Biography.* https://doi.org/10.1093/ref:odnb/7629 (accessed 14 July 2020).

Freind, John. 1725. *The history of physick; from the time of Galen, to the beginning of the sixteenth century [. . .]*, 2 vols. London: J. Walthoe Jr.

Getz, Faye Marie. 1990. Charity, translation and the language of medical learning in medieval England. *Bulletin of the History of Medicine* 64: 1–17.

Green, Monica H. 2008. *Making women's medicine masculine: The rise of male authority in pre-modern gynaecology.* Oxford: Oxford University Press.

Hamond, Walter. 1617. *The method of curing vvounds made by gun-shot also by arrowes and darts, with their accidents. Written by Ambrose Parie of Laual, counsellor and chiefe chirurgean to the French King. Faithfully done into English out of the French copie, by Walter Hamond chirurgean.* London: Isaac Jaggard.

Hamond, Walter. 1640. *A paradox prooving that the inhabitants of the isle called Madagascar, or St. Laurence, (in temporall things) are the happiest people in the world. Whereunto is prefixed, a briefe and true description of that island: the nature of the climate, and condition of the inhabitants, and their speciall affection to the English above other nations. With most probable arguments of a hopefull and fit plantation of a colony there, in respect of the fruitfulnesse of the soyle, the benignity of the ayre, and the relieving of our English ships, both to and from the East-Indies*. London: Nathaniell Butter.

Hamond, Walter. 1643. *Madagascar, the richest and most frvitfvll island in the world wherein the temperature of the clymate, the nature of the inhabitants, the commodities of the countrie and the facility and benefit of a plantation by our people there are compendiously and truely described: Dedicated to the Honourable Iohn Bond, governour of the island, whose proceeding is authorized for this expedition, both by the king and Parliament*. London: Nicholas Bourne.

Hellinga, Lotte (ed.). 1999. *The Cambridge history of the book in Britain*, vol. III: *1400–1557*. Cambridge: Cambridge University Press.

Heyworth, Peter. 2004. Humfrey Wanley (1672–1726). *Oxford Dictionary of National Biography*. https://doi.org/10.1093/ref:odnb/28664 (accessed 14 July 2020).

Hunt, Arnold. 2012. Sloane as a collector of manuscripts. In Michael Hunter, Alison Walker, & Arthur MacGregor (eds.), *From books to bezoars: Sir Hans Sloane and his collections*, 190–207. London: British Library.

Jackson, Deirdre. 2011. Humfrey Wanley and the Harley collection. *Electronic British Library Journal*, 2011: article 2.

Jones, Peter Murray. 1987. 'Sicut hic depingitur …': John of Arderne and English medical illustration in the 14th and 15th centuries. In Wolfram Prinz & Andreas Beyer (eds.), *Die Kunst und das Studium der Natur vom 14. zum 16. Jahrhundert*, 103–26. Weinheim: Acta Humaniora.

Jones, Peter Murray. 1989. Four Middle English translations of John of Arderne. In Alistair Minnis (ed.), *Latin and vernacular: Studies in late medieval manuscripts*, 61–89. Woodbridge: Boydell and Brewer.

Jones, Peter Murray. 1990. British Library MS Sloane 76: A translator's holograph. In Linda L. Brownrigg (ed.), *Medieval book production: Assessing the evidence*, 21–39. Los Altos Hills, CA: Anderson-Lovelace, Red Gull Press.

Jones, Peter Murray. 1994. John of Arderne and the Mediterranean tradition of scholastic surgery. In Luis Garcia-Ballester, Roger French, Jon Arrizabalaga, & Andrew Cunningham (eds.), *Practical medicine from Salerno to the Black Death*, 289–321. Cambridge: Cambridge University Press.

Jones, Peter Murray. 2002. Staying with the programme: Illustrated manuscripts of John of Arderne, c. 1380–c.1550. In A. S. G. Edwards (ed.), *English manuscript studies 1100–1700*, vol. 10: *Decoration and illustration in medieval English manuscripts*, 204–27. London: British Library.

Jones, Peter Murray. 2004. Arderne, John (*b.* 1307/8, *d.* in or after 1377), surgeon and author. *Oxford Dictionary of National Biography*. https://doi.org/10.1093/ref:odnb/636 (accessed 16 July 2020).

Jones, Peter Murray. 2015. Language and register in English medieval surgery. In Mary Carruthers (ed.), *Language in medieval Britain: Networks and exchanges*, 74–89. Harlaxton medieval studies XXV. Donington: Shaun Tyas.

Jones, Peter Murray. 2019. *Experimenta*, compilation and construction in two medieval books. *Poetica: An International Journal of Linguistic-Literary Studies* 91 & 92: 61–80.

Lindberg, David C., & Michael H. Shank (eds.). 2013. *The Cambridge history of science*, vol. 2: *Medieval science*. Cambridge: Cambridge University Press.

McCall, Taylor. 2016. *Reliquam dicit pictura*: Text and image in a twelfth-century illustrated anatomical manual (Gonville and Caius College, Cambridge, MS 190/223). *Transactions of the Cambridge Bibliographical Society* 16(1): 1–22.

McConnell, Anita. 2004. Walter Hamond, *d.*1648. *Oxford Dictionary of National Biography*. https://doi.org/10.1093/ref:odnb/12167 (accessed 14 July 2020).

Moshenka, Joe. 2017. *A stain in the blood*. London: Windmill Books. www.penguin.co.uk/books/1097776/a-stain-in-the-blood/9780099591764.html (accessed 14 July 2020).

Nance, Brian. 2001. *Turquet de Mayerne as baroque physician: The art of medical portraiture*. Amsterdam; New York: Rodopi.

Nuvoloni, Laura. 2008. The Harleian medical manuscripts. *Electronic British Library Journal*, 2008: article 7.

O'Doherty, Mary. 2013. The Lentaigne Manuscript. *Heritage Collections of the Royal College of Surgeons in Ireland*. https://rcsiheritage.blogspot.com/2013/11/the-lentaigne-manuscript.html (accessed 14 July 2020).

Park, Katharine, & Lorraine Daston (eds.). 2006. *The Cambridge history of science*, vol. 3: *Early modern science*. Cambridge: Cambridge University Press.

Power, D'Arcy (ed.). 1910. *Treatises of fistula in ano haemorrhoids, and clysters by John Arderne from an early fifteenth-century manuscript translation*. London: Early English Text Society.

Power, D'Arcy. 1913. *The lesser writings of John Arderne*. https://archive.org/details/b21463724 (accessed 14 July 2020).

Rampling, Jennifer M. 2020. *The experimental fire: Inventing English alchemy 1300–1700*. Chicago: University of Chicago Press.

Read, John. 1588. *A most excellent and compendious method of curing woundes in the head, [...] With a treatise of the fistulae in the fundament, and other places of the body, translated out of Iohannes Ardern [...]*. London: T. East.

Royal College of Physicians of London. 1632. *Pharmacopoeia Londinensis in qua medicamenta antiqua et noua vsitatissima, sedulò collecta, accuratissime examinata, quotidianâ experientia confirmata describuntur [...]*. London: John Marriott.

Sharpe, Richard. 1997. *A handlist of the Latin writers of Great Britain and Ireland before 1540*. Turnhout: Brepols.

Skemer, Don C. 2006. *Binding words: Textual amulets in the Middle Ages*. University Park: Pennsylvania State University Press.

Svenberg, Torgny, & Peter Murray Jones (eds.). 2014. *De arte phisicali et de cirurgia by John Arderne: From a new digital version of the Stockholm roll*. Stockholm: Hagströmer Biblioteket.

Symons, John. 2004. John Read (*fl.* 1588), surgeon. *Oxford Dictionary of National Biography*. https://doi.org/10.1093/ref:odnb/23217 (accessed 14 July 2020).

Talbot, C. H., & E. A. Hammond. 1965. *The medical practitioners in medieval London: A biographical register*. London: Wellcome Historical Medical Library.

Tavormina, M. Teresa (ed.). 2006. *Sex, aging, & death in a medieval medical compendium: Trinity College Cambridge MS R.14.52, its texts, language and scribe*, 2 vols. Tempe, AR: ACMRS.

Thomson, R. M. 2011. *A descriptive catalogue of the medieval manuscripts of Corpus Christi College Oxford*. Woodbridge: D. S. Brewer.

Trevor-Roper, Hugh. 2006. *Europe's physician: The various life of Sir Theodore de Mayerne*. New Haven, CT; London: Yale University Press.

Watson, Andrew G. 1979. *Catalogue of dated and datable manuscripts c. 700–1600 in the Department of Manuscripts: The British Library*, 2 vols. London: British Library.

Watson, Andrew G. 1985. Robert Green of Welby, alchemist and Count Palatine c.1467–c. 1540. *Notes and Queries* 32: 312–13.

Widdess, J. D. H. 1943. Practica magistri Johannis Arderne (an account of an early 15th century manuscript in the Library of the Royal College of Surgeons in Ireland). *Irish Journal of Medical Science* 18: 77–81.

Young, John, & P. Henderson Aitken. 1908. *A catalogue of the manuscripts in the Library of the Hunterian Museum in the University of Glasgow*. Glasgow: James Maclehose and Sons.

CHAPTER 3

John Mirfield's Gouernayl of Helþe

Lori Jones

> Now that I have [. . .] set downe & declared certayne rules and observations with other things pertayninge unto the Regiment of Healthe [. . .].
>
> (Wellcome Collection MS 674: p. 55, hereafter WC674)[1]

An anonymous author offers the above-noted preface to his book of medicines, midway through the later sixteenth-century WC674.[2] The first part of the 138-leaf manuscript contains several treatises, the health regimen, two unique versions of John of Burgundy's plague tract, and recipes for plague medicines and preservatives (Jones 2018).[3] Following the book of medicines are many pages of recipes for ointments, plasters, and oils against poison, venom, and sores, plus instructions for identifying and healing broken bones and injuries. Thereafter follows a surgical antidotary and more treatments for wounds, swellings, sores, bruises, boils, and apostumes. The writer notes with admiration that John Arderne – 'an excellent chirurgion in his tyme' (WC674: fol. 2) – had proved some of the very same treatments.[4] An unfinished herbal ends the contemporary part of the manuscript.

At first glance, this unprepossessing English medical manuscript – its original limp vellum cover and some of its bindings and ties still intact, its

[1] The first half of the manuscript is paginated 13–60 (the initial pages are missing); midway through some recipes a different hand switches to foliation (1–113). For accuracy, I follow this dual system, using p. and fol., respectively.

[2] The Wellcome Collection catalogue proposes a production date of 1625–1682, following marginal notations and annotated receipts from fol. 96r forward. Palaeographical analysis shows that all of the treatises and most of the recipes before fol. 96r are written in the same Tudor Secretary hand of the mid to later sixteenth century. I am grateful for Alpo Honkapohja's assistance with dating, using the website *English Handwriting 1500–1700: An Online Course*, www.english.cam.ac.uk/ceres/ehoc/index.html (accessed 23 April 2022).

[3] On John of Burgundy's plague tract, see Chapter 5 in this volume and Jones (2021).

[4] On John Arderne's *Surgery*, see Chapter 2 in this volume. The recipe for *flos unguentorum* Mirfield attributes to Arderne is not in fact one of his recipes (personal correspondence with Peter Murray Jones, 2 June 2020).

often untidy and ink-blotted hand consistent throughout – is similar to other contemporary survivals. It includes familiar medical treatises deemed essential knowledge for someone offering medical care. Much of the manuscript's contents relate specifically to surgery and wound management, suggesting that the unidentified Wellcome compiler was perhaps a surgeon, apprentice, or cleric interested or involved in providing healing care.

Given the manuscript's emphasis on identifying and treating acute external bodily ailments, the presence of the *Regiment of Health* – a genre of medical advice literature concerned with the preservation and maintenance of physical and mental health 'under normal circumstances' (Cavallo & Storey 2017b: 24) – is noteworthy. The regimen is, like the other treatises in the compilation, a one-off modernisation of a popular centuries-old work. In this case, the Wellcome author revised the *Gouernayl of Helþe* written by late fourteenth-century London clerk John Mirfield (also spelled Mirfeld). Mirfield's regimen circulated in the fifteenth century in both Latin and English translation before William Caxton slightly modified and printed the English version around 1489. A flood of modern regimens eclipsed Mirfield's treatise by the mid-sixteenth century and it passed out of wide circulation. Instead of turning to these recent works, however, the Wellcome author updated Mirfield's regimen to reflect the priorities of his own time and place.

Mirfield's *Gouernayl of Helþe* made the transition from manuscript to print and then was appropriated by early modern manuscript culture. It offers further evidence of how medieval ideas of healthiness changed over time, and how later writers modernised medieval medical texts to reflect new ways of life. Tracing the substantive changes that subsequent producers made in this regimen highlights which aspects of health culture they identified as needing revision in late fifteenth-century England and then again a century later, notably which spheres of life (non-naturals) they deemed most important and what they regarded as harmful or beneficial to health.

3.1 Methodological Approach

This chapter examines the enduring influence of medieval medical genres and the extent to which knowledge was enriched, in the age of print, as it circulated back and forth between printed and manuscript compilations (Jones 1995; Leong 2018). It builds on existing scholarship on the emergence and vernacular evolution of medical genres (Taavitsainen 2006), the role of regimens in medical discourse and knowledge transmission (Gil-Sotres 1998; Nicoud 2007; Cavallo & Storey 2017a), and their material transition (Cavallo & Storey 2013). It extends A. R. D. Kiernander's (1980) preliminary comparisons between extant medieval English manuscript copies of Mirfield's regimen and its printed versions (c. 1489–1530) by analysing the structural and conceptual changes the Wellcome writer made while modernising Mirfield's work. Finally, it considers the significance of those changes to evolving attitudes about what constituted a healthy regimen in sixteenth-century England.

3.2 Regimens of Health: A Medieval Medical Genre

Medieval regimens of health evolved from a long tradition of governance advice and Hippocratic dietetic medicine that simultaneously sought to conserve or regulate the health of the body politic and the human body (Hardingham 2005: 2). In its oldest medical sense, the Greek *dietetic* referred primarily to appropriate food intake while accounting for the broader set of actions or habits necessary for managing healthy physical, mental, and spiritual lifestyles. In Hippocratic medicine, this meant the essential balance between diet and exercise. Galenic medicine added four further non-naturals (external factors whose maintenance affects health): sleep/wakefulness, passions/emotions, air, and excretion. In his ninth-century *Isagoge*, the Arabic translator Hunayn ibn Ishaq (Johannitius) incorporated sexual activity and bathing into the non-naturals. He and other medieval Arabic writers then began to organise medical thought around causes of illness that were natural (internal bodily processes), non-natural, and contra-natural (pathological factors). Medieval regimens of health – *Regimina sanitatis* – emerged from dietetic doctrines translated from Arabic into Latin after the eleventh century (Nicoud 2007; Cavallo & Storey 2013: 3–4).

Among early and influential works were Latin translations of the dietary regimen in the long pseudo-Aristotelian *Secretum secretorum* and Ibn Zuhr's (Avenzoar) *Liber de regimine sanitatis*, as well as the didactic verse *Regimen sanitatis Salernitanum* (or *Flos medicinae*). More important to the lasting formation of the medieval regimen genre were the subsequent works of thirteenth- and fourteenth-century university-trained physicians, surgeons, scholars, and clerics such as Aldobrandin of Siena, John of Toledo, William of Salicet, Petrus Hispanus, Taddeo Alderotti, Arnold of Villanova, Bernard de Gordon, and Maino de Maineri, among others. While inherently heterogeneous in their aims, intended audiences, and attention given to individual non-naturals, taken together their crucial interventions include extending the concept of dietetics to encapsulate not only health maintenance but also prevention and therapy. In expanding the parameters of dietetics, they also facilitated its incorporation into learned university discourse. Some works, like Aldobrandin of Siena's *Régime du corps*, were composed in the vernacular, and this too had significant implications for the regimens' longer-term influence. While still especially popular among the wealthy elite, regimens of health moved outside the court environment targeted by the *Secretum secretorum* and appealed to an educated but non-Latinate audience that sought medical and lifestyle guidance in the vernacular (Demaitre 1980: 67–9; Gil-Sotres 1998; Nicoud 2007).

The popularity, reach, and vernacularisation of health regimens expanded considerably following the Black Death (c. 1346–1353) through plague treatises, which discussed causes of plague, offered personal and environmental preventive advice (i.e. a regimen of health), and recommended treatments and cures (Jones 2022: 25–26). The many hundreds of surviving regimens, in both manuscript and early modern print, differ in their writing style, their organisational frameworks, and their cultural concerns. Tessa Storey (2017), for example, points to features rooted in national and religious contexts that distinguish early modern printed English regimens from their Italian counterparts. Perhaps most obvious are the Protestant identity that permeates most English regimens after the 1530s and the shift toward Hippocratic rather than Galenic medicine. The more direct incorporation of the Hippocratic *Airs, Water, Places* tradition established, in England, 'a singular "English" climate [. . . and] a single English body', while in Italy it gave rise to a plethora of 'local bodies' requiring regimens distinguished by geography (Storey 2017: 214–15). Sandra Cavallo and Storey (2013) likewise trace ideological changes in Italian regimens to sociocultural transformations among Italy's elites and the Counter-Reformation's effects, while Andrew Wear (2000: 154–209) and Eleanor Barnett (2020) note the increasing Protestant moralisation embedded in early modern English regimens alongside attempts to separate English practices and ideals from European Catholic ones.

Chief among most regimens' concerns, regardless of authorship or place of production, were food and drink; exercise was the next most commonly addressed non-natural. While the majority of regimens targeted general audiences, others concentrated on specific bodies, including pregnant women, babies and wet-nurses, the convalescent, labourers, armies, or travellers (Weiss-Amer 1993; Adamson 2004, 2010: 428; Newton 2017).

Still others dealt with spiritual matters (Yoshikawa 2013) or institutional needs (Hardingham 2005: ch. 3).

3.3 John Mirfield's *Gouernayl of Helþe*

3.3.1 Mirfield's Work in the English Regimen Corpus

Latin and vernacular regimens of health circulated in hundreds of manuscripts and multiple versions in late medieval England (Hardingham 2005: 261–5; eVK2 2019). Around the turn of the fifteenth century, John Mirfield produced yet another within his larger *Breviarium Bartholomei* that collated the works of previous authorities. Mirfield was well placed to produce this work. Although not a formally trained physician, by 1395 he was an ordained (but unbeneficed) priest and chaplain at St Bartholomew's Hospital, Smithfield (London), and in that role witnessed, if not actively provided, healing care for sick poor patients (Hartley & Aldridge 1936: 4–7; Getz 1985: 24). Certainly, the *Brevarium* was meant for use within the hospital and its attached priory. In Mirfield's own words, it targeted people without the financial means to consult a trained physician or medical books. Indeed, Faye Getz (2010: xxiii) notes that Mirfield used *De regimine sanitatis* to call attention to one of the key difficulties of dietetic medicine: the fact that the poor lacked the necessary lifestyle options to partake of 'a well-regulated regimen of health'.

Mirfield's regimen largely relied upon the *Regimen sanitatis* in Bernard de Gordon's 1308 *Liber de conservatione vite humane* for its content and the *Secretum secretorum*'s regimen for its structure (Hardingham 2005: 69). It was subsequently extracted from the *Breviarium* and circulated on its own, in both Latin (*Tractatus nobilis de regimine sanitatis*) and English translation (*Gouernayl of Helþe*). A new introduction severed its tie to the *Brevarium* and to Mirfield. The excerpted regimen ultimately proved to be more popular than the broader compilation: only two copies of the full *Breviarium Bartholomei* survive, compared to at least a dozen copies each of the Latin regimen and its English translation.[5] No excerpted regimen mentions Mirfield, but some are attributed erroneously to others.[6]

5 Kiernander (1980: 1) identified eight English copies. Hardingham (2005: 71–2) adds one, while eVK2 (2019) notices three more. Latin versions are found, among others, in six codices known as the Voigts–Sloane sibling group (Honkapohja 2017: 10–11) and in a professionally illuminated manuscript made for Lady Margaret Beaufort (Cambridge, Fitzwilliam Museum MS 261, fol. 19–20).

6 One attribution each to John of Bordeaux and to "Barthoēi" led nineteenth-century bibliographer William Blades (1858: 4–5) to mistakenly assign authorship to these men.

Around 1489, William Caxton printed a slightly revised version in English titled, like its source, *The Governayle of Helth*. This was among the earliest medical books printed in England. Caxton's successor Wynkyn de Worde printed two subsequent editions c. 1506 and c. 1528–1530. An excerpt from Lydgate's *Dietary* appears at the end of all three printed editions. Before the early 1600s, more English regimens of health appeared in print, often in multiple editions over years or decades. Some were translations of long-standing manuscript texts, such as Thomas Paynel's *Regimen sanitatis Salerni* (1528), or of printed Continental books like Thomas Phayer's *Regiment of Lyfe* (1543) and Sir John Harington's *The Englishmans Docter* [sic] (1607). Others were relatively original English productions that nevertheless overlapped significantly – sometimes verbatim – with each other and their predecessors, including works such as Sir Thomas Elyot's *Castel of Helth* (1539), Andrew Boorde's *Compendyous Regyment or Dyetary of Helth* (1547), William Bullein's *Gouernment of Health* (1558), Thomas Cogan's *Haven of Health* (1584), and Francis Bacon's *Of Regiment of Health* (1598). Paul Slack's (1979: 243) and Mary Fissell's (2011: 421) respective examinations of English medical printing rank regimens at about 20 per cent of total output until the 1660s.

3.3.2 Contents of Mirfield's Regimen

Mirfield's eight-chapter *Gouernayl of Helþe* claims to offer 'summe þinges þat longen to bodily helpe [. . . for] hym þat wele haue long lyf' (British Library Additional MS 29301: fol.89v in Kiernander 1980: 37, hereafter Add. 29301). Purportedly quoting Galen, the first chapter begins by summarising the advantages of 'holsom gouernaunce'. Mirfield touches briefly on each of the six non-naturals, noting for example that one should eat and drink moderately and at suitable times; exercise until winded or sweating; sleep until awoken 'by þin owne wille'; avoid cold or hot air after bloodletting; eat only in joy and eschew wrath, anger, and heavy thoughts; and, finally, not force or hinder defecation and 'hold noȝt þi pisse'. In short, he says, 'Kepe wel þees þre: gladnes in mende, trauayl in mesure and rewle of mete and drink' (Add. 29301: fol. 90r–v). Yet the primary focus of Mirfield's regimen is the Hippocratic *dietetic* – that is, food and exercise – and the subsequent chapters primarily address those two non-naturals. The chapter headings likewise concern only either food/drink or exercise. Although Mirfield briefly discusses sleep, emotions, air, and excretion elsewhere in the regimen, he does so almost exclusively as they relate to exercise or diet. He offers no separate advice, for example, to rectify the air or to improve one's frame of mind; nor does he do so for excreta or bedding. For him, the Hippocratic balance between diet and exercise is paramount in governing health; the other non-naturals play a supportive role rather than having intrinsic value of their own.

Chapters 2–4 focus largely on exercise and movement. The first actions to be taken each morning after awakening include stretching, combing one's hair to draw out vapours that filled the head during sleep, and washing. Evacuation is encouraged: 'put out þe superfluitees [. . .] [by] seeginge, pissyng, coghyng and spittyng' (Add. 29301: fol. 90r). The best exercises for health are voluntary and wilful. The involuntary manual labour and walking associated with carpenters, ploughmen, merchants, burgesses, and monks ('cloystrerers'), by contrast, do not count as 'excercyse of lechecraft' (Add. 29301: fol. 90v).[7] Exercises are offered both for those with financial resources (such as horse riding) and that can be done by people of limited means (such as carrying stones or holding one's breath). For lusty young men, Mirfield recommends, among other exercises, 'tempred flescly companyng' (i.e. moderate sex) with women, since it helps to govern their health and, supporting other non-naturals, enables them to better eat and sleep (Add. 29301: fol. 91r). Referencing Fulgencius and Galen, Mirfield states that wilful exercise not only improves humoral balance, sleep, excretion, appetite, and overall health, but also drives away vice and brings joy to one's mind. In other words, exercise both replaces all other medicines, including bloodletting, bathing, laxatives, and vomitories, since it 'fulfilleþ þe fawtes of alle othir' remedies, and ensures the proper maintenance of other non-naturals.

Chapters 5–7 turn to diet, providing instructions for when, how often, how much, and under what conditions one should eat and drink, as well as appropriate pre- and post-eating activities. Long lists of suitable foods appear, alongside warnings about which foods might endanger health. Singular care must be taken to avoid eating too many diverse foods at the same time, and certain pairings are dangerous: taken together, milk and fish, or milk and wine, cause leprosy, for example (Add. 29301: fol. 91v).[8] Mirfield suggests foods appropriate for people of different social standings and temperaments, but for all he counsels light exercise after eating, followed by sleep. Sleep, undertaken appropriately and in the right

[7] Mirfield takes this emphasis on voluntary exercise from Gordon; it stems from 'an Aristotelian understanding of leisure as a state of freedom from the necessity to work' (Hardingham 2005: 117).

[8] The same warning appears in the *Secretum secretorum*.

position, helps digestion and mitigates the effects of gluttony; too much or too little sleep, though, or sleeping at the wrong time, 'is noȝt gode' because it interferes with digestion, undoes the benefits of exercise, and causes weakness (Add. 29301: fol. 92v).

The final chapter chastises people who not only eschew good governance but also 'scorn leches and othir wyse men þat vse gode gouernaunce' by claiming that their customary habits – eating the wrong foods, sleeping too little, exercising inappropriately, or suffering heat or cold – do them no wrong (Add. 29301: fol. 93r). Every day, Mirfield says, such people inch closer to becoming leprous or dying suddenly.

3.3.3 Caxton's Amendments

Caxton's *The Governayle of Helth* is largely true to Mirfield's work. The latter's emphasis on diet and exercise over other non-naturals remains intact and, echoing Mirfield, Caxton has nothing further to say about sleep, air, excretions, or emotions aside from their relationship to diet and exercise. Nevertheless, concerning wine consumption (food/drink) and sexual activity (exercise), the printed version shifts markedly from the intention of Mirfield's advice. Where Mirfield advises the sparing use of strong drinks, from which he excludes wine given his numerous recommendations to drink it, Caxton says the opposite: 'eschew and spare stronge drynkes and *namely of wyne*' (emphasis added; c. 1489: A3v). He specifies that 'grete & hihe myghty or hihe coloured' (c. 1489: B1v) wine in particular, when mixed with milk, causes leprosy. Caxton's aversion to dark wine is evidenced throughout in the regimen, as he consistently alters Mirfield's wording to discuss its dangers. Caxton clearly preferred a lighter, clearer wine and only agrees with Mirfield about wine in terms of 'grete myghty coloured wyne' being appropriate for the 'coleryk mannys stomak' (Kiernander 1980: 81).

Second, Caxton adds a more detailed description of the type of women suitable for Mirfield's 'tempred flescly companyng wiþ womman' (Add. 29301: fol. 91r): 'wyth a yo[n]g broun woman is goode in wynter and wyth a yonge white woman ys goode in somer' (c. 1489: A7v–A8r). Such advice appears in the popular medieval encyclopaedic poem *Sidrak and Bokkus* with a full humoral explanation that Caxton omits: 'brown' women exude more heat, which men need in the cold winter.[9] The 'exercise' of sex, then, benefits men if done with appropriate kinds of

[9] I thank Alpo Honkapohja for bringing this to my attention.

women. Caxton further extends Mirfield's mild admonishment about the dangers of too much sex by adding a spiritual component. Mirfield contends that such exercise helps to govern health, but Caxton insists that while sex may help govern the *body*'s health, it does 'not to soule' (c. 1489: A8r). He also implies that simply engaging with women is both harmful and dangerous. In this way, Caxton foreshadows the English Protestant tendency to temper the benefits of moderate sexual intercourse that the medieval regimens promoted.

3.4 Wellcome Collection MS 674's *Regiment of Health*

3.4.1 Recalibrating the Non-naturals in Late Tudor England

The Wellcome *Regiment of Health* also largely copies the *Gouernayl of Helþe*, but uses modernised phraseology and considerably streamlines, condenses, and reconfigures the content. It begins by listing Mirfield's eight chapters but abandons the effort after the sixth chapter, leaving the seventh and eighth unrecorded. More importantly, the target audience transforms: while Mirfield's regimen addresses St Bartholomew's Hospital inmates and other low-resource people, including perhaps the priory monks and hospital workers, the Wellcome regimen clearly pursues a wealthier audience.

First, Mirfield specifies that horse riding 'is for riche men' and then offers a wide range of exercises for others (Add. 29301: fol. 90r). The Wellcome author proposes essentially the same range of outdoor–indoor exercises, but for him the distinction is not resources but rather 'yf a man can neyther ryde nor go abroad *by reason of the fowleness of the weather*' (emphasis added, WC674: p. 49). The weather dictates the suitability of exercises, not one's ability to afford them. Hardingham (2005: 122) notes that few general medieval regimens qualified their advice by recognising that horse riding was beyond the means of their readers, while Wear (2000: 160–1) similarly remarks that their recommended exercises show that early modern regimens appealed to 'the middling and upper ranks of society'. Mirfield's work is relatively unique in that it accounts for the capacities of all segments of society. Yet in remaking the regimen, the Wellcome author deliberately reorients its target audience and omits the features that made Mirfield's work more widely relevant.

Second, the Wellcome author recognises that some cannot afford to eat or drink whatever they wish. However, instead of discussing foods suitable for those of little means, as Mirfield does, he states: 'These rules therfore serve for such as may make choyce in their dyett and live in plentie' (WC674: p. 50). In other words, as with his exercise advice, the Wellcome author assumes his readers have the necessary resources to follow the proffered advice and that Mirfield's alternatives for different socioeconomic groups are unnecessary or inappropriate. Omitted too is Mirfield's advice to visit the poor, presumably as an act of charity. These are significant departures from Mirfield's original intention and point to the very different milieus in which the two writers lived, worked, and wrote: Mirfield among the sick poor, the Wellcome author perhaps for a clientele wealthy enough to pay for his services.[10]

The Wellcome regimen also modifies Mirfield's work in a way that illustrates changing ideas of healthiness and the relative importance of the six non-naturals. In the three chapters on exercise, perhaps minor revisions include the complete deletion of 'flescly companyng' as a recommended exercise and of 'cloystrerers' from the list of labourers whose non-voluntary exercise is 'immoderate and troublesome' (WC674: p. 47). For the former, the *Regiment* simply advises readers to 'flee unmeasureable exercyse of venerie' (WC674: pp. 49–50). No further mention of coitus appears, despite its elaboration in Caxton's version and the greater attention given to the act by other sixteenth-century English regimens (Storey 2017: 225–6). Without knowing the identity of the Wellcome author, it is difficult to assess if this exclusion represents a personal belief or is couched in some wider social meaning. The latter omission, by contrast, clearly reflects the suppression and closure of monasteries, priories, and convents earlier in the century following King Henry VIII's Act of Supremacy.

A much more significant change in this part of the regimen concerns a non-natural to which Mirfield pays little attention: the air and the surrounding environment. Relying on Hippocratic and Galenic tradition, medical writers had long blamed environmental features such as stagnant bodies of water, damp enclosed spaces, human and animal waste, or industrial by-products – anything that emitted foul odours – for generating diseases such as plague. Recurrent outbreaks also spurred continued attempts to cleanse and improve disease-ridden (natural and built) environments (Jones 2016). Like other regimen writers, Mirfield entreats readers to exercise 'in clene places' where they can enjoy the 'clene eir and delyte in seyng fer and ner, on water and on lond, heuen and erþe, grene and falow' (Add. 29301: fol. 90v). A new and substantial ecological

[10] The question of whether the Wellcome author intended to publish his work is beyond the scope of this chapter.

description in the Wellcome regimen highlights the much greater relevance being attributed to the quality of the environment in safeguarding health by the later sixteenth century, as London's rapidly increasing population and greatly expanded urban boundaries, for example, not only altered the urban environment but enabled more devastating outbreaks of disease than the city had seen for almost a century.[11] To the Wellcome author, potentially disease-ridden urban environments means that labour and exercise

> is a verie good recreation for the bodye *yf it be done* in sweete and drye places and holsome ayres where a man may take pleasure and delight to see goodlye trees and plantes, pleasant countryes, delectable fields meadows and pastures, delightfull streames of running waters, and especyally in such places wher he may take the sweete sent and odour of most flagrant & odoriferous flowers and most holsome hearbes in well tilled, dressed and manured lands and by the viwe therof and by the delectation and sweete contentment he shall receyve therby his mynd may contynually be stirred upp to give laud and prayse to our good and gracious lord God and Saviour. (emphasis added, WC674: p. 48; see Figure 9 in the Image Gallery)

Where Mirfield recommends exercising in 'clene eyer', the Wellcome author insists that for exercise to be truly beneficial for body, mind, and spirit, it must be done in a salubrious environment that evokes a true sense of pleasure, positively stirs one's emotions, and delights one's senses of sight, hearing, and smell. While Mirfield calls on exercisers to praise God for the sights they witness, the Wellcome author shifts agency to the environment itself, seeing in it the power to invoke such 'sweete contentment' that the exerciser's mind is emotionally and mentally moved to praise God for bestowing such benefits upon humankind. This shift in intent adds a medical aspect to Alexandra Walsham's (2011: 566) observation that the Reformation 'upheld the idea that God used nature as a supplementary text of revelation and that He emblazoned trees, springs, and other natural and preternatural phenomena with moral and spiritual lessons.' They also had health-giving benefits. The Wellcome writer further links action and environment elsewhere in the regimen, emphasising that walking and riding should only be done 'in cleane places, and hight and in pure ayres and not to come amongst muckhills or marishes'

[11] Although plague is not mentioned in the regimen, the Wellcome author's inclusion of two plague treatises in the manuscript points to immediate concerns with the disease.

(WC674: p. 47) or 'in sweete ayres drye and cleane places free from evill savours and from filthie marishe waters *as is before rehearsed*' (emphasis added, WC674: p. 49). In each instance, he turns Mirfield's simple direction to exercise in 'clene places' into an elucidation of the environment's intrinsic value in governing and promoting physical, spiritual, and mental health.

The influential Hippocratic *Airs, Waters, and Places* tradition suggested a relationship between particular geographies, topographies, climates, and their diseases. After its translation into Latin in 1525, a renewed interest in Hippocratic ideas influenced early modern English thinking about which environments were healthy or unhealthy (Wear 2008). There already existed a long-standing assumption that the countryside was cleaner – and thus healthier – than the city, and that city living itself was deleterious to health (Wear 2000: 155–209). Yet the Wellcome author's long addition also accords with recent research (Cavallo 2016; Cavallo & Storey 2017a) on the growing attention paid in sixteenth- and seventeenth-century Italy to the explicit importance of good air quality and sound ecologies for maintaining health. Represented here by wholesome airs, sweet running streams, odiferous flowers, and delectable meadows, these ideas clearly reached England. Most sixteenth-century English regimens that addressed the environment, however, focused primarily on air temperature or climate – or on the filth of cities – rather than on the health-giving visual, auditory, and olfactory aspects of the natural environment that the Wellcome writer emphasises. On this point, he seems to have been ahead of his local contemporaries, not only in recognising the wider role of the environment in human health but also in noticing its reciprocal role with several non-naturals: exercise, air, and emotions.

The Wellcome regimen likewise gives more detailed attention than Mirfield to the eating/drinking non-natural, in particular to food choices in a new eighth chapter, and blends both food and drink together (whereas Mirfield allocates separate chapters to them). One set of differences, namely the items included in or omitted from lists of healthy and unhealthy nourishments, most likely reflects the evolution of food availabilities, preferences, customs, and taboos – including the greatly increased use of and taste for sugar in the sixteenth century – both society wide and among the specific socioeconomic and religious audiences targeted by the two versions of the regimen (Thirsk 2006; Barnett 2020). Joan Thirsk argues that larger quantities and more varieties of meat and fowl appeared on English tables during the Tudor decades. Her observation that 'hardly a bird in the sky was not eaten' (2006: xi) is borne out by the Wellcome list.

Whereas Mirfield considers that wholesome meats include a wide range of birds 'of þe feld and of þe wode *but no3t of þe water*' (emphasis added, Add. 29301: fol. 91v), the Wellcome inventory comprises thirty-two different bird species, many of which are waterfowl. Also notable in terms of changing tastes is the list of fish that once played a significant role in the English diet that now are no longer deemed to be palatable or wholesome: 'cunger, dogge ffishe, raye, freshe salmon, Thornebacke, herringe, makarell, porpus, seale [. . . and] all muddye fishe that are slymye as Eales, Tench, Roche' (WC674: p. 53). By contrast, other foods once deemed unappetising or unhealthy, such as fruits and vegetables, increasingly find their way into English dietaries. Wear (2000: 169–78) notes the centrality of food, its relationship to health and illness, and the connections made between cooks and physicians in early modern English regimens. Many of the contemporary printed regimens with which the Wellcome writer was likely familiar also included long discussions of healthy and unhealthy foods. While those texts offered detailed analyses of the health benefits of individual foods and linked them to humoral complexions, however, the Wellcome text does little more than offer a list of approved or disapproved foods.

In some ways, the Wellcome text is more like its medieval source than its contemporaries. Yet the Wellcome regimen moves away from Mirfield in terms of what Barnett calls 'Protestant perceptions of food and eating in Reformation England' (Barnett 2020: 507–8). Mirfield offers an extended discussion of the harms caused by Lenten foods, namely the costive nature of fish and peas pottage, and provides instructions to safely ease one's digestion through fasting periods (Add. 29301: fol. 93v). Although the English Church continued to enforce what were essentially Catholic fasting practices until the mid-seventeenth century, Protestant writers desacralised food and recast the fasting habit as both a secular one designed to benefit commercial and military needs and a godly one that evoked obedience to princely (not popish) laws (Barnett 2020: 515–17). The Wellcome author does not go so far as some of his fellow regimen writers in discussing the godly significance of fasting or of food, remaining focused instead on the agreeableness of food and eating habits with one's 'constitutio[n], and for the healthe of his bodye' (WC674: p. 50). He does, nevertheless, erase all mention of Lent, fasting, and peas pottage from his version of the regimen, rendering invisible Mirfield's original Catholic assumptions.

The Wellcome author enhances Mirfield's discussion of the other non-naturals by giving more direct notice to sleep and emotions (but not to excretion). Rather than simply embedding sleep within the chapter 'What schold be do [sic] aftir mete' (Add. 29301: fol. 92r), for example, the Wellcome regimen states explicitly: 'The seventhe chapter teachethe certayne rules to be observed [. . .] about sleepinge good for the preservation of the healthe of man' (WC674: p. 51). Like Mirfield and following medieval tradition, the Wellcome author recommends sleeping first on the right side, and then on the left. He then diverges from Mirfield's advice: instead of advising the sleeper to return to the right side and to sleep slightly curled up or on the stomach but never upright – since doing so turns superfluities into wicked evils – the Wellcome writer instructs 'lye at yor ease *soe yo^{u} lye not on the backe*, for that causethe the superfluities to drawe unto the hearte' (emphasis added, WC674: p. 52). Wear (2000: 178) notes that all early modern English regimen authors forbade sleeping on the back; in interpolating this notion into Mirfield's regimen, the Wellcome author brought the medieval advice up to date and dispensed with what no longer held value.

In condensing Mirfield's longer preliminary discussion of wholesome governance, the Wellcome writer likewise adds an early modern recognition that emotions reside in both the mind and the heart:

> Gallion & Constantyne affirme that measurable Abstinency is the most p[ro]fitable medycyne to eschue cares and penssiveness heviness and dulness, wrathe and anger [. . . the best advice is] keepe yor hart merrye and yor mynd ioyfull. (WC674: p. 46)

A similar point is made about the value of a morning walk: it enables one to be 'honestlye merrye' and 'doe much comfort and glad the heart' at the same time that it 'consume[s] evill and grosse humors in the bodye'. Walking in a salubrious environment likewise 'ingendre[s] ioye comfort and consolation' and 'comfortethe all the members and parts of the bodye' (WC674: pp. 47–9). Mirfield does not make such a direct connection between exercise and emotions, nor does he extend merriness to the heart – and thus, presumably, to the soul, as Protestant writers later declare.

The final section of the Wellcome regimen corresponds with Mirfield's original eighth chapter, focusing on people's customary poor regimental habits related to diet, exercise, sleep, and air temperature. The primary turn here comes in how the Wellcome author describes the impact of immoderation: instead of Mirfield's stroke of death, it would 'spoyle a mans complexion, waste nature [and] destroye his livelie spirits' (WC674: p. 53). The phrase 'livelie spirits' is one that the Wellcome writer uses throughout the manuscript, including in his version of John of Burgundy's plague tract and numerous recipes, and which he typically associates with 'spiritual members' (WC674: p. 40), or the soul. By 'keepinge the bodye in good governement free from excesse', he claims that one is 'more fitt to serve God and to mannage worldlye affayres'. This, it seems, may be the ultimate purpose of the Wellcome regimen.

3.4.2 *The Wellcome Regimen: Protestant Undertones*

As the last quote suggests, the Wellcome writer put significantly more emphasis on the link between a healthy regimen and serving God than did Mirfield. Performing one's 'duties in his devotions towards Almightie God' (WC674: p. 47) should occur first each day before any other activity, and all actions thereafter are to be done while 'servinge God contynually'. Furthermore, the Wellcome regimen ends with this summary: 'And soe to conclud lett us ever more give laud and thanks unto Almightie God & gratious Lord wch hath given to man remedyes for all sicknesses & diseases' (WC674: p. 54). Although Mirfield was a cleric and priest, his regimen is less overtly religious than the Wellcome *Regiment*. Instead, acknowledging Christ's help, making reference to God and his angels, and advising that one should pray and praise God garner no more emphasis than washing one's face or drinking good wine. The Wellcome author wrote during an era of religious upheaval in England, and early modern regimens embodied the increasingly moralising tone that appeared in other contemporary writing (Wear 2000: 178–84; Barnett 2020).[12]

A century earlier, Caxton had inserted moral judgement into Mirfield's regimen related to the issues of drinking and sex; at the very least, his amendments reflected personal preferences that remained intact in de Worde's subsequent editions. As Kiernander notes (1980: 80), Caxton's 'attempt to edit and update the text and make it more suitable for and accessible to a wider readership' surely must have reflected changing attitudes and dispositions. Late fifteenth-century English plague treatises also started to adopt a moralistic tone, and religious rhetoric was a common feature of sixteenth- and seventeenth-century tracts (Slack 1985: 228–47; Jones 2022). Like plague treatises, early modern regimens increasingly reflected what George Keiser (2003: 292) calls the 'religious, moral, and medical concerns of early modern England'. Many of the authors and translators of English regimens were directly tied to the church

[12] The Wellcome author made similar religious and audience shifts in rewriting a centuries-old plague treatise. See Jones 2021.

or 'were deeply religious men' (Cavallo & Storey 2017b: 32). Although the author of the Wellcome text is rather less moralistic or condemnatory than the regimens published by some of his contemporaries – who often invoked biblical verse from the Geneva Bible to reinforce their anti-excess messages (Wear 2000: 182–4) – he nevertheless raises the importance of 'Almightie God' to a level seen in neither Mirfield's original work nor Caxton's later version.

In an era when humanist medicine generated a new reverence for ancient authorities, perhaps the most striking among the many omissions that the Wellcome author made in adapting Mirfield's regimen is the near-erasure of the traditional medical figures on whose authority much of the advice was based. This too may result from the regimen's more religious tone. Although a few mentions do remain, most of Mirfield's references to Galen, Aristotle, Avicenna, and Constantine – or even to general 'leches' – are gone. In the place of these canonical medical authors and third-person advice, the author instead speaks directly to the reader. Where Mirfield says 'a general reule of alle leches is þat þin oure be of etynge when þou hungrest' (Add. 29301: fol. 91r), for example, the Wellcome text reads 'eate not without an Appetite' (WC674: p. 50). This directness mimics in many ways the biblical verses cited in Elyot's *Castel of Helth* (1539), Boorde's *Compendyous Regyment or Dyetary of Helth* (1547), and Cogan's *Haven of Health* (1584), suggestively placing the Wellcome author in the milieu of Protestant reforming culture.

3.5 Conclusion

Cavallo and Storey (2013, 2017a) point to significant developments in the health regimen genre by the early modern era. First, as humoral theory evolved, so too did ideas about what constituted healthy living, a healthy body, and a healthy environment. Second, the holistic nature and interdependence of – and reciprocity between – the six non-naturals became somewhat clearer. Third, national and religious identities became increasingly evident. In copying and modernising Mirfield's *Gouernayl of Helþe*, the Wellcome author straddles medieval tradition and early modern innovation. Although created in the same temporal and religious context as its English contemporaries, the Wellcome regimen's reliance on a late fourteenth-century work sets it somewhat apart from its printed counterparts. Its wealthier target audience, emphasis on the natural environment, greater attention to all the non-naturals (aside from excretion), and religiosity – both explicit and implicit – are evident departures from Mirfield's regimen, revealing how the author adapted an old work to suit his modern setting. On the one hand, the Wellcome author's revisions reflect English attention to the Hippocratic *Airs, Waters, Places* tradition and the ways in which an emerging Protestant identity recast ideas about what was regarded as harmful or beneficial to health. Yet, on the other hand, he does not take his revised regimen further along the path established by writers such as Elyot, Bullein, or Cogan, who shifted English regimens' focus in the sixteenth century from the six Galenic non-naturals to the 'Hippocratic Five' and placed much greater emphasis on sexual intercourse (Storey 2017). The Wellcome manuscript regimen thus remains in a transitional position, not quite medieval and not quite (early) modern. Despite Wear's contention (2000: 155) that English regimens represent '*l'histoire immobile*', the Wellcome *Regiment of Health* provides a window into evolving conceptions of health culture and points to the ongoing relevance of medieval ideas and works in an era of considerable social change.

REFERENCES

Primary Sources

London, British Library, Additional MS 29301.

London, Wellcome Collection MS 674.

[No author]. 1489–90. *The Governayle of Helth*. London: William Caxton.

Bacon, Francis. 1598. *Of Regiment of Health*. London: John Windet.

Boorde, Andrew. 1547. *Compendyous Regyment or Dyetary of Helth*. London: William Powell.

Bullein, William. 1558. *Gouernment of Health*. London: John Day.

Cogan, Thomas. 1584. *Haven of Health*. London: Henry Midleton.

Elyot, Thomas. 1539. *Castel of Helth*. London: Thomas Berthelet.

Harington, John. 1607. *The Englishmans Docter. Or, The Schoole of Salerne*. London: William Jaggard.

Paynel, Thomas. 1528. *Regimen sanitatis Salerni*. London: Thomas Berthelet.

Phayer, Thomas. 1543. *Regiment of Lyfe*. London: Edward Whytchurch.

Secondary Sources

Adamson, Melitta Weiss. 2004. Baby-food in the middle ages. In Richard Hosking (ed.), *Nurture: Proceedings of the Oxford symposium on food and cookery 2003*, 1–11. Bristol: Footwork.

Adamson, Melitta. 2010. Bernard de Gordon and Arnald de Villanova: A tale of two regimes. In Andreas Speer & David Wirmer (eds.), *1308: Eine*

Topographie historischer Gleichzeitigkeit, 419–35. Berlin; New York: Walter de Gruyter.

Barnett, Eleanor. 2020. Reforming food and eating in Protestant England, c.1540–c.1640. *Historical Journal* 63(3): 507–27.

Blades, William. 1858. *The gouernayle of helthe: With the medecyne of ye stomacke. Reprinted from Caxton's editio, (circa m.cccc.xci), with introductory remarks and notes*. London: Blades, East, & Blades.

Cavallo, Sandra. 2016. Health, air and material culture in the early modern Italian domestic environment. *Social History of Medicine* 29(4): 694–716.

Cavallo, Sandra, & Tessa Storey. 2013. *Healthy living in late renaissance Italy*. Oxford: Oxford University Press.

Cavallo, Sandra, & Tessa Storey (eds.). 2017a. *Conserving health in early modern culture: Bodies and environments in Italy and England*. Manchester: Manchester University Press.

Cavallo, Sandra & Tessa Storey. 2017b. Regimens, authors and readers: Italy and England compared. In Cavallo, Sandra, & Tessa Storey (eds.), *Conserving health in early modern culture: Bodies and environments in Italy and England*, 23–52. Manchester: Manchester University Press.

Demaitre, Luke E. 1980. *Doctor Bernard de Gordon: Professor and practitioner*. Toronto: Pontifical Institute of Mediaeval Studies.

eVK2. 2019. An expanded and revised version of Linda Ehrsam Voigts and Patricia Deery Kurtz, *Scientific and Medical Writings in Old and Middle English: An Electronic Reference*. Ann Arbor: University of Michigan Press.

Fissell, Mary. 2011. Popular medical writing. In Joad Raymond (ed.), *Oxford history of popular print culture*, vol. 1, 418–31. Oxford: Oxford University Press.

Getz, Faye. 1985. John Mirfield and the *Breviarium Bartholomei*: The medical writings of a clerk at St Bartholomew's Hospital in the later fourteenth century. *Society for the Social History of Medicine Bulletin* 37: 24–6.

Getz, Faye. 2010. *Healing and society in medieval England: A Middle English translation of the pharmaceutical writings of Gilbertus Anglicus*. Madison: University of Wisconsin Press.

Gil-Sotres, Pedro. 1998. The regimens of health. In Mirko D. Grmek (ed.), Antony Shugaar (trans.), *Western medical thought from antiquity to the middle ages*, 291–318. Cambridge, MA: Harvard University Press.

Hardingham, Glenn James. 2005. The regimen in late medieval England. PhD dissertation, University of Cambridge.

Hartley, Sir Percival Horton-Smith, & Harold Richard Aldridge (eds.). 1936. *Johannes de Mirfield of St Bartholomew's, Smithfield: His life and work*. Cambridge: Cambridge University Press.

Honkapohja, Alpo. 2017. *Alchemy, medicine, and commercial book production: A codicological and linguistic study of the Sloane manuscript group*. Turnhout: Brepols.

Jones, Lori. 2016. The diseased landscape: Medieval and early modern plaguescapes. *Landscapes* 17(2): 108–23.

Jones, Lori. 2018. Unrecorded versions of John of Burgundy's plague tract and identifying 'lost' copies of the same. *Notes and Queries* 65(1): 14–17.

Jones, Lori. 2021. Itineraries and transformations: John of Burgundy's Plague Treatise. *Bulletin of the History of Medicine* 95(2): 277–314.

Jones, Lori. 2022. *Patterns of plague: Changing ideas of plague in England and France, 1348–1750*. Montreal: McGill-Queen's University Press.

Jones, Peter Murray. 1995. Reading medicine in Tudor Cambridge. In Vivian Nutton & Roy Porter (eds.), *The history of medical education in Britain*, 153–83. Amsterdam: Rodopi.

Keiser, George R. 2003. Two medieval plague treatises and their afterlife in early modern England. *Journal of the History of Medicine and Allied Sciences* 58(3): 292–324.

Kiernander, A. R. D. 1980. The Governal of health. PhD dissertation, University of Auckland.

Leong, Elaine. 2018. *Recipes and everyday knowledge: Medicine, science and the household in early modern England*. Chicago: University of Chicago Press.

Newton, Hannah. 2017. 'She sleeps well and eats an egg': Convalescent care in early modern England. In Sandra Cavallo & Tessa Storey (eds.), *Conserving health in early modern culture: Bodies and environments in Italy and England*, 104–32. Manchester: Manchester University Press.

Nicoud, Marilyn. 2007. *Les régimes de santé au Moyen Âge*. Rome: Publications de l'École française de Rome.

Slack, Paul. 1979. Mirrors of health and treasure of poor men: The uses of the vernacular medical literature of Tudor England. In Charles Webster (ed.), *Health, medicine and mortality in the sixteenth century*, 237–74. Cambridge: Cambridge University Press.

Slack, Paul. 1985. *The impact of plague in Tudor and Stuart England*. London: Routledge & Kegan Paul.

Storey, Tessa. 2017. English and Italian health advice: Protestant and Catholic bodies. In Sandra Cavallo & Tessa Storey (eds.), *Conserving health in early modern culture: Bodies and environments in Italy and England*, 210–34. Manchester: Manchester University Press.

Taavitsainen, Irma. 2006. Medical discourse: Early genres, 14th and 15th centuries. In Keith Brown (ed.), *The encyclopedia of language & linguistics*, 2nd ed., 688–94. Oxford: Elsevier.

Thirsk, Joan. 2006. *Food in early modern England: Phases, fads, fashions, 1500–1760*. London: Hambledon Continuum.

Walsham, Alexandra. 2011. *The reformation of the landscape: Religion, identity and memory in early modern Britain and Ireland*. Oxford: Oxford University Press.

Wear, Andrew. 2000. *Knowledge and practice in English medicine, 1550–1680*. Cambridge: Cambridge University Press.

Wear, Andrew. 2008. Place, health, and disease: The *Airs, waters, places* tradition in early modern England and North America. *Journal of Medieval and Early Modern Studies* 38(3): 443–65.

Weiss-Amer, Melitta. 1993. Medieval women's guides to food during pregnancy: Origins, texts, and traditions. *Canadian Bulletin of Medical History* 10(1): 5–23.

Yoshikawa, Naoë Kukita. 2013. The translation of the *Regimen Sanitatis* into a handbook for the devout laity: A new look at the Kalender of Shepherds and its context. In Alessandra Petrina (ed.), *The Medieval translator / Traduire au Moyen Age: In principio fuit interpres*, 303–15. Turnhout: Brepols.

CHAPTER 4

Surgical Handbooks Translated into Low German

Chiara Benati

Hieronymus Brunschwig's *Buch der Cirurgia* (Johannes Grüninger 1497, reprinted in Klein 1911) and Hans von Gersdorff's *Feldtbuch der Wundarzney* (Schott 1517) are the first two surgical handbooks printed in the High German language area. During the early modern age these texts enjoyed great popularity, as witnessed by the high number of editions after the first ones and by the existence of, respectively, English and Dutch and Dutch and Latin (?)[1] translations.

Moreover, these two surgical compendia also became popular in the northern part of present-day Germany: in 1518, a complete Low German translation of Brunschwig's *Cirurgia* – the *Boek der Wundenartzstedye* – was produced and printed by Ludwig Dietz in Rostock, while some twenty years later a large portion of a Low German version of Hans von Gersdorff's *Feldtbuch der Wundarzney* was included – under the title *Dat velt bock* – in the manuscript miscellanea of medical texts known as Copenhagen, Kongelige Bibliotek, GKS, 1663 4to (fols. 1r–86v).

Despite the similarity of the High German sources and the identity of the target language – Low German, a cognate[2] vernacular[3] – the *Boek der Wundenartzstedye* and the *Velt bock* represent two different and, in many ways, opposite forms of the translation and reception of a medical text.

[1] It is uncertain whether any Latin translation of the text really existed. A Latin edition of the *Feldtbuch* dating to 1551 is mentioned in the late eighteenth-century bibliographical repository *Biblioteca chirurgica* by Albrecht von Haller (1774: 176). Frederiksen (1983: 627) refers to two different Latin editions of the surgical handbook printed in Strasbourg by Schott in 1542 and in Frankfurt by Gülfferich in 1551. Since no surviving copies of these exist and no Latin translation of von Gersdorff's work is recorded among the texts produced by either Schott or Gülfferich, we can assume that these indications were based on some kind of misunderstanding, e.g. a 1532 Albucasis edition containing some of the woodcuts used in the *Feldtbuch* could have been mistaken for a Latin translation of the surgical handbook. See also Panse (2012: 154).

[2] On the linguistic peculiarity of scientific translation between cognate languages, see Benati (2018).

[3] In the sixteenth century translations from one vernacular into another were still quite rare, especially in the field of medicine and science in general, which continued to be informed by the Latin–vernacular bilingualism. See also Pantin (2007: 165).

4.1 Aims and Methods

The present chapter aims to show, on the basis of two case studies, how High German surgical texts were not only translated but also transformed and adapted to new modes and circumstances of use as they travelled northward and reached the Low German language area, and how the medium (print vs manuscript) and expected readership are reflected in the text genre, conventions, structure, and authors' attitude towards their work.

To do this, the 1518 printed *Boek der Wundenartzstedye* (edited in Benati 2012) and the *Velt bock* (edited in Benati 2017a) transmitted in Copenhagen, GKS 1663 4to, are systematically compared with their respective High German sources on both a macroscopic (genre, structure, medium of transmission) and a microscopic level (pragmatically determined variants in the Low German rendering of the single passages and prescriptions). The results of this collation are not seen exclusively as translation decisions, but are evaluated within a broader theoretical framework constituted, first of all, by Irma Taavitsainen's (2006) classification of the medieval genres of medical discourse and also by the history of commonplace books in practice (Havens 2001) and, since manuscript commonplace books such as the Copenhagen one are written extensions of reading (Havens 2001: 9), by the history of reading and of medical knowledge in use (Andersen & Sauer 2001; Sherman 2001; Sherman 2009; Leong 2018). Since the main focus of these studies is constituted by English medical texts, this chapter fundamentally applies their epistemic models to a different language area; that is, the German one.[4]

4.2 The Low German Texts

4.2.1 *Dat Boek der Wundenartzstedye. yn latin geheten Cirurgia*

At the beginning of the sixteenth century, Brunschwig's handbook reached the Low German language area, where it was translated and printed in Rostock by Ludwig Dietz in 1518. The text, of which three copies are known (Berlin, Staatsbibliothek, Jg 3484; Schwerin, Landesbibliothek von

[4] For a detailed description of the two High German handbooks, see Benati (2012: 7–10) and Benati (2017a: 8–10), respectively.

Mecklenburg-Vorpommern, Rara HSt VII 745; Copenhagen, Kongelige Bibliotek, barcode 20002339), appears under the title *Dat Boek der Wundenartzstedye. yn latin geheten Cirurgia.* This title appears on the work's first page together with a woodcut representing the so-called wound man (German *Wundenmann*) (see Figure 10 in the Image Gallery).

The name of the Low German translator is never mentioned in the text or in the preface, where we find the name of the Strasbourg surgeon ('Hieronimus Brunswyck bőrdich va*n* Straßeborch'; see Benati 2012: 15). According to Lisch (1839: 154), the High German surgical manual could have reached Rostock through the court physician Dr Rembertus Giltzheim, who, in 1519, published with Ludwig Dietz the *Liber collectionum Aphorismorum Hypocratis* (Lisch 1838: 64).

Apart from the anatomical addendum (*Von der Anathomi*), the Middle Low German handbook preserves the structure of the High German original, which is divided into seven treatises (Benati 2012: 11):

1. wat eyneme yewelke*n* wundenartzste*n* in steede*n* vn*d* wesen notrostich js (What every surgeon needs);
2. va*n* alle*n* wunde*n* yn eyner gemeyne*n* lere / wo de gescheen to heele*n* vnd to curere*n* (On all wounds in general, how to heal them where they are);
3. va*n* alle*n* wunde*n* yn eyneme yewelke*n* besundere*n* gelede van deme hőuede beth to de*n* vőte*n* (On all wounds in a specific part from head to heel);
4. van Valle*n*. Slån. Stően / bynnen edder buten lyues: van em suluen gescheen edder dorch andere minschen (On falls, blows, and hits both inside and outside the body which happen alone or are caused by other people);
5. wo du de brőke der been va*n* dem*e* hőuede beth vp de vőte richte*n* vn*d* bynde*n* schalt (How you should treat and bandage fractures from head to heel);
6. van den lederen. Enkelen vn*d* bőgen yn to theen de dar sint vorrůcket ynt ghemeyne van deme hőuede beth to den vőten (On sprained joint and ankles in general from head to heel);
7. vynden eyn yslick stůcke des du yn desseme werke nottrofftich bist / ghescheeten Anthidotarius sere kort begrepen (How to find the remedies which are mentioned in this work, a very short antidotary).

Apart from the woodcut of the 'wound man' on the title page, the 1518 Low German print includes only another large (fol. XIXr) and twelve smaller images (fols. LXXIIIr, LXXIIIv, LXXIIIIr, LXIIIIv, CXXIIr, and

CLr)[5] that represent surgical instruments and the procedure to reduce mandibular fractures, though none of the original woodcuts of the surgeon teaching his students has been reproduced.

4.2.2 Dat velt bock *in Copenhagen, Kongelige Bibliotek, GKS 1663 4to*

A fragment of the only known Low German translation of Hans von Gersdorff's *Feldtbuch der Wundarzney* is transmitted in the early sixteenth-century (probably before 1540)[6] parts of Copenhagen, Kongelige Bibliotek, GKS 1663 4to.[7]

As far as its contents are concerned, the manuscript may be defined as a collection of Middle Low German medical texts including:

- the fragment of a Low German translation of Hans von Gersdorff's *Feldtbuch der Wundarzney* known as *Dat velt bock* (fols. 1r–86v);
- *Dat kinder bock* (fols. 87r–146r);[8]
- a collection of recipes for the preparation of unguents (fols. 146v–58r);
- a detailed explanation of some common medical verbs deriving from Latin (fols. 158v–66v);
- two paragraphs about anthrax, which probably constitute an addition to what comes after (fol. 170v);
- an alphabetical glossary on surgically treatable pathologies (fols. 171r–7v);
- an alphabetical glossary on medical terms and phrases (fols. 179r–204r; on this, see Benati 2016b);
- a *practica* (fols. 226r–7r);

[5] Some of these images are extremely similar to those included in the High German first edition of Brunschwig's work, e.g. a perspective of a table on which many surgical instruments are placed in fol. XIXr, which seems to be indebted to the one in the Strasbourg edition, even though they cannot possibly have been printed using the same woodblock. See also Benati (2012: 12).

[6] The Roman digits *MDXL*, which can be found on the lower margin of fol. 227r and are repeated in fol. 241v, can be interpreted as the possible year of the manuscript's completion. See also Borchling (1900: 57).

[7] In its present form the manuscript is constituted by three parts that were bound together in modern times: fols. 1–206, in quarto, early sixteenth century, probably before 1540, written by a single hand (H 1) most likely in the region south of Lüneburg; fols. 207–25, end of the fifteenth century, written by another, neater, and more regular hand (H 2) and provided with red rubrics and initials; and fols. 226–41, in duodecimo, written by H 1, in the same irregular *cursiva*. See also Borchling (1900) and Panse (2012: 154).

[8] This Middle Low German handbook, preserved exclusively in GKS 1663 4to, consists of a treatise on phlebotomy, an incomplete calendar, and a series of prescriptions for pathologies, which are ordered from head to heel, and has been identified as a Middle Low German translation of the Latin treatise *Liber de aegritudinibus infantium* by Cornelius Roelans van Mecheln (1486). On this, see also Benati (2017b), Lindgren (1983: 1148–9), and Malm (2015: 1460–2).

- a *practica*, mentioning the twelve months as well as the hours of the day (fols. 227v–40r).[9]

Moreover, the analysis of the alphabetical glossary on fols. 179r–204r and of the cross-references constituting some of its glosses proves that the manuscript, in its original form, included at least two other large works (over 400 leaves altogether) – most likely a surgical manual (*Ciurgia*) and a herbal (*Herbariuß*) – which are now lost. The presence of the latter in the original construction of this medical commonplace book is also confirmed by the otherwise quite surprising absence of pharmacobotanical terms in the glossary (Benati 2016b: 7).

The fragment of the Low German translation of Hans von Gersdorff's *Feldtbuch der Wundarzney*, whose title – *Dat velt bock* – appears in fol. 1r (see Figure 11 in the Image Gallery), together with that of the second text contained in the manuscript – *Dat kinder bock* – and repeated in fol. 15r, is preceded by a short note on how to perform medicine correctly and on the impossibility of fully mastering this art, two paragraphs containing therapeutic indications (fol. 2r), an analytical index to the text (fols. 3r–12v; Benati 2013: 298), and a short glossary of Latin terms (fols. 13r–14r; Benati 2013: 300; Benati 2022b: 406).

The actual fragment transmits a series of apparently randomly ordered thematic chapters from the High German handbook, whose beginning is usually marked by bold-written keywords. These deal, *inter alia*, with phlebotomy (*Ader latende*, fol. 15r), zodiac signs (*Van den teken*, fol. 20v), fistula (*Fistel*, fol. 21r), carbuncle (*Carbunculuß*, fol. 23v), anthrax (*Antrox edder Antrax*, fol. 24v), ulcerated cancer (*Cancer ulceratum*, fol. 26r), estiomenus (*Estiomenuß*, fol. 28r), stemming blood flow (*Blot stillen*, fol. 33v), leprosy (*Lepra*, fol. 34v), morphea (*Morphea*, fol. 35v), the various remedies a surgeon has to know and use (*Medicina*, fol. 38v), head wounds (*Houet dat vorwundet iß*, fol. 45v), wounds to internal organs (*Ingeweyd vorwüntinge*, fol. 56r), and haemorrhoids (*Von den flot*, *Emorroidarum*, fol. 61r; Benati 2017c: 508–9).

4.3 Two Different Paths of Knowledge Dissemination: Translation versus Transformation (and Translation) of Medical Discourse

The *Boek der Wundenartzstedye* and the *Velt bock* represent two different and, in many respects, opposite forms of translation and, more generally,

[9] As for those included in other essays of mine on the topic, this description of the Copenhagen manuscript is a synthesis of the one included in Benati (2017a: 11–12).

the reception of medical discourse. The very role of the translation – that is, of the language code switching between High and Low German – in the two texts appears to have been extremely different. While the publication of the *Boek der Wundenartzstedye* was mainly motivated by the wish to make Brunschwig's surgical compendium accessible to the northern German public, the Low German rendering of the prescriptions inserted in Copenhagen, GKS 1663 4to, is complementary to the transformation of von Gersdorff's handbook into part of a medical commonplace book. The *Velt bock* is, in fact, primarily this and thus resembles other – High German – manuscript witnesses of the *Feldtbuch der Wundarzney*, for example the eighteenth-century Lucerne, ZHB, Pp 27 4to,[10] which can be inserted into the 'dynamic dialogue' between manuscript and printed cultures described by Leong (2018: 170).

4.3.1 Medium of Transmission and Expected Readership

The first element contributing to determining this different approach to the source text is constituted by the medium of transmission: while the Low German version of Brunschwig's *Buch der Cirurgia* is transmitted in print, the fragment of Hans von Gersdorff's *Feldtbuch der Wundarzney* is inserted into a manuscript medical miscellanea.

The choice of different mediums is closely connected with the expected readership of the two translations. Printed texts such as the *Boek der Wundenartzstedye* were meant to be for sale and, therefore, for a wide circulation among practitioners and other medically concerned readers with a highly differentiated spectrum of interests. For this reason, its High German source has been translated integrally, from the first page to the last, without operating a selection of specific topics.

On the other hand, the fragmentary nature of the *Velt bock* included in Copenhagen, Kongelige Bibliotek, GKS 1663 4to, is the direct result of the specific time and circumstances in which this medical commonplace book came into being. In this historical moment, when writing by hand no longer represented the main form of large-scale knowledge dissemination,

[10] Lucerne, Zentral- und Hochschulbibliothek, Pp 27/4, has never been described scientifically nor studied in depth. According to the database zbh-script 2000 of the University Library in Lucerne, the manuscript was compiled around the year 1700. At the beginning of the manuscript (fol. 1r), which was written by a single hand, we find a note placing the medical collection in the monastery of Werthenstein in the canton of Lucerne in 1731, when it would have belonged to a certain brother Jacob Meyer ('Dises Büöchlein gehört dem bruder Jacob Meyer in dem Convent Werdenstein 1731'). See also Panse (2012: 158).

the very existence of a medical collection of this kind appears justified on an exclusively personal (or local) level as a scrapbook of a person somehow competent and active in medical practice, who wants to keep a record of what he considers to be the most interesting and useful indications he has found in various sources (see Taavitsainen 2006: 692). The very fact that the anonymous compiler of the Copenhagen manuscript refrained from having his work printed suggests that he was not interested in making it available for the larger public. Not only does this free him from the conventions required by the market (e.g. paratextual elements, such as prefaces and colophons), but it also automatically excludes a linear, from-the-first-to-the-last-page reception of von Gersdorff's *Feldtbuch*, opening the way to the free selection of individual topics and prescriptions within it.

4.3.2 *Structure and the Translator's Attitude towards His Work*

The different mediums of transmission and expected readership not only influence the structure of these Low German translations in terms of indiscriminate or selective approaches to the source, but also determine the text (in)stability and the translator's attitude towards his work. While the *Boek der Wundenartzstedye*, once printed, can be considered a stable text that can be revised by the author only in the case of a new edition, the *Velt bock* – as with all the texts in Copenhagen, Kongelige Bibliotek, GKS 1663 4to – is an object of continuous revision and re-elaboration by its author.

This constant reworking of the Low German manuscript is witnessed by a great number of interlinear glosses and marginalia partially emending the original diction. Many of these emendations are of a terminological nature and can be explained with the precariousness of vernacular surgical terminology in general and with the challenge represented by translating it from one vernacular to another.

As the contrastive analysis of the specialised terminology in the *Boek der Wundenartzstedye* and in its High German source has shown (Benati 2018), Giltzheim (or whoever translated Brunschwig's surgical handbook) only replaced the High German term if the Low German language had a consolidated alternative to it, for instance in the semantic field of anatomy. If, on the other hand, no such consolidated term existed in Low German (or if it coincided, at least etymologically, with the High German one), the original diction had to be borrowed, phonologically – and graphemically – adapted to the target language, and, if necessary, clarified through juxtaposition with a synonym and/or a paraphrase (Benati 2018: 81–4).

A very similar approach was applied by the scribe of Copenhagen GKS 1663 4to, who, despite the differences in the medium of transmission and expected readership, certainly shared with the translator of the *Boek der Wundenartzstedye* a concern for the risks connected with the arbitrariness of the specialised terminology in early sixteenth-century Low German. Moreover, since the Copenhagen manuscript was the work of a lifetime for him and was never released for autonomous circulation, for example in printed form, its author continued to have access to his own work to revise previous terminological choices, which, at the moment of the first translation, must have appeared adequate and unequivocal, but, at a later consultation, no longer appeared so clear (Benati 2020: 33–4). In these cases, a different adaptation of a loanword (1), a synonym (2), or a paraphrase (3) was inserted between the lines or on the margin:

(1) dat vor herte ^{harden} den stem (Benati 2017a: 22)
'this hardens the voice'

(2) wente ith sint pustule ^{blaszen} (Benati 2017a: 32)
'because these are pustules'

(3) En secret $^{\text{hemelik dyngh}}$ to deme Creuethe (Benati 2017a: 36)
'A secret about cancer'

A further witness of the *Velt bock* and, in general, of Copenhagen GKS 1663 4to being a perpetual 'work in progress' is provided by the numerous additions to the High German text of von Gersdorff's *Feldtbuch*, as well as by the deletion of both single words and entire prescriptions. The former situation, which is witnessed – among others – by short prescriptions on the treatment of fistulas and synovitis hastily written in fol. 21r between two passages from von Gersdorff's chapter on fistulas (Benati 2017a: 28) and on the Longinus blood-staunching blessing in fol. 34r (Benati 2017a: 49; Benati 2016a), is to be ascribed to the author's wish to update his previous work on the basis of the reading of new sources. The latter circumstance can, on the other hand, be considered the result of both an attentive and critical reflection on the operative instructions found in his readings of medical texts and his own activity as practitioner.

The critical approach to the source is witnessed in the passage on the use of phlebotomy as a therapy for the quartan ague, in which the scribe of the Copenhagen manuscript corrected a mistake present in the 1517 first Strasbourg edition of the *Feldtbuch* and repeated in all the subsequent printed editions; namely, that the *vena salvatella* must be punctured between the middle finger and the ring finger and not between the middle finger and the little finger, as stated in the prints (Benati 2014: 13–14). On the other hand, the scribe's medical practice, which had proven certain remedies to be ineffective, is most likely at the basis of the rejection of the recipes previously inserted in the manuscript (Benati 2014: 14).

In this respect, the Low German scribe of the Copenhagen manuscript is at the same time the author and the consumer of his own work: his first draft was later revised, emended in both language and content, and integrated with new information, which was no different from what (early) modern readers did (and still do) by annotating printed texts on the margins (see also Leong 2018: 161). Another form of interaction with the previously written text is possibly represented by the underlining of specific passages and prescriptions and the insertion of manicules pointing at them (see Sherman 2009: 25–52). Even though we cannot know for sure that these markings can be ascribed to the same hand that wrote the main text, this assumption seems to be consistent with the above-described continuous reworking of the manuscript: as ineffective remedies were deleted, those that had proved to be particularly useful were underlined or marked in some other way.

As we have seen, the compiler of the Copenhagen manuscript freely selected single passages from the High German surgical handbook on the basis of their potential relevance to his own practice. Furthermore, the manuscript's medium and limited intended readership of the *Velt bock* also determine the author's attitude towards these portions of text. Not only does he, in fact, almost exclusively translate prescriptions and praxis-oriented passages (see Panse 2012: 158), but – within these pragmatic parts – he also systematically omits all those elements simply aimed at legitimising the message or providing 'bibliographical' references for it.

In the High German originals, both Brunschwig and von Gersdorff needed to convince any potential reader that he or she should follow their instructions, entrusting someone's life to them. This aim is pursued in different ways throughout the two sources: both authors refer – though with different emphases – to their own personal experience (*experientia*; see also Toellner 1984: 164) and to universally acknowledged medical authorities (*auctoritates*). Single remedies and procedures are usually first ascribed to one or another authority, and then their efficacy is assessed through the surgeon's experience. In some cases, a logical explanation (*ratio*) for a procedure is provided.

The need for legitimation was shared by Giltzheim (or whoever translated the *Boek der Wundenartzstedye*), who, consequently, followed the conventions of printed texts and adopted the same legitimation strategies as Brunschwig. The preface to the *Boek der Wundenartzstedye*, which begins with the usual dedication to God, the Virgin, and the Saints, revolves around Brunschwig's diligence in collecting the teaching of the most eminent masters of the past in order to prevent damage possibly arising from unexperienced surgeons and barbers:

(4) Wente wor vmme / vele der minschen schaden nemen van den yungen angåanden Meyster der scherer vnd wundenartzsten / de syk vnderwinden vnd angån sodanes des se nicht geleret hebben / vnd nycht wetten den anfank / middel noch ende [. . .] O gy yngen angånden Meystere vnd Knechte der scherer vnd wundartzsten / nemet war vnd merket mit flyte vp dit kleene boek dat dy Hieronimus Brunswyck / boͤrdich van Straßeborch / mit flite vnd ernst tosamende brocht heft van vele gelereden vnd guden meysteren / vnd hebbe gedacht an dat wort dat de olden gesproken vnd ok geleret hebben segghende. (Benati 2012: 15; see also Klein 1911: 4)

Because many people are damaged by young barbers and surgeons who operate despite not having studied and do not know where to start [. . .]. You, young prospective masters and barber's and surgeon's apprentices, take good notice of this small booklet which I, Hieronymus Brunschwig born in Strasbourg, have carefully compiled on the basis of many learned and good masters thinking of the words pronounced and taught by the old masters.

Writing for himself, the scribe of Copenhagen, GKS 1663 4to, does not need to explain the reason why he started his personal scrapbook, nor does he need to 'promote' his work to potential readers and buyers. Consequently, he can omit the preface singing the praises of Hans von Gersdorff and of his forty-year experience in the field of surgery (von Gersdorff 1517: preface); moreover, the Strasburgian surgeon is never mentioned in the manuscript. The only mention of the High German field surgery manual is represented by the translation of its title – *Dat velt bock* – appearing in fols. 1r and 15r, which should not be considered a real bibliographical reference, but rather a tool allowing easier and quicker consultation of the prescriptions collected in his commonplace book, as witnessed by the cross-references included in the glossary in fols. 179r–204r (see Benati 2016b).

Similarly, the Copenhagen scribe does not need to justify his selection of texts or display his erudition by dropping the names of recognised medical authorities and summarising their position in the medical debates of the time. He is exclusively interested in doses, remedy ingredients, and operative instructions. This approach is perfectly exemplified by the Low German scribe's rendering of this passage on the treatment of the wounds of the intestines, where both Albucasis's rejection of ant suture[11] and Rogerius's suggestion to lay elder pith in the intestine to prevent infections are completely glossed over:

(5) Die dårme soltu auch gewarsamlich heruß zyehen / vnd hefft oder någ sye noch ir notturfft / mit einer nodt als ein kürßner macht / vn*d* mit omeyßen håubtere*n* / als die gemeinen hafften. wan*n* sye vnnutz vnd verdrüsszlich seint / als Albucasis spricht. Rogerius vn*d* etlich mer die raten / d*az* man in die verwundten dårm vnder die hafften holder rôrlin leg / d*az* die håfft nit ful werden. (von Gersdorff 1517: fol. XXXIr)

You should carefully extract the intestine and stitch or sew it up according to necessity with a suture as those made by furriers and not with an ant suture, as is common. These are, in fact, unnecessary and useless as Albucasis says. Rogerius and many others suggest to lay elder pith in the wounded intestine under the suture, so that it does not become infected.

(6) Item de dermen scaltu neygen myt ener nat also de korsinerß edder pelserß negen. (Benati 2017a: 85)

You should sew the intestine with the kind of suture used by furriers.

Since the references to von Gersdorff's personal experience have lost their function as knowledge legitimation, all anecdotes are omitted, and all first-person passages are rephrased in a more impersonal form (usually the third-person indicative or the second-person imperative). In this way, 'Wann ich ein fystel gereiniget hett' ('Once I had cleaned the fistula') is rendered as 'Wen de fisteln gereyniget iß' ('Once the fistula is clean') and 'so hab ich sye geheylt' ('then I healed them') is rendered as 'dar na hele se' ('Then, heal them') (von Gersdorff 1715: fol LXIIr; Benati 2017a: 29). The same logic applies to introductory passages, general recommendations to the reader (e.g. to be careful when performing a procedure), and efficacy statements (see also Benati 2020: 37–8).

An analogous reduction of purely conventional discursive elements in favour of praxis-oriented indications can be found in another, later medical

[11] This particular technique consists of bringing together the two edges of the wounds and placing a series of ants on them, so that they can bite the edges and keep them together even after their heads have been cut, with them remaining there until the wound is healed. See Köhler (1901: 73–4).

commonplace book in which fragments of Hans von Gersdorff's *Feldtbuch der Wundarzney* are transmitted (Lucerne, ZHB, Pp 27 4to), and such a reduction seems to be typical of this kind of transformation of medical discourse.[12]

4.4 Concluding Remarks

In this study, two Low German translations of High German surgical handbooks were contrasted and discussed to highlight how different the path of diatopic knowledge dissemination can be. Despite the typological, linguistic, and chronological affinity of the High German sources – Hieronymus Brunschwig's *Cirurgia* (Strasbourg 1497) and Hans von Gersdorff's *Feldtbuch der Wundarzney* (Strasbourg 1517) – their Low German reception diverges in many respects.

First and foremost, the label 'translation' perfectly fits the Low German edition of Brunschwig's *Buch der Cirurgia* printed by Dietz in Rostock in 1518, while it only partially describes the transformation undergone by von Gersdorff's medical discourse in Copenhagen, Kongelige Bibliotek, GKS 1663 4to. The former is nothing more than a translation of the source, whereas the latter is also a translation of the original surgical handbook, which, in the Copenhagen manuscript, is transposed into a new medical genre – the commonplace book – and translated. In this respect, the *Velt bock* combines two different means of knowledge travel and dissemination.

This is primarily ascribed to the medium of transmission of the two Low German texts: print for the *Boek der Wundenartzstedye* and manuscript for the *Velt bock*. The different mediums were determined by the expected readership of the translations, and both were closely connected to the texts' structures, as well as to the translators' attitude towards their work.

On the one hand, the *Boek der Wundenartzstedye* was an integral translation of the High German source and was aimed at wide circulation among practitioners and surgeons-to-be. To attain this objective, the Low German translator had to conform to the conventions imposed by the editorial market of the time and to convince his potential readers that he

[12] See, for example, von Gersdorff (1517: fol. XLIIv): 'vnd lege es also warm doruff als du es erlyden magst. Kein gewisszers hab ich gesehen dann diß / das hab ich ritteren / edelen vnd vnedelen gebrucht / vnd hab es gerecht erfunden' ('And lay this on it as warm as you can stand it. I have seen nothing surer than this, which I have used treating knights, noble and humble people and I have found it right') vs Lucerne (ZHB, Pp 27 4to, fol. 24r): 'vnd leg disu darüber alß warmß leiden magst, kain gewisserß' ('And lay this on it as warm as you can stand it, nothing surer than this'). See also Benati 2022a.

could be trusted and that his handbook was worth buying and reading. Therefore, he faithfully reproduced the rhetoric strategies of knowledge legitimation already present in Brunschwig's original.

On the other hand, the *Velt bock* was part of a private scrapbook of a medically competent individual taking notes to keep record of the most interesting and useful indications found in a wide spectrum of sources. The sole criterium for insertion in the manuscript was the scribe's discernment, which automatically validated all remedies and prescriptions in the collection and made all original references to von Gersdorff's experience and to eminent physicians and surgeons of the past unnecessary.

This selective approach to the source is associated with a high degree of textual instability. The scribe of the Copenhagen manuscript, in fact, continued to have access to his own work to revise, improve, and integrate it on the basis of further readings, personal reflection, and experience. A high number of interlinear and marginal glosses, deletions, emendations, additions to the main text, and markings testify that the compiler of Copenhagen, Kongelige Bibliotek, GKS 1663 4to, used his work in his everyday medical practice and was simultaneously the author and the consumer of the text. A further witness of the pragmatic purpose of the manuscript collection is constituted by the insertion, in the Latin–Low German glossary in fols. 179r–204r, of a set of cross-references aimed at facilitating consultation of the work. Allowing quicker access to single prescriptions within the manuscript may represent the only reason for the quotation of the title of the High German surgical handbook.

In this respect, the Low German commonplace book, which is a 'map' of the individual compiler's own reading universe (Havens 2001: 65), provides interesting insights into the history of surgical knowledge in use in early sixteenth-century northern Germany. For example, it is worth noting that specifically field-surgical topics such as amputations are not included in the Copenhagen manuscript, possibly because its author considered them scarcely useful in his everyday practice. Along with the investigation of the additions to the *Velt bock* in the first part of the commonplace book (see Benati 2017a and 2017c), this datum suggests that its anonymous scribe was consulted for wounds and traumata, but also for other medical conditions not requiring proper surgical procedures.

In conclusion, the two Low German texts discussed in this study exemplify two possible itineraries of knowledge dissemination. The *Boek der Wundenartzstedye* is a vernacular–vernacular translation that fundamentally reproduces, in a different linguistic form, its High German sources and addresses the same social and cultural reservoir of (potential) readers; that is, practitioners, barbers, and surgeons-to-be. The *Velt bock*, on the other hand, is a translation combined with a radical transformation of the original field surgery manual into a commonplace book, tailored to the interests and professional needs of a single expert in the field. On the basis of these interests and needs it is also possible to describe the *Velt bock* as domestication of a handbook born on the battlefields that became the everyday companion of an individual more often consulted to treat stinky feet rather than to perform trepanation of the skull.

REFERENCES

Andersen, Jennifer, & Elizabeth Sauer. 2001. Current trends in the history of reading. In Jennifer Andersen & Elizabeth Sauer (eds.), *Books and readers in early modern England: Material studies*, 1–20. Philadelphia: University of Pennsylvania Press.

Benati, Chiara. 2012. Dat Boek der Wundenartzstedye *und der niederdeutsche chirurgische Fachwortschatz*. Göppingen: Kümmerle.

Benati, Chiara. 2013. Surgeon or lexicographer? The Latin-German glossaries in Addendum to Hans von Gersdorff's *Feldtbuch der Wundarzney*. *Linguistica e filologia* 33: 35–57.

Benati, Chiara. 2014. Zur Überlieferung von Hans von Gersdorffs *Feldtbuch der Wundarzney*: Die Handschrift Kopenhagen GKS 1663 4to und ihr Verhältnis zu den Druckfassungen. *Filologia germanica – Germanic Philology* 6: 1–20.

Benati, Chiara. 2016a. Eine neue niederdeutsche Fassung des Longinussegen zur Blutstillung. *Zeitschrift für deutsches Altertum und deutsche Literatur* 145: 89–97.

Benati, Chiara. 2016b. A medical dictionary for personal usage: The Latin–Low German glossary on fol. 179r–204r of Copenhagen, Royal Library, GKS 1663 4to. In Maria Victoria Domínguez-Rodríguez, Alicia Rodríguez-Álvarez, Gregorio Rodríguez Herrera, & Verónica C. Trujillo-González (eds.), *Words across history: Advances in historical lexicography and lexicology*, 54–66. Las Palmas: Servicio de Publicaciones y Difusión Científica.

Benati, Chiara. 2017a. *Die niederdeutsche Fassung des* Feldtbuchs der Wundarzney *in Kopenhagen, Kongelige Bibliotek, GKS 1663 4[o]. Edition und Kommentar.* Göppingen: Kümmerle.

Benati, Chiara. 2017b. *Dat kinder bock*: A Low German pediatric medical book in Copenhagen, Kongelige Bibliotek, GKS 1663 4to. In Sibylle Jefferis (ed.), *Medieval German Tristan and Trojan war stories: Interpretations, interpolations, and adaptations*, 273–308. Kalamazoo papers 2015–2016. Göppingen: Kümmerle.

Benati, Chiara. 2017c. The field surgery manual which became a medical commonplace book: Hans von Gersdorff's *Feldtbuch der Wundarzney* (1517) translated into Low German. In Albrecht Classen (ed.), *Bodily and spiritual hygiene in medieval and early modern literature. Explorations of textual presentations of filth and water*, 501–27. Berlin; Boston, MA: de Gruyter.

Benati, Chiara. 2018. Coping with a foreign language for specific purposes in the early sixteenth century: The Low German translation of Hieronymus Brunschwig's *Buch der Cirurgia*. In Nolwena Monnier (ed.), *Languages for specific purposes in history*, 74–93. Newcastle upon Tyne: Cambridge Scholars Publishing.

Benati, Chiara, 2022a. Die handschriftliche Überlieferung des Feldtbuchs der Wundarzney: Luzern, Zentral- und Hochschulbibliothek, Pp 27 40. *Filologia germanica - Germanic Philology Supplemento* 3: 53–71.

Benati, Chiara. 2022b. Preventing Miscommunication: Early Modern German Surgeons as Specialized Translators. In Albrecht Classen (ed.), *Communication, Translation, and Community in the Middle Ages and Early Modern Period*, 393–413. Berlin; Boston, MA: de Gruyter.

Benati, Chiara. 2020. The translations of Brunschwig's *Cirurgia* and von Gersdorff's *Feldtbuch der Wundarzney* into Low German: Reception and transmission of scientific texts in 16th-century Germany. In Manuel Bellmunt Serrano & Joan Mahiques Climent (eds.), *Literature, science & religion: Textual transmission and translation in medieval and early modern Europe*, 23–42. Kassel: Edition Reichenberger.

Borchling, Conrad. 1900. *Mittelniederdeutsche Handschriften in Skandinavien, Schleswig-Holstein, Mecklenburg und Vorpommern. Zweiter Reisebericht.* Göttingen: Lüder Horstmann.

Frederiksen, Jan. 1983. Johannes (Hans) von Gersdorff (Schielhans). In Kurt Ruh, Gundolf Keil, Werner Schröder, Burghart Wachinger, & Frank Josef Worstbrock (eds.), *Die deutsche Literatur des Mittelalters. Verfasserlexikon*, vol. 4, 626–30. Berlin; New York: de Gruyter.

Haller, Albrecht von. 1774. *Biblioteca chirurgica. Qua scripta ad artem chirurgicam facientia a rerum initiis recensentur*, vol. 1. Bern: Johannes Schweighauser.

Havens, Earle. 2001. *Commonplace books. A history of manuscripts and printed books from antiquity to the twentieth century*. New Haven, CT: Beinecke Rare Book and Manuscript Library, University Press of New England.

Klein, Gundolf (ed.). 1911. *Das Buch der Cirurgia des Hieronymus Brunschwig.* Munich: Kuhn.

Köhler, Albert. 1901. *Grundriss einer Geschichte der Kriegschirurgie.* Berlin: August Hirschwald.

Leong, Elaine. 2018. *Recipes and everyday knowledge: Medicine, science and the household in early modern England.* Chicago; London: University of Chicago Press.

Lindgren, Agi. 1983. Dat Kinderbock. In Kurt Ruh, Gundolf Keil, Werner Schröder, Burghart Wachinger, & Frank Josef Worstbrock (eds.), *Die deutsche Literatur des Mittelalters. Verfasserlexikon*, vol. 4, 1148–9. Berlin; New York: De Gruyter.

Lisch, Georg Christian Friedrich. 1838. Schweißsucht in Mecklenburg im Jahre 1529 und der fürstliche Leibartz, Professor Dr. Rhembertus Giltzheim.

Jahrbücher des Vereins für Mecklenburgische Geschichte und Altertumskunde 3: 60–83.

Lisch, Georg Christian Friedrich. 1839. *Geschichte der Buchdruckerkunst in Mecklenburg bis zum Jahre 1540*. Schwerin: Stiller.

Malm, Mike. 2015. Kinderbock. In Wolfgang Achnitz (ed.), *Deutsches Literatur-Lexikon. Das Mittelalter. Autoren und Werke nach Themenkreisen und Gattungen*, vol. 7: *Das wissensvermittelnde Schrifttum im 15. Jahrhundert*, 1460–2. Berlin; Boston, MA: De Gruyter.

Panse, Melanie. 2012. *Hans von Gersdorffs 'Feldbuch der Wundarznei'. Produktion, Präsentation und Rezeption von Wissen*. Wiesbaden: Reichert Verlag.

Pantin, Isabelle. 2007. The role of translations in European scientific exchanges in the sixteenth and seventeenth centuries. In Peter Burke & R. Po-chia Hsia (eds.), *Cultural translation in Early Modern Europe*, 163–79. Cambridge: Cambridge University Press.

Sherman, William H. 2001. What did Renaissance readers write in their books? In Jennifer Andersen & Elizabeth Sauer (eds.), *Books and readers in early modern England: Material studies*, 119–37. Philadelphia: University of Pennsylvania Press.

Sherman, William H. 2009. *Used books: Marking readers in Renaissance England*. Philadelphia: University of Pennsylvania Press.

Taavitsainen, Irma. 2006. Medical discourse: Early genres, 14th and 15th centuries. In Keith Brown (ed.), *Encyclopedia of language & linguistics*, 688–94. Amsterdam: Elsevier.

Toellner, Richard. 1984. Zum Begriff der Autorität in der Medizin der Renaissance. In Rudolf Schmitz & Gundolf Keil (eds.), *Humanismus und Medizin*, 159–79. Weinheim: Acta Humaniora.

von Gersdorff, Hans. 1517. *Feldtbuch der Wundarznei*. Strasbourg: Schott.

CHAPTER 5

Tracing the Early Modern John of Burgundy

Alpo Honkapohja[*]

The most widely copied plague tract in medieval England was *John of Burgundy's Treatise* (henceforward JoBT). It survives in more than one hundred manuscript copies, including several Latin and Middle English versions. Despite such widespread medieval dissemination, JoBT never appeared as an English early modern printed edition,[1] although material derived from JoBT was published within a collection called *Myrour or Glasse of Helthe*, which was reprinted some twenty times and was attributed to the Dominican friar Thomas Multon.

Nevertheless, despite the lack of a printed edition, post-1500 manuscripts of JoBT survive. This chapter's purpose is to describe the manuscript context of these late and neglected witnesses of JoBT, demonstrating the text's ongoing and substantial societal impact.

George Keiser (2003: 311) argued that Multon's treatise superseded JoBT because it 'anticipated the terms in which plague would be explained, constructed, and argued through the latter part of the sixteenth and early seventeenth centuries'. Keiser identified as crucial in this regard Multon's moralising frame, as opposed to JoBT's astrological-medical approach:

> Moulton begins his treatise with a moral statement concerning plague as divine retribution for sin, deferring the astrological material found at the beginning of the source to a secondary position. This cultural construction

[*] I am grateful to the British Academy, which awarded me a Neil Ker Memorial Fund grant, which made possible the underpinning library work for this chapter. I am also grateful to Lori Jones, my collaborator in an ongoing project on tracing all copies of JoBT and determining their stemmatic relations, as well as Peter Murray Jones and Linda Voigts for their comments, Jeremy Smith for the peer review, and Alberto Tanturri for information about surgical practice during the Italian plague epidemics. Needless to say, all remaining mistakes are my own.

[1] A Dutch printed edition attributed to 'Ioannes van Bourgondien anders metten barde ghenaemt een borghere van Luydick' did appear as part of a medical compendium between 1530 and 1622 (cf. Honkapohja & Jones 2020: 19).

> of plague was common in moral writings and sermons from the time of the Black Death. It is, however, unprecedented in the various forms of the John of Burgundy treatise. (Keiser 2003: 300–1)

However, examination of the later witnesses for JoBT, based on an exhaustive textual and codicological examination, allows us to revise Keiser's views. To that end, this chapter's main research questions are:

(1) In what kind of manuscript context did JoBT survive in the post-1500 world?
(2) If plague treatises took a more moralising and religious turn, do copies of JoBT display evidence of this?
(3) Are there any changes in medical discourse in copies of JoBT?
(4) If changes occur, how do they relate to ongoing changes in medical discourse regarding the causes and transmission of the disease?

5.1 John of Burgundy: The Author and His Treatise

JoBT underpinned the understanding and treatment of plague in England for close to two hundred years. Yet its origins are in continental Europe.

The author known as John of Burgundy was active in the city of Liège, at the time in the Duchy of Burgundy (present-day Belgium), in the 1360s. The treatise was written in the aftermath of the second outbreak of bubonic plague in 1361–1362: the *pestis secunda* ('second plague') or *pestis puerorum* ('the plague of children') rather than the original Black Death (Matheson 2006: 569). The exact year of composition, based on information in the earliest dated copy, is likely to have been 1365. The author is known by several aliases in addition to the name now generally used, including 'John with a beard' (*Jehan à la barba*, *Johannes cum barba*, *Johannes von barba*, *Ioannes metten barde*) and 'John of Bordeaux', and indeed the text is often ascribed to other writers altogether. However, the earliest copies are consistent in calling him John of Burgundy (see Honkapohja & Jones 2020 for fuller discussion).[2]

Reasons for the medieval demand for copies of JoBT were its attractive compactness, the lack of competition, and its adaptability. According to Matheson (2005: 26), 'it offered a short, practical set of rules, especially

[2] Another layer of confusion is added by a long-running tradition according to which John of Burgundy was confused with the historical John of Mandeville, author of *Mandeville's Travels*; a confusion already found in the French translation of 1371 (see Honkapohja & Jones 2020).

after the astrological introduction had been cut and the structure simplified into four chapters'. It could be added to collections or copied as a booklet. It also lacked, in England, native competition, since the medical profession was less developed there than on the continent (cf. Jones 2022); the medical faculties at Oxford and Cambridge were by continental standards small.

JoBT was continuously edited and reorganised by copyists and readers, as was customary at the time. Keiser (2003: 300) gives credit to Multon for recognising 'the inefficiency and repetitiveness of his source' and 'vastly' improving its 'organisation', but his point of comparison is British Library, MS Sloane 3449, which according to him (2003: 300) and Waley Singer (1916: 163–9) is very close to the earliest dated copies of a 'long' JoBT. As Keiser himself acknowledges (2003: 299): '[i]n English, the shorter and better organised treatise is by far the more popular'. Many of the simplifications already took place in the increasingly abbreviated English and Latin copies of the 'short' version, including organisation into three chapters. The short version is also found in all of the eight manuscripts discussed in this chapter.[3]

5.2 Manuscript Descriptions and Methodology

5.2.1 The Corpus: An Overview of Post-1500 Copies of JoBT

There are at least eight post-1500 manuscript copies of the English short version of JoBT. In addition, one copy of the Latin short version survives on flyleaves of a printed book, alongside a recipe explicitly attributed to John of Burgundy (Bodleian Library, 4° A. 14Med). Table 5.1 lists the manuscript copies in rough chronological order alongside scribes and owners (where known), and the English incipit/attribution. Some copies can be dated exactly, but other datings are based on palaeographical/codicological evidence.

A noteworthy feature of the incipits is that the majority attribute the tract to 'John of Bordeaux'. This is a feature inherited from the Middle English short version. Five early modern copies contain an attribution to *Maister Joh̄n Burdeux*,[4] *Iohn of bvrdewise*, *John a Burdewe*, *John of Burdewe*,

[3] There are also copies of the Middle English long version (Trinity O.8.29) and a Latin epistolary version (Fitzwilliam 261), but space does not permit discussing and analysing them in the scope of this chapter, or of a few recipes copied in an early printed book.

[4] The bar over the *n* could indicate an abbreviation for 'Johannes'.

Table 5.1 *Post-medieval manuscripts: owners, scribes, related manuscripts (MSS), and incipits*

MS	Time	Owner(s) and scribes	Related MSS	Incipit/attribution
Fitzwilliam 261	Before 1509	Owner: Lady Margaret Beaufort (1443–1509)		*Here begynneth a nobyll tretyse . made by a right worthy physician named Maister Johñ Burdeux*
Rawlinson A.393	c. 1528–1529	Owner: the Findern family Scribe: Sir John Reed, a parson of Nether Broughton, Leicestershire, and vicar of Melbourne, Derbyshire[a]	Lincoln Cathedral MS 91	*her ffol̄oith a good medicyn against pestilence* *in tyme off seknez . noblely devidedj in iiijth* *chapitrej. afft⁹ one mañ opynioū*
Sloane 776	1532	Owner: Charles White, a barber-surgeon in London Scribe: Nicholas Browne, a professional London scribe	Cambridge, Emmanuel College MS 69	*here begynnythe a Noble* *treatẜ made of a good physycyan callyd Iohn* *of bvrdewise medysyns & gou⁹naūce agaynst* *the pestylence euyll*
Trinity O.8.29	Sixteenth century	Unknown	Trinity College Cambridge O.2.13	*Heáre beginneth a noble practise of a good phisission .* *John a Burdewe for medicine a gainste the pestillence* *euill*
Sloane 2507	Sixteenth century	Unknown – owned by the Guide family prior to coming to the possession of Sir Hans Sloane[b]	British Library, Harley 3383 Cambridge, Magdalene College, MS Pepys 878 Trinity College Cambridge O.2.13 Wellcome 674	*A noble tretys or . Rewle . to p⁹serve . a maū or* *womaū from the . jnfeccoū of the plage* *or Pestilence and wheñ any maū hath ytt* *be cured of yt . [. . .] by the - noble . phicysioū.* *Iohñ of Burgoū*

Table 5.1 (*cont.*)

MS	Time	Owner(s) and scribes	Related MSS	Incipit/attribution
Wellcome 674	Late sixteenth century	Unknown (see Chapter 3 in this volume)	British Library, Harley 3383 Cambridge, Magdalene College, MS Pepys 878 Trinity College Cambridge O.2.13 British Library, Sloane 2507	*A Treatise of medicynes good agaynst yͤ pestilence devided into three parts*
Lansdowne 285	Sixteenth/ seventeenth centuries	Owner(s): Sir Thomas Wriothesley (1505–1550), Sir William Dethick (1542–1612)	Yale, Center for British Art, Paul Mellon Collection, John Porter MS	*Here beginnethe a noble tretis made by the ordvnaunc⁹ of a great clark m⁹ John Bordewe at the prayer of king Ric⁹ & other the Lordꝭ for Pestelence*
Sloane 1588[c]	Sixteenth/ seventeenth centuries	Owner: Sir Edmund King (fl. 1630–1709)	Wood MS D.8	*Here beginnethe a noble treatise made by a* *good phisison Iohn of Burdeewxe, for medi* *cines against the pestellence, whiche treatise ys diuised into fowre ptꝭ.*

[a]See Keiser (1980).
[b]British Library catalogue, http://hviewer.bl.uk/IamsHViewer/Default.aspx?mdark=ark:/81055/vdc_100000000040.0x00011c&_ga=2.54829099.1402931959.1598093060-1809094398.1598093060 (accessed 23 April 2022).
[c]The BL catalogue dates the manuscript to the seventeenth century, but an earlier date is suggested by Rand (2006).

and *John of Burdeewxe.*[5] On the other hand, Sloane 2507 is attributed to *Iohn̄ of Burgoū*, which could refer to Bourgogne, the French name for Burgundy. Two are anonymous. Rawlinson A.393 introduces the text as *after one man's opinion.* Wellcome 674 introduces the text as *A Treatise of medicynes good agaynst yͤ pestilence devided into three parts.*

A second noteworthy feature is that despite this homogeneous (mis) attribution, nearly all early modern copies of JoBT descend from different exemplars.[6] Two manuscripts were copied directly from extant medieval exemplars. The early modern continuations in Lansdowne 285 were copied directly, probably by Sir William Dethick (see Section 5.2.2), from a mid-fifteenth-century manuscript, the so-called John Porter manuscript, copied and owned by John Porter (fl. 1445–1485), an MP from Worcester. Another instance appears in Trinity College, Cambridge O.8.27, itself a miscellany of the type Hanna (1986) calls 'binding accidents'. Its Middle English contents were copied directly from the late medieval Trinity College, Cambridge, MS R.14.52, a large volume that continued to be annotated in the sixteenth and seventeenth centuries (see Chapter 2 in this volume).[7]

While other manuscripts do not have extant medieval exemplars, they have evident textual affiliations with medieval copies. Sloane 776 is related to Cambridge, Emmanuel College MS 69.[8] Sloane 1588 is related to Wood MS D.8. However, most early modern copies are not closely linked in textual affiliation. The only instance where two early modern copies can be said to belong to the same family are Sloane 2507 and Wellcome 674

[5] The only copies of the Middle English short version that attribute the text to Burgundy rather than Bordeaux are ones containing interpolations characteristic of John Shirley, who is generally considered a reliable biographer of, for example, Chaucer or Lydgate (cf. Connolly 1998; Honkapohja & Jones 2020: 19). Moreover, Latin, French, and Dutch versions attribute the tract to Burgundy, clearly suggesting that this was the original. Matheson (2005, 2006) argues that the confusion originates as a mistake. Jones (2022) argues that it could be a conscious effort to connect the treatise with Bordeaux, which had positive associations during the early part of the Hundred Years' War. Richard II, during whose reign the English translation may originate, was also known as 'Richard of Bordeaux'. An entirely different approach to weighing the merits of John's two alleged home regions is advocated by Buck (1961: 453): '[t]o distinguish between Burgundy and Bordeaux is a case, according to a French judge quoted by the well-known vinologist Frank Schoonmaker, "in which the evidence on both sides is so interesting that one might spend most of his life examining it, and allow his decision to be made public only after his death."'

[6] These groupings are based on the preliminary ones made by Lori Jones, to which I am indebted.

[7] R.14.52, which Tavormina (2006: xii) describes as 'an unusually ambitious instance of vernacularization of medical and scientific writings in late medieval England', was subject to an extensive collection of articles edited by Tavormina (2006; see especially Voigts and Deery-Kurtz 2006: 50–2). The JoBT copies in it were edited by Matheson (2006).

[8] The same manuscript also contains copies of closely related texts by John of Arderne (see Chapter 2 in this volume).

(see also Chapter 3 in this volume), as both share two errors ('fever acute' for 'fever ague' and 'vein tocall/focall').[9] However, these errors are also found in three medieval copies: Trinity College Cambridge O.2.13; British Library, Harley 3383; and Magdalene College Cambridge Ms Pepys 878. Consequently, very few of the post-1500 copies belong to the same subgroup.

5.2.2 Early Modern Owners and Their Reasons for Owning a Copy of John of Burgundy

The early modern owners and scribes of several manuscripts are known. Two scribes have been identified with certainty, while five manuscripts can be linked to known sixteenth- and seventeenth-century persons. Three of these five individuals were fairly high on the social ladder, in one case royalty.

The earliest manuscript included in this study is Fitzwilliam 261, a small but suitably luxurious book, once belonging to Margaret Beaufort, mother of Henry VII (Powell 1998: 199–200; see Figure 12 in the Image Gallery). All its contents are related to the plague.[10] The appearance of the treatise in a deluxe collection is part of a larger trend, as JoBT is also found in several other high-end books copied between 1475 and 1509.[11] Upper-class audiences continued to provide a market for luxurious hand-copied books even after the printing press had made books available for the middle classes (cf. Smith 1996: 30, 76). The manuscript is from very early

[9] Lori Jones, personal communication.

[10] The volume is a thematically unified collection on the theme of plague, containing medical texts, hymns and prayers, and regimens of health. This thematic focus makes it unlike not only all other post-1500 copies of JoBT but also medieval ones, as the treatise is usually joined with other types of texts. Fitzwilliam 261 contains the following texts: f.1r 'Canutus' plague treatise (Latin), f.9v Canutus plague treatise (English), f.19r–f.20r a Latin regimen beginning *Aristoteles autem scribens Alexandro magno* (Latin), f.20r–23r JoBT (Latin, epistolary version), f.23r–f.26v JoBT (English short version), f.27r–29r prayers and hymns for plague, f.29r a regimen, f.0v Lydgate's dietary.

[11] These are finely decorated volumes copied on parchment, during a period when paper was available much more cheaply and Caxton had started the first printing press in Westminster. Deluxe copies of JoBT include a copy of the John or Shirley version in a pocket-sized book, Sloane 965, which has gilded initials. They also include the last copes of the Voigts-Sloane Sibling Set Text, a medical anthology in Latin and English that found its way in nearly identical order to six manuscripts copied in London or its vicinity between the 1450s and 1490s. Voigts (1990) christened these 'the second generation of a family that grew prosperous'. A copy of JoBT was also included in a medical anthology in the guild book of barber-surgeons of York, a finely decorated volume that seems to have been used mainly for ceremonial purposes. All these other deluxe manuscripts are from the late fifteenth century, and consequently outside the scope of this chapter, but some of them contain evidence of continued use after the Middle Ages.

on in our period, as both Lady Margaret and Henry VII passed away in 1509.

Two other manuscripts, also owned by prominent figures, contain JoBT. One is Lansdowne 285, which was owned by two sixteenth-century heralds at the courts of Henry VIII and Elizabeth I, respectively: Sir Thomas Wriothesley (1505–1550) and Sir William Dethick (1542–1612). The manuscript is a well-known collection copied in 1468 for Sir John Paston (II), who refers to it as his 'Great Book' (see Doyle 1956; Lester 1984, 1987); the two early modern heralds made continuations in empty and attached leaves at the book's end. The copy of JoBT appears as the last item of post-medieval continuations, probably made by Dethick from the John Porter MS, which he also owned (see Table 5.1). Sir John Paston's 'Great Book' contains much information about nobility in the fifteenth century, making it of interest to both heralds. It is less easy to see, however, why Dethick chose to add JoBT. The motive can hardly have been heraldic.[12] Perhaps Dethick's interest in the treatise was topical, relating to the recurrence of early modern plague epidemics, including epidemics in 1603 and 1610.

A third copy of JoBT connected to a prominent individual appears in Sloane 1588. The manuscript was owned and annotated by Sir Edmund King (c. 1630–1709), one of the most prominent surgeons of his day, whose patients included the Archbishop of Canterbury and Charles II, who knighted the surgeon as a reward in 1676. King was an active experimental anatomist, who dissected both humans and animal corpses. He was also an early user of the microscope, collaborating with Robert Hooke (cf. Jardine 2004), and experimented with blood transfusion into calves, publishing his work in the *Philosophical Transactions*. In this case, a JoBT copy was thus owned by a medical practitioner, who was very much part of the emergence of the 'new science'.[13] King made notes and copied medical receipts in blank spaces of the recipe book between

12 According to the incipit, the treatise was copied *by the ordvnauncꝰ of a great clark mꝰ John Bordewe at the prayer of king Ricꝰ & other the Lordꝭ for Pestelence*. The wording is almost identical to that found in the Porter MS, except the latter reads *King Ricꝰ & other* $g^{e}t$ *lordez*. Both abbreviate the name of the monarch and neither gives regnal year or specifies which Richard (although, as the Porter MS was copied in c. 1450, the reference could not have been to Richard III). The main alteration is an unwitting copying error, as the only change made by Dethick is reproducing the abbreviated word $g^{e}t$ ('great') as *the*. His exact reproduction of the monarch's abbreviated name and the unwitting alteration of 'the' for 'great' suggest he did not take interest in the incipit or year of composition for JoBT.

13 Another example would, of course, be King's contemporary Sir Hans Sloane, in whose possession this volume later ended up along with several other copies of JoBT.

1664 and 1684. His annotations, however, provide no evidence of interest in the fairly short plague tract in Sloane 1588, which is a thick volume.

King was also a surgeon, and surgeons are well represented in the provenance of surviving manuscript witnesses. Wellcome 674 was possibly copied by a surgeon or an apprentice (see Chapter 3 in this volume). Moreover, Sloane 2507 may also have been copied by someone similar, judging by the inclusion of Lanfrank's surgery. Sloane 776 was commissioned by the London-based barber-surgeon Charles White, and copied for him by Nicholas Browne in 1532. This last manuscript also contains a copy of John Arderne's *Fistula in ano*, discussed in Chapter 2 of this volume. In his will, White referred to this manuscript as 'the John of Ardren' (cf. Chapter 2). JoBT is the last text in the manuscript and is undecorated.

JoBT's appearance in a compilation belonging to a barber-surgeon is perhaps significant: 'given its emphasis on bloodletting, barber surgeons would have found the work useful' (Matheson 2005: 25). Furthermore, surgeons also had important roles in treating plague: 'Surgery was [. . .] especially associated with the most serious and deadly phase of the disease [. . .]. When the plague affected the skin, then the surgeon appeared on the scene' (Wear 2000: 344–5). Tasks such as applying cataplasms, medicating ulcerations and wounds, incising buboes, bleeding, or performing enemas belonged to surgeons, barbers, and practitioners, who lacked academic training and came from the lower or middle classes (cf. Tanturri 2018).[14]

5.2.3 Evidence of Use

There is also evidence of use in post-medieval copies of JoBT. One of the clearest instances comes from Rawlinson A.393. This northern manuscript was copied by Sir John Reed, a parson of Nether Broughton, Leicestershire, and vicar of Melbourne, Derbyshire (cf. Macray 1862–1900). The copy of JoBT in the manuscript is closely related to Lincoln Cathedral MS 91, the famous 'Lincoln Thornton', a personal anthology of vernacular literature followed by medical texts, copied by Robert Thornton (1418–1456), a member of the landed gentry in Yorkshire.[15] According to Keiser (1980: 445), 'the greater part of [Rawlinson A.393] is derived ultimately from the same manuscript that

[14] This often led to higher mortality among surgeons. In the case of the Noja plague in Italy, all the doctors remained unharmed, and none of them contracted the disease. Conversely, the twelve inmates used as attendants in the *lazzaretto* were all sick with plague, and six died. Three gravediggers also became infected, one of whom died (Tanturri 2018).

[15] The medical contents, including JoBT, were edited by Ogden as *Liber de diversis medicinis* (1938).

Robert Thornton used'. However, Reed's copy contains a couple of marginal notes, which are missing from the Lincoln Thornton and other post-1500 JoBT copies.

The most interesting notes in Rawlinson A.393 are in the bottom right corner of the first leaf, apparently summarising Reed's practice of treating the bubonic plague, based on his reading of JoBT and possibly other sources. These notes suggest that when you feel *it prick and stir* under the ear, arm, or between the thighs, you need *to go to hym þ*^{t} *can lett blod* or to use a laxative medicine. After twelve hours, the recommendation is to *lax þ*^{e} *bett*^{9} ('lax thee better') and to take a drink of treacle. The comment also recommends not sleeping for twenty-four hours, which matches fairly well the standard recommendations for treating the plague, including not sleeping, which is mentioned for example in Multon's adaptation, in which the recommendation is *take good hede that thou slepe not after thy bloude lettyng of .xiii. houres* (f.B7v). To the left of the first marginal comment, Reed has added another that says: when you need to lie down, take a warm drink. Very interestingly, the marginal note finishes with the words *& w*th *godſ g*^{a}*ce þ*^{u} *shall scaip*[?] *sepi9 probatū bo*^{m} ('and with God's Grace, you shall escape. Often tried. Good'). Elsewhere in the manuscript, Reed is in the habit of recording which cures he has tried himself; the phrasing suggests he treated the disease several times and believed the cure to be effective, if God was merciful.

Further evidence of early modern use of JoBT comes from Bodleian Library, 4° A. 14Med, a printed book in which someone copied, by hand, a Latin long version of the work. There are also several copies of recipes against the plague copied by the same hand, one deriving from JoBT, flagged by the heading. Further evidence for continued use and relevance for JoBT can also be found in Sloane 1588 and Sloane 2507, which both contain detailed early modern indexes, including folio numbers, that cover JoBT.

5.3 Changes in Discourse

5.3.1 Methodology

The aim of this section is to analyse changes in vocabulary in the JoBT tradition. Are there notable trends in medical discourse in the various versions? Research questions here addressed are:

- Do the JoBT copies display evidence of a more moralising and religious turn?

- Are there any changes in medical discourse in copies of JoBT?
- If changes occur, how do they relate to ongoing changes in medical discourse regarding the causes and transmission of the disease?

However, some things need to be taken into account first. The manuscript transmission of a tract like JoBT is very complicated. The Latin version was modified throughout its period of transmission. Moreover, it seems to have been translated several times. There are also several different subgroups of the English short version, which all the manuscripts studied in this chapter represent. Therefore, one must be careful when looking at linguistic developments in the early modern versions of the short JoBT. Since the surviving copies represent different subgroups, it is possible that differences between them are inherited from earlier copies rather than new developments. To overcome this problem, I compared each copy with an earlier related manuscript. If differences in terminology are mainly between different post-1500 copies, but a term is the same between a closely related pre-1500 and post-1500 one, then it is to be explained by differences in the treatise's subgroups. If, on the other hand, more than one post-1500 copy change a term from the related medieval manuscript, then we can conclude that it may be due to some development or change of terminology.

I considered the possibility of looking at diachrony within the period; however, the problem with this approach is that the precision with which the manuscripts can be dated varies. Some, such as Rawlinson A.393 or Sloane 776, can be dated to an exact year, whereas others can only be dated palaeographically or codicologically (and are thus datable rather than dated). The manuscripts were therefore only divided into two groups: those probably copied before 1550, and those probably copied after, enabling comparison between them.

The terminology deployed is compared in several ways. One of the main points of comparison is the *Early Modern English Medical Texts* (EMEMT) corpus (Taavitsainen et al. 2010). There are four plague treatises in EMEMT from the 1500–1600 period to which the JoBT manuscripts can be dated: Multon's *Myrrour or Glasse of Healthe* (1539 edition), Brasbridge's *Poore Man's Iewel* (1578), Balmford's *Plagues Infection* (1603), and Lodge's *Treatise of the Plague* (1603). Three of these are written by religious practitioners: Multon (a fifteenth-century friar), and Brasbridge and Balmford, who were active in the post-Reformation world. Lodge, on the other hand, introduces himself as a 'Doctor of Physick' and his treatise is a very thorough examination of the topic. For lexical comparison I also use the *Oxford English Dictionary* (OED) and the *Historical Thesaurus of English*.

5.3.2 *Framing the Treatise: From Astrology to Morality?*

Little astrology remains in the English short version of JoBT, most having been dropped from manuscripts earlier. As Matheson (2005: 18) puts it, the likely reason is that the 'astrological section' was 'considered too time specific for later texts', since university-trained physicians believed a deadly triple conjunction of Mars, Saturn, and Jupiter in 1345 had created a lethal miasma leading to the original Black Death.

No substituting moralizing framework appears in JoBT to the same extent as in Multon's adaptation. However, since JoBT is fairly short, it is sometimes combined with religious tracts in the miscellanies, which may offer moralizing interpretations. A prime example is Fitzwilliam 261, in which JoBT is followed by hymns and prayers specifically related to plague. Moreover, many copies contain small insertions, flagging a change in attitudes. For instance, John Reed, the scribe of Rawlinson A.393, has inserted a phrase extolling how all health lies in God, in a passage otherwise concerned with bleeding:

(1) And bledyng be tyme on? vaynez þ^t j shall tell her afft^9 *shall help itt. And: wth þ^e g^ace and licence of god in whom all helth lyth.* itt shall haue ye seknez away (Rawlinson A.393, emphasis added)

The earlier copy reads:

(2) And bledy(n)g in tymes on vaynes yat I sall telle aft^9 sall helpe & haste it awaye (Lincoln Cathedral MS 91, f.301v)

Another small addition can be found in Sloane 776, which ends by evoking St Roch:

(3) and throughe outte the /// grace of god / *and saynte roke* he shall be frome that syknesse kepte / and de lyueryd (Sloane 776, emphasis added)

The phrase is lacking from the earlier, medieval copy:

(4) and thorough the grace of god he shal be for that sekenes kepte and delyu(er)ed (Cambridge, Emmanuel College MS 69)

St Roche had contracted the pestilence while taking care of the sick in Italy. He recovered, but died later after he was falsely imprisoned as a spy. His cult spread in Italy in the fifteenth century (cf. Horrox 1994: 97). His appearance in Sloane 776 may indicate that the cult was spreading in England.

5.3.3 Sexual Terminology

Sexual terminology was a challenge for early modern puritans, and Outhwaite (2018: 251) noted changes in the vocabulary used for male genitalia in two copies of compilation known as *Practica physicalia*. There

> a reader has ruled through the word *pyntell* (penis) in the title with a thick black ink, so that only the tips of the ascenders and descenders are visible. *Pyntell* is replaced with the Latin equivalent *veratrum*. (Outhwaite 2018: 252)

It might be anticipated that late copies of JoBT would censor some sexual references.

JoBT includes several candidates for censorship. One activity JoBT flags as risking infection is sexual intercourse, which opens the body's pores, causing 'venomous air' to enter. Another relates to a principal plague symptom, buboes, when lymph nodes became tender and swollen with bacterial matter; the groin, which JoBT interprets as a cleansing place of the liver, is uncomfortably close to the genitalia. Such passages seem to be especially susceptible to change, as listed in Table 5.2.

Some copies address the difficulty through Latin code switching, often indicated by a change of script or rubrics. Others refer to *lechery* or *venery*. In most cases, however, early modern scribes use the same strategy for sexual content as their exemplar. Rawlinson 393 uses the same Latin phrasing as the related earlier Yorkshire 'Lincoln Thornton' manuscript. Sloane 2507 and the closely related Trinity O.2.13 and Harley 3383 all use the same Latin phrases, while Sloane 776, Trinity O.8.29, and Lansdowne 285 all use the English term *lechery* without modification.

The only instance where the phrasing is revised is in Sloane 1588, which introduces *Therfor take hede I saie, of the much vse of womon* in preference to the earlier *And specyally bewar off ffleschly delyng be twen man & woman þ^t sesone* in Wood MS D.8. This an objectifying change to a male perspective, since 'use of women' may be a reference to use of prostitutes.[16]

The most common revision was, perhaps unsurprisingly, with reference to genitalia. Nearly all late medieval copies refer to 'privy things', whereas

[16] While it is difficult to establish exact figures, the number of prostitutes in the early modern period is likely to have been high. The sixteenth and seventeenth centuries were a period of social turmoil and religious tension and saw large-scale migration of unskilled people into cities. According to McEnery and Baker (2017: 34), 'There was already a rudimentary poor relief system in place at the beginning of the seventeenth century [. . .]. If a woman was single, childless and physically able to work, as many prostitutes were, local officials considered her responsible for her own economic well-being and were almost always unwilling to provide outdoor relief.'

Table 5.2 *Genitalia and sexual intercourse in copies of John of Burgundy*

Manuscript	Sexual intercourse	Sexual intercourse in earlier MSS	Genitalia	Genitalia in earlier MSS
Early sixteenth century				
Fitzwilliam 261	*specialy hauntyng of lechery*		*the pryue member^9*	
Rawlinson 393	*Et super om̄ia nocet coitus /. & acceleret ad hūc morbū . q2 maxīe aperit poros & distruit spc̄ vitales /*	*super omnia alia nocet coitus* (Lincoln MS 91)	*þi p^9vay membr̄s*	*preue thynge* (Lincoln MS 91)
Sloane 776	*And // sou^9aynly hauntynge of lecherye*	*lecherye* (Cambridge, Emmanuel College MS 69)	*the prevey thy̅g*	*ye privy thyng* (Cambridge, Emmanuel College MS 69)
Trinity O.8.29	*and in especiall lecherie for that enfebleth the kinde*	*And in especiall lechery for that enfebleth the kind* (Trinity R.14.52)	*in the Inner side by the privie placꝭ, the privie pártes*	*In the jnner side bi the prevy thynges* (Trinity R.14.52)
Late sixteenth or early seventeenth century				
Sloane 2507	*Et sup om̄ia alia nocet coit9 & accelerati ad hūc morb̄m & maxime Apit poros & distruit spirrit vitales*	*et super omnia alia nocet coitus* (Trinity O.2.13) *et super omnia alia nocet coitus* (Harley 3383)	*the p^9vy thyngꝭ, thy p^9vyties*	*preu(ey) thyngg(is)* (Trinity O.2.13) *p(i)uy thynggys* (Harley 3383)
Wellcome 674	*And principallie to eshue and avoyde the often use of venerie*		*the privie members*	
Lansdowne 285	*vse no lechery*	*vse no lecherie* (Porter MS)	*the pryvise*	*ye p^iue thing* (Porter MS)
Sloane 1588	*Therfor take hede I saie, of the much vse of womon*	*And specyally bewar off ffleschly delyng be twen man & woman þ^t sesone* (Wood MS D.8)	*the priuie place, on the inner side by the priuie member*	*in the inner sid, by the p^ivy member* (Wood MS D.8)

most early modern scribes revise this usage variously to 'privy member' (Fitzwilliam 261; Rawlinson 393; Wellcome 674; Sloane 1588), 'privy places' (Trinity O.8.29; Sloane 1588), 'privy parts' (Trinity O.8.29), or the 'privies/privates' (Sloane 2507; Lansdowne 285). This is a small but interesting change, implying that 'privy thing' had somehow become less acceptable, perhaps comparable with *pintell* (see Outhwaite 2018: 251). It may be that what was considered a 'relatively neutral anatomical label' (Outhwaite 2018: 251) had become obscene or old-fashioned, and/or not part of a medical register.[17]

5.3.4 Medical Discourse

Names for body parts, names for veins, names for fever, and references to patients all display lexical variation, but the distribution of variants seems to be related to textual affiliation rather than diachrony. However, as shown in Table 5.3, diachronic variation was found in two lexical items, that is, references to (1) the sickness as a general name, and (2) the mixture that is created when poisonous air mixes with blood:

> And thus poisonous air, when it has been mixed with blood, immediately seeks the heart, the seat of nature, to attack it. [. . .] By means of these events, which are signs to the physician, it is possible to tell where the poisonous matter is lurking and by what vein it ought to be drained. (Horrox 1994: 188)

John, likening the mixture of poisonous air and blood to the venom of a snake, claims the body tries to expel in the same way as the snake expels venom.

The results reveal some diachronic differences. Two copies probably owned by medical practitioners, Sloane 2507 and Wellcome 674, refer to *infection of the plague*. The *pestilence evil*, in which the *evil* means 'sickness', on the other hand, is not used in later copies, even though the adjective 'evil' is used referring to the *evil blood* (Wellcome 674). This change relates to contemporary debates on the concept of contagion.

The traditional scholastic/Hippocratic/Aristotelian/Galenic model was paradigmatic throughout the period when copies of JoBT were being made. However, this model in principle had difficulty explaining the

[17] Interestingly, the *Historical Thesaurus* offers little clue to this change, as it lists *privy member* (1297–1660), *privy members* (1297–1681), *thing* (c. 1386–), *privities* (c. 1375 Scots, c. 1386–1822/1834), *(privy) harness* (1382–1600), *privy parts* (1556), *privacies* (1656), and *private parts* (1785–), as well as *privates* (1940–). According to this list, *privy member(s)*, *thing*, and *privities* were all acceptable expressions during this period.

Table 5.3 *Names for pestilence in copies of John of Burgundy*

Manuscript (MS)	Name of the disease	Name of the disease in earlier MSS	Name of the matter	Name of the matter in earlier MSS
Early sixteenth century				
Fitzwilliam 261	*Malady of the pestilence, sekenesse, sykenesse, pestilence, euyll*		*Venome, the mater*	
Rawlinson 393	*Pestilence, seknez, sekenez*	*Ye pestilence, sekenes* (Lincoln MS 91)	*Matt(er), venome*	*Venomous mater, matir* (Lincoln MS 91)
Sloane 776	*The pestylence euyll, pestylence, euyll, syknes, syknesse*	*Pestilence yvell, ye yvell* (Cambridge Emmanuel 69)	*Venyme, the matter*	*Ye venyme, ye mater* (Cambridge Emmanuel 69)
Trinity O.8.29	*The pestillence euill, pestilence, this evill, this sickeness*	*The pestilence evill, sikenes* (Trinity R.14.52)	*Venime, venome, the matter, the mater*	*Matier* (Trinity R.14.52)
Late sixteenth or early seventeenth century				
Sloane 2507	*the . jnfeccoū of the plage or Pestilence, the sicknes, this sicknes of the plage or pestilence*	*ye pestelance* (Trinity O.2.13)	*Yat venimous matter, the matter*	*venemous mater* (Trinity O.2.13)
Wellcome 674	*Ye pestilence, the said sicknes, this contagious disease, the sicknes*	*Pestilence* (Harley 3383)	*The evill blood, the matter, infection, the corruption, infection and venom*	*The mat(er)* (Harley 3383)
Lansdowne 285	*Pestelence, pestilence, dissease*	*Pestilens, sikenes*	*The matter, the corrupt matter*	*The mat(er)*
Sloane 1588	*Pestellence, siknes, siknesse, in this feuer*	*The pestilence, pestlens, seknes*	*Venimes, matter*	*The veneme, the mater*

plague, since it considered sickness to result from the imbalance of the body's elements. Plague could be transmitted from one person to another.

Nevertheless, there were changes in views on plague. For example, the Council of London in 1543 'pinned the responsibility for infection firmly on the disorders of the infected [. . .]. Any passive deductions drawn from concepts of miasma were censured, since plague increased "rather by the negligence, disorder and want of charity in such as have been [. . .] infected [. . .] than by corruption of the air"' (Slack 1985: 203). One EMEMT author in particular, James Balmford (1603), focuses on infection. In his tract *A Short Dialogve Concerning the Plagves Infection*, which takes place between a professor and a preacher, the latter, given more convincing arguments, discusses the disease's infectiousness and advocates measures of social distancing. (Balmford himself did not flee the plague, but remained in the city to look after infected poor.)

(5) The hert kyndely casteth fro hym that ys contrary ageynst hym / and putteth *the venome* that ys entered in to his clensyng place (Fitzwilliam 261, emphasis added)

(6) the harte being thus infected infec teth and destroyethe what soever is obvious unto it striving to expell [pb/] expell *this contagion* at this clensing place (Wellcome 674, emphasis added)

The shift to *infection* or *contagion* may indicate changes in understanding the disease, moving from the earlier astromedical framework, a development also reflected in the way Wellcome 674 and Sloane 2507 refer to contagion instead of venomous matter. The lexis used in discussing infection was apparently changing because of massive practical experience with bubonic plague, even though it would take decades before scholastic medical theory was eventually abandoned.

5.4 Conclusions

As Guttmann (1903: 5) puts it, the name Jean à la Barbe, Johannes cum Barba, or indeed John of Burgundy is not found in most works on medical history.[18] Yet the many surviving manuscripts speak of JoBT's widespread

[18] *Jean à la Barbe, auch Johannes cum Barba oder Johannes de Burgundia geheißen, gehört zu denjenigen Ärzten des Mittelalters, welche in keinem der bekannten größeren oder kleineren Werke der Medizin einen Platz gefunden haben* ['Jean à la Barbe, also known as Johannes cum Barba or Johannes de Burgundia, belongs to those medical practitioners of the Middle Ages who did not find a place in any of the bigger or smaller known books of medicine'].

circulation and major cultural impact well after the time of original composition.

As with their medieval predecessors, and as we have seen in this chapter, early modern copies of JoBT appear in very heterogeneous manuscript contexts, with owners ranging from royalty to clergy. And this medieval treatise had an ongoing afterlife, continuing to be copied and used until the end of the seventeenth century and the emergence of modern science, when copies of JoBT were owned by active Royal Society members such as Sir Edmund King or Sir Hans Sloane.

Four out of eight post-1500 copies of JoBT were probably owned by surgeons, attracted doubtless by the work's emphasis on bloodletting. One was commissioned for a barber-surgeon (Sloane 776), and another survives in what was possibly a surgeon's commonplace book (Wellcome 674; see Chapter 3 in this volume). In two manuscripts, Sloane 1588 and 2507, JoBT appears in medical miscellanies with sophisticated indexes, the former being annotated by Sir Edmund King, and the latter too probably owned by a surgeon (it also contains a copy of Lanfrank's antidotary).

The afterlife of JoBT sheds further light on the evolution of the medical lexicon during the period, offering evidence of the text's continued use and adaptation. For instance, in at least two later copies the terms *pestilential matter* and *venomous matter* are replaced by the more precise *infection* and *contagion*, a change that can be paralleled in treatises such as Balmford's (1603), and correlating with the Council of London's recommendations for 1543 (cf. Slack 1985: 203). While there was not a major upheaval in theoretical understanding of the plague even during the great (and final) epidemic of 1665–1666 (cf. Slack 1985; Wear 2000), such terminological changes flag how JoBT was modified as scholastic explanations of poisoned air were gradually abandoned. Comparable changes may be detected in terminology for genitalia, as *privy thing* is replaced by alternatives. Perhaps surprisingly, passages containing sexual references resist puritanical censorship.

This study has not challenged the view that Multon's tract replaced JoBT because the former aligned better with contemporary moralising tastes. However, Lori Jones (2022) has suggested that the appearance of Multon's work in print related to close connections between its printers, rather than the cultural displacement of JoBT, whose early modern ownership by distinguished individuals attests to its ongoing societal impact. Jones (2022: 129) argues that 'Moulton's tract—and the larger miscellany of which it was a part—might be better considered as standard house stock that was passed down (or "borrowed") from one printer and bookseller to another than as a work that was repeatedly reprinted solely because of customer demand and "popularity"'.

Indeed, JoBT is by no means the only scientific/medical treatise that survives in many manuscript copies, but never as a printed edition. Another example is the *Wise Book*, which Griffin (2013: xlvi) considers 'a medieval "bestseller" that is suspiciously and conspicuously absent from the canon of early printed works'. Griffin speculates that this work may have 'come to be regarded as a folkloric', suited only for antiquarian tastes (Griffin 2013: xlvi). With JoBT this was not the case, given evidence of its early modern use, such as marginal comments in Rawlinson A.393, which finish with a phrase indicating that JoBT's recommended remedy was successfully used several times. The same is suggested by the hand-copied recipes attributed to John of Burgundy found in an early printed book (Bodleian Library, 4° A. 14Med). Terminological updating of JoBT (e.g. *contagion*, *infection*) suggests continued use rather than being a mere historical curiosity of antiquarian interest. All this evidence points to the continued use and relevance of JoBT, as an important bridge between the medieval and early modern understandings of plague.

REFERENCES

Primary Sources

BL Lansdowne MS 285, date: late 16th/early 17th century (catalogue)
BL Sloane MS 1588, date: late 16th century (Rand 2006); 17th century (catalogue)
BL Sloane MS 2507, date: 16th century (catalogue)
BL Sloane MS 776, date: c. 1532 (catalogue)
Bodleian Library, 4° A. 14Med
Bodleian Library Rawlinson MS A.393, date: 1528–9 (Keiser 1980); early 16th century ('about the beginning of Henry VIII's reign' – catalogue)
Fitzwilliam Museum MS 261, date: c. 1485–1509 (Rand 2006); c. 1500, before 1509 (catalogue)
Trinity College MS O.8.29, date: 16th century (catalogue; Matheson)
Wellcome Western MS 674, late 16th century (based on script)

Secondary Sources

Buck, Robert W. 1961. Doctors afield: Sir John Mandeville: John (with the Beard) de Bourgogne. *Medical Intelligence* 264(9): 451–55.
Connolly, Margaret. 1998. *John Shirley: Book production and the noble household.* Farnham: Taylor & Francis.

Doyle, A. I. 1956. The work of a late-fifteenth century English scribe, William Ebesham. *Bulletin of the John Rylands Library, Manchester* 39: 298–325.

Griffin, Carrie. 2013. *The Middle English* Wise Book of Philosophy and Astronomy: *a parallel-text edition*. Heidelberg: Winter.

Guttmann, Georg. 1903. *Die Pestschrift des Jean à la Barbe (1370): zum ersten Male herausgeben, übersetzt und erklärt*. Berlin: Universitäts-Buchdruckerei von Gustav Schade (Otto Francke).

Hanna, Ralph, III. 1986. Booklets in medieval manuscripts: Further considerations. *Studies in Bibliography* 39: 100–11.

Historical Thesaurus of English, The. Glasgow: University of Glasgow. https://ht.ac.uk (accessed 15 May 2021).

Honkapohja, Alpo, & Lori Jones. 2020. From *Practica Phisicalia* to *Mandeville's Travels*: Untangling the misattributed identities and writings of John of Burgundy. *Notes and Queries* 67(1): 18–27.

Horrox, Rosemary. 1994. *The Black Death*. Manchester Medieval Sources Series. Manchester: Manchester University Press.

Jardine, Lisa. 2004. *The curious life of Robert Hooke: The man who measured London*. New York: HarperCollins.

Jones, Lori. 2022. *Patterns of plague: Changing ideas about plague in England and France, 1348–1750*. Montreal: McGill-Queen's University Press.

Keiser, George R. 1980. MS. Rawlinson: Another Findern manuscript. *Transactions of the Cambridge Bibliographical Society* 7(4): 445–8.

Keiser, George R. 2003. Two medieval plague treatises and their afterlife in early modern England. *Journal of the History of Medicine* 58: 292–324.

Lester, G. A. 1984. *Sir John Paston's 'Grete boke': A descriptive catalogue, with an introduction, of British Library MS Lansdowne 285*. Cambridge: D. S. Brewer.

Lester, G. A. 1987. The books of a fifteenth-century English gentleman, Sir John Paston. *Neuphilologische Mitteilungen* 88(2): 200–17.

Macray, W. D. 1862–1900. *Catalogi codicum manuscriptorum Bibliothecæ Bodleianæ…viri munificentissimi Ricardi Rawlinson, J.C.D., codicum…complectens*, Quarto Catalogues V, 5 fascicles. Oxford: Oxford University Press.

Matheson, Lister M. 2005. Médecin sans frontières? The European dissemination of John of Burgundy's plague treatise. *ANQ: A Quarterly Journal of Short Articles* 18: 17–28.

Matheson, Lister M. 2006. JoBT: Treatises on plague. In Teresa Tavormina (ed.), *Sex, aging, & death in a medieval medical compendium: Trinity College Cambridge R.14.52, its texts, language, and scribe*, 569–602. Tempe, AZ: Arizona Center for Medieval and Renaissance Studies.

McEnery, Anthony, & Helen Baker. 2017. *Corpus linguistics and 17th-century prostitution: Computational linguistics and history*. London: Bloomsbury Academic. www.bloomsburycollections.com/book/corpus-linguistics-and-17th-century-prostitution-computational-linguistics-and-history/ch2-life-as-a-17th-century-prostitute (accessed 15 May 2021).

Ogden, M. S. (ed.). 1938. *The 'Liber de diversis medicinis' in the Thornton manuscript (MS. Lincoln Cathedral A.5.2), EETS, o.s. 207*. London: Oxford University Press.

Outhwaite, Patrick. 2018. Two manuscripts of the *Practica Phisicalia Magistri Johannis de Burgundia* and their censorship. *Journal of the Early Book Society* 21: 251–8.

Powell, Susan. 1998. Lady Margaret Beaufort and her books. *The Library. Sixth Series* XX(3): 197–240.

Rand, Kari Anne. 2006. A previously unnoticed fragment of John of Burgundy's plague tract and some connected pest regimens. *Notes and Queries* 53: 295–7.

Slack, Paul. 1985. *The impact of Plague in Tudor and Stuart England*. London: Routledge & Kegan Paul.

Smith, Jeremy. 1996. *An historical study of English: Function, form and change*. London; New York: Routledge.

Taavitsainen, I., P. Pahta, T. Hiltunen, V. Marttila, M. Mäkinen, M. Ratia, C. Suhr, & J. Tyrkkö. 2010. *Early Modern English Medical Texts: The Corpus of Early Modern English Medical Writing*. Amsterdam: Benjamins.

Tanturri, Alberto. 2018. *'Il soffio avvelenato del contagio'. La peste di Noja del 1815–16*. Milan: Edizioni Unicopli.

Tavormina, Theresa M. (ed.). 2006. *Sex, aging, & death in a medieval medical companion. Trinity College Cambridge MS R.14.52, its texts, language, and scribe*. Tempe, AZ: Arizona Center for Medieval and Renaissance Studies.

Voigts, Linda Ehrsam. 1990. The 'Sloane Group': Related scientific and medical manuscripts from the fifteenth century in the Sloane Collection. *British Library Journal* 16: 26–57.

Voigts, Linda Ehrsam, & Patrizia Deery-Kurtz. 2006. Contents, unique treatises, and related manuscripts. In Theresa M. Tavormina (ed.), *Sex, aging, & death in a medieval medical companion*, 19–54. Tempe, AZ: Arizona Center for Medieval and Renaissance Studies.

Waley Singer, Dorothea. 1916. Some plague tractates (fourteenth and fifteenth centuries). *Proceedings of the Royal Society of Medicine* ix: 159–212.

Wear, Andrew. 2000. *Knowledge and practice in English medicine, 1550–1680*. Cambridge: Cambridge University Press.

CHAPTER 6

The Plague in Southern Italy in 1815–1816

Alberto Tanturri

In 1815, the plague arrived in Noja (now called Noicattaro), a small town in southern Italy, near Bari. A number of epidemic outbreaks had appeared as early as 1812, initially in the eastern Mediterranean and subsequently in the high, medium, and low Adriatic, as well as in the Ionian and Aegean Seas. For eight months, between November 1815 and June the following year, the disease raged within Noja's town walls, killing – according to the most reliable statistics – 716 inhabitants out of a population of approximately 5,300. Such figures make this epidemic one of the major late manifestations of the plague in continental Europe.[1]

The newly restored Bourbon government confronted the disease with a typically repressive and military approach, as was common practice in European states of the time. As soon as the disease emerged, the small town was surrounded by a cordon sanitaire divided into two ditches, buttressed by chevaux de frise and staffed by some 1,200 fully armed garrison troops. Moreover, in order to preempt the transmission of the infection by sea, a maritime cordon sanitaire was set up along the entire coastline of the Kingdom of the Two Sicilies, whose overall length was 1,134 miles (2,115 kilometres), consisting of a guard post every mile, overseen by conscripted armed civilians. It was a massive and clearly very costly deployment of men and equipment.

Università Cattolica del Sacro Cuore contributed to the funding of this research project.

[1] The Noja plague has been the subject of several historiographic treatises. The first studies were published in the years immediately following the plague outbreak and, despite being diverse in content, they united in praising the Bourbon government: Della Valle (1816), [Bozzelli] (1816), D'Onofrio (1817), and Morea (1817). The only local narrative highly critical of the government, to which it paid tribute for having circumscribed the epidemic while emphasising the terrible suffering inflicted on the inhabitants of the small town, was only released many years after the events. It was written by Tagarelli (1934). More recently, however, the topic has continued to engage scholars, albeit with minor studies only; a select list includes Petraccone (1977), Da Molin (1983), and Valerio (2011).

The present study does not, however, intend to examine the strategy chosen by the government to try to contain the disease and preempt its spread in the territory of the Kingdom. Rather, it focuses on the response that contemporary medical science developed against the plague. The Noja epidemic raised lively medical and scientific debate concerning the nature of the disease and its feasible cures, as well as enabling the field testing of distinct therapeutic approaches. Hence, the intention in the following pages is, on the one hand, to review some of the most significant doctrinal positions on the plague that emerged within the southern European medical profession and, on the other, to analyse the therapies used by the team of doctors who found themselves operating in the infected town.

6.1 The Medical Debate on the Plague

The first voice reported from southern Italy at the outbreak of the Noja epidemic is that of Francesco Romani, author in 1816 of a treatise entitled *Ricordi su la peste redatti in un sistema teorico–pratico*. With the initial aim of identifying the nature of the disease, Romani follows to the letter the innovative nosographic parameters set by the Scottish physician John Brown.

Towards the end of the eighteenth century, Brown's views ('Brunonianism') had stirred widespread interest throughout Europe and in the Italian states, also thanks to the work of effective (though not entirely orthodox) disseminators, such as Pietro Moscati and Giovanni Rasori (Frasca 2014). Based on the identification of a rather vague key characteristic of human beings known as 'excitability', Brown had emphasised the sensitivity of the body to outside stimuli such as air, food, state of motion or rest, sleep or wakefulness, and the very passions of the soul. Accordingly, all pathological processes could fall into two major categories: 'asthenic' diseases (divided in turn into directly or indirectly asthenic), characterised by understimulation, and 'sthenic' diseases, which appeared as overstimulation (Brown 1803: 114). According to Brown, statistically the great majority of diseases (about 97 per cent) were asthenic, whereas only a small minority (3 per cent) were sthenic.[2] Brown's simplifying framework resulted in the need to use two distinct therapeutic modalities: for asthenic diseases, 'excitant' drugs and treatments that would reinvigorate the body, whereas for sthenic ones it was appropriate to administer

[2] Cf. Cosmacini (1987: 259).

'anti-excitants' suitable for the mitigation of overexcitement (Brown 1803: 124–5).

According to Romani, the plague was a disease that could manifest itself in either the asthenic or sthenic form. The symptoms of the former were prostration and weakness, cadaveric lividity, blurred vision, sadness, vertigo, drowsiness, weak or intermittent pulse, swallowing difficulties or inability to swallow. The symptoms of the sthenic form were restlessness, cephalalgia, hectic frenzy, accelerated pulse rate, burning thirst, and epistaxis. Therapies clearly varied depending on the type of symptoms: in the case of asthenic plague, it was necessary to administer medicines to which the traditional pharmacopoeia ascribed invigorating properties, primarily opium, camphor, musk, ether, ammonia, and sulphuric acid. Other invigorators identified by Romani, albeit less effective, were strong wines, Virginia serpentary, infusion of chinchona bark, and angostura. If, on the other hand, the plague manifested itself in the sthenic form, in cases of moderate excitement it was necessary to turn to citrus fruit such as oranges and lemons, light emetics, and refreshing beverages. In more serious cases remedies to be used included antimony potassium tartrate and oroxyd of antimony combined with sulphur (Romani 1816: 74–5). In all cases, however, the most effective remedy for this type of plague – considered 'vital' when symptoms were particularly acute – was still bloodletting, followed by the administration of emetics and cold baths, or full-body ice rubbing. For topical medication of buboes, which one could turn to in all cases, the author recommended the application of ointments, so as to facilitate the suppuration process, followed by incision and the use of cicatrising substances.

Brown's taxonomic criteria, evidently considered of undisputed authority on the subject, were acknowledged also by Luigi Smith, the author of a work in two volumes with the title *Della peste. Trattato completo* (Naples, 1817). Smith, however, took a more straightforward approach than Romani did. In Smith's opinion (1817, II:62), the plague was a disease that was 'absolutely asthenic, epidemic, extremely contagious and considerably acute'. Hence, one had to reject completely therapies recommended by traditional pharmacopoeia, such as Andromachus's theriac, which had the sole effect of sitting heavy on the stomach and worsening the patient's general malaise, or bezoar powder, which was 'much vaunted only by its sellers' (Smith 1817, I:166–7).[3] If the plague

[3] *Andromachus's theriac*, according to tradition, was invented by Andromachus the Elder, Nero's doctor, and had been used since ancient times as a remedy for several illnesses. Theriac's market

was indeed an asthenic disease, as Smith claimed, the cure should be sthenic or excitant. Making use of debilitating remedies (mainly phlebotomy) was in Smith's view a serious mistake, given that it would remove from the body the means used to confront the onslaught of the disease.

The best antidotes to the disease were rather, according to Smith, acids, which had the power to counteract the septic action of the 'poison' circulating in the body. Thus, to cure the plague, administering acid substances, albeit in extremely small doses, sufficed. Hence, an excellent remedy was the Gloutton tincture, a preparation made from sulphuric acid and muriatic acid, which also included excellent tonics such as angelica root, cardamom, and Virginia serpentary. (The therapeutic properties of this third tonic were substantiated by the fact that the indigenous people of Virginia and Pennsylvania used it to counter the effects of rattlesnake bites, which produced symptoms similar to those of plague.) Spiritus mindereri and emetic tartar, combined with nitre, camphor, or acids, were equally valid; James's powder, together with castoreum and musk, was also recommended; and among the preventive remedies were included tobacco smoke and ointments with warm olive oil. Moreover, in line with his innovative positions, Smith (1817, I:137) argued that the opinion of those who considered Jenner's smallpox vaccine effectual in securing persons from the plague was not unfounded.[4] Nevertheless, he added, with flawless syllogistic reasoning, that if inoculating someone with cowpox immunised the body against smallpox, likewise inoculation with rinderpest would produce the same effects against human plague.

price was particularly high; therefore the poorest classes – luckily for them – were excluded from consuming this medicine, now considered a poison, a useless drug, or at best a placebo. The first severe blow to the drug's reliability was delivered in 1745 with the work of the Scottish doctor W. Heberden, Sr., *Antitheriaca: An essay on mithridatium and theriaca*. Nevertheless, theriac continued to be sold and consumed for a long time. See inter alia Griffin (2004), Nockels-Fabbri (2007), Catellani and Console (2007), Bonnemain (2010), Chast (2010), and Karaberopoulos, Karamanou, and Androutsos (2012). *Bezoar* was a mass that formed in the digestive system of certain ruminants, to which Arabic medicine had ascribed therapeutic properties with respect to many diseases since the eighth century. According to the *Oxford English Dictionary*, the term in several European languages derives from Arabic *bāzahr* or *bādizahr*, cf. Persian *pādzahr* ('antidote, counterpoison'). Like theriac, bezoar also had great prominence within modern (not only European) pharmacopoeia until the end of the eighteenth century: see Williams (1986), Sanders (2004), Do Sameiro Barroso (2014), and Espinoza González (2016).

[4] These are certainly not isolated doctrinal stances: for example, a treatise published in the United States in 1803 considered the vaccine 'effectual in securing persons from the plague' (Scofield 1803: 65). This is somewhat naive optimism, which is nevertheless understandable in view of the increasingly clearly proven preventive effectiveness of Jenner's method against smallpox. On the success of the smallpox vaccine in southern Italy, see Tanturri (2014) and Tisci (2015).

Another interesting voice in the doctrinal debate on this subject was that of Sicilian doctor and priest Pasquale Panvini, author of *Chiara dimostrazione de' veri preservativi della peste, e de' rimedj che distruggono il contagio* (Naples, 1816). As opposed to the treatises mentioned above, Panvini's was free of classificatory concerns as he focuses mostly on therapeutic modalities, although in some cases incidentally showing some agreement with Smith's theories. In Panvini's opinion, the safest way to destroy the plague is using oxygen, proven by the fact that prolonged exposure of infected goods to air purifies them thoroughly. Since acid substances are rich with oxygen, they have the power of breaking down and destroying the pestilent poison. When treating a patient affected by the plague, doctors must set themselves two objectives: first, to keep the fever under control and preserve the strength of the diseased; and second, to eliminate infection. Given that bloodletting is of limited use as a remedy for fever, Panvini recommends using medicaments such as antimony potassium tartrate instead. For regaining strength, drugs such as Virginia serpentary, camphor, valerian, angelica root, and *Arnica montana* flowers, besides the familiar musk, opium, and castoreum, are recommended. In order to eliminate the infection, Panvini (1816: 60–2) considers nothing more suitable than using 'mineral acids', and he accompanies this therapeutic suggestion with several precise prescriptions of doses: the person infected with plague should be administered twenty-five drops of sulphuric acid every half hour, dissolved in sugar water or in a sage or camomile infusion. Nitric acid must be ingested in the same dosage, whereas muriatic acid, being 'less caustic than the first two', can be administered in much higher doses (Panvini 1816: 62). Once the diseased, due to such cures, showed signs of improvement, Panvini considered it necessary to reduce the dosage and to proceed with baths in herbal decoctions, for instance sage, camomile, laurel, and rosemary, or with the rubbing of camphor spirit. These herbs, and camphor as well, contain oxygen, the most reliable destroyer of the plague. As for the buboes, suppuration should be facilitated through the application of specific ointments; then they should be cut open through incision or cauterised with fire (the latter option was preferred), finally facilitating the cicatrisation process. In addition to therapeutic prescriptions, Panvini added instructions on carrying out fumigations in order to purify spaces such as hospital rooms or warehouses containing goods infected by the plague, or liable to be so. The method consisted in leaving to evaporate solutions made from nitric acid and sulphuric acid, which would result in a healthy disinfestation in any room. However, as a precautionary measure, it was necessary to ensure that the rooms were cleared out, given that both substances attacked the lungs, causing a severe whooping cough (Panvini 1816: 68). Panvini (1816: 36) concludes by recommending preventive measures, including tobacco smoke and the application of oil all over the body, observing that during several pestilences 'oil sellers escaped the disease in the midst of infected people'.[5]

Another doctrinal study worthy of interest is the work of Giuseppe Zocchi, author of the brief but original *Pensiere sulla peste* (Naples, 1816). Like Panvini, he does not seem to be excessively concerned about defining the nature of the disease; rather, he focuses on testable therapeutic opportunities. For this purpose, he starts from the observation that the plague and syphilis have one thing in common, namely, that they mainly attack the endocrine and lymphatic system; it follows that the treatment methods used for the two diseases may be validly assumed to be similar. In those days, the basis of the most common anti-syphilitic therapies consisted in preparations made from mercury, even though doctors debated whether it was appropriate to administer this substance by rubbing it on the skin, orally, or by means of fumigation.[6] Hence, given that mercury, argues Zocchi (1816: 19), 'admirably destroys, and heals syphilis when used wisely and according to need', nothing makes more sense than that this substance may have just as outstanding healing effects with respect to the plague. With this remedy, 'one day we may have the pleasure of seeing the taming of the plague, just as we luckily see that of the venereal disease' ([Zocchi] 1816: 21). Among the most commonly used mercurial preparations, the most suitable in the case of the plague is, according to Zocchi, undoubtedly mercury sublimate, which ought to be administered as follows: a granule of this substance should be dissolved in an ounce of guaiac or sarsaparilla decoctions or distilled water (with the addition of a

[5] As for tobacco smoke, doctrinal opinions were far from in agreement. Its anti-plague properties were endorsed by the renowned Dutch doctor Isbrand van Diemerbroeck in his treatise *De peste libri quatuor, truculentissimi morbi historiam ratione & experientiâ confirmatam exhibentes* (Arenaci, 1646). Similarly his English colleague Thomas Willis (1691: 21), referring to the London plague of 1665, asserted that the circumstance that 'in the last great plague no tobacco-shop was infected' was not a coincidence. Richard Bradley (1721: 48–9) was even more explicit: 'in the time of the last plague in London, anno 1665, that distemper did not reach those who smoak'd tobacco every day'. On the other hand, Nathaniel Hodges, a doctor also active in the London plague of 1665, was strongly against tobacco smoke; he believed that by using it 'the aptitude of the pestilential poison might be drawn into the lungs that much more easily' (see Duffin 2016: 34). By contrast, opinions with respect to oil's preventive properties were unanimously favourable. For example, doctor Francesco Grassi (1843: 34) wrote that during the plague 'one can see water carriers [. . .], oil sellers, fryers etc. [. . .] if not completely immune, the least affected'. Lastly, doctor Thomas Hancock (1821: 63) observed that, during the London plague of 1665, professional groups such as 'tanners and oil-sellers escaped the disease'.

[6] See Kampmeier (1976), Del Lungo (1983), O'Shea (1990), and Tilles and Wallach (1996).

syrup, so as to make it less unpalatable). The diseased should then be made to swallow it in small and repeated doses. The precise dosage of the drug must in any case be decided by the doctor, according to the age, gender, and general state of health of the diseased, as well as to the individual response to the therapy. Indeed, should the diseased experience abdominal cramps and diarrhoea (symptoms that are not caused by the plague but by an excessive dose of the sublimate), pain might be relieved through the administration of opium or of a nutritious liquid substance, such as a good broth ([Zocchi] 1816: 30). Should the diseased be totally intolerant of the drug, one could turn to mercurous chloride (or calomel) – also an excellent anti-syphilitic – either by oral administration or, after mixing it with a greasy substance, through rubbing. The effectiveness of this substance is similar to that of mercury sublimate, even preferable insofar as it causes hypersalivation (an effect that Zocchi clearly considered beneficial). However, the plague – Zocchi adds – like smallpox, measles, syphilis, and also petechial haemorrhage itself is a protean disease. Hence, although in the great majority of cases it causes a depression of vital forces, at times it may manifest itself as a 'vigour disease' ([Zocchi] 1816: 41). In such circumstances, using an 'excitant' remedy such as mercury could even have lethal effects: it will instead be advisable to reduce the excitement through anti-excitant treatments, also taking into account the possibility of bloodletting. Zocchi concludes that mercury remains the best antidote to the plague. It can be used without limits with persons infected with the plague who show dejection and weakness. However, should they manifest 'irritation and sthenic orgasm', this substance 'will have to be used with some reservations, together with other medicines, that would limit and gently calm the irritated forces and the tumultuous excitement' ([Zocchi] 1816: 47–8).[7]

We conclude this review of doctrinal opinions with a voice that, differently from those considered so far, is extraneous to the southern context, yet that, due to its acknowledged prestige, was recognised also in this geographical area. It is that of the Lombard doctor Giuseppe Giannini, tied by common interest to the entourage of Rasori and Moscati, and author of a weighty treatise entitled *Della natura delle febbri e dei metodi di curarle* (Milan, 1805–9), which also includes some therapeutic advice related to the plague. Giannini begins with the remark that countless

[7] It should be pointed out that the use of medicaments made from mercury against the plague had been recommended by some medical treatises since the middle of the seventeenth century (see Conforti 2006: 143).

methods of treatment have been experimented with for this disease; however, none has enjoyed universal acclaim, since none has ever derived from a precise knowledge of the plague's aetiology and nature.

The best therapy for persons infected with the plague is, Giannini considers, to take cold baths; a remedy that he almost saw as a universal panacea. Baths are particularly effective if they are taken as soon as the febrile symptom appears, and if they are repeated each time it reappears. Should immersion in cold water not manage to disperse all the excess heat, one can turn to rubbing with ice.

Giannini's bath-based remedy applies to routine cases. There are, however, a minority of cases in which the acuteness of the condition portends a fatal outcome right from the start. In such circumstances one must turn to extraordinary measures, such as full-body mercurial rubbing, in exceptionally high doses, and right from the first day of the illness. The rubbing should be coupled with the administration of calomel and, naturally, cold baths (Giannini 1805: 379–81).

Doctrinal opinions at the time when the plague broke out in Noja were, therefore, mixed; we shall now look at the therapies actually implemented by those who had to confront the epidemic.

6.2 The Therapies Tested in Noja

The earliest approaches were eclectic, since there was an ignorance – later widely acknowledged – of the root causes of the disease. A decree of the Naples Magistrate for Health dated 3 January 1816 suggested the use of antiseptic and moderately diaphoretic drugs, revealing therein the legacy of the traditional Hippocratic view that believed plague to be the effect of a 'poison' circulating in the body, and thus postulated that it should be expelled by sweating.[8] In addition to these medicines, others appeared that had vaguely exotic names, such as serpentary, musk, and thebaic tincture, whose anti-plague properties had already been praised, as outlined above, by numerous scientific treatises. There were also dietary, rather than pharmacological, prescriptions, such as the administration of good wine in 'moderate doses', of acidic beverages, and of 'some weak broth'. As regards the medication of the most characteristic symptom of the plague,

[8] See Archivio di Stato di Bari, *Sanità pubblica – Intendenza*, b. 5, f. 30, *Istruzioni temporanee pe 'l trattamento interno della città di Noja*, of 3 January 1816, art. 9. The quotations that follow in the text are taken from this document.

namely the bubo, the use of cataplasms, which were suitable for facilitating suppuration, was recommended.

By and large, those treating the illness were groping in the dark, as can be inferred also from a report, dated 12 January, by the doctors of the internal medical committee, a subgroup of a larger provincial body. Committee members noted that there was continuous experimentation of different treatments on the infected, who were administered diaphoretics, evacuants, or invigorators, while nonetheless admitting that all these medicines 'were scarcely or not at all effective' (Morea 1817: 75). On the basis of this report, the subgroup first classified the diseased into three categories according to severity. Moreover, since all the diseased without exception manifested 'weakness' and 'lack of vitality', the disease had to qualify as 'directly asthenic in nature', and was as such susceptible to undergoing an 'invigorating' treatment (Morea 1817: 76). Accordingly, the report reiterated the pharmacological prescriptions recommended in the treatises discussed above, namely musk, castoreum, thebaic tincture, camphor, ether, and infusions of chinchona bark; it also recommended resorting to mercurial rubbing, so dear to Giuseppe Zocchi.

Naturally, not even these treatments delivered any useful results, a circumstance that was also immediately obvious to the government. At the end of January, it was decided to consider the proposal that Domenico Cotugno, one of the most distinguished representatives of southern medical culture, put forward during a meeting of the Magistrate for Health on 29 January.[9] Cotugno, in view of the observed worthlessness of the experimental cures hitherto attempted, suggested assigning a specific share of the sick to each doctor present in Noja. Distinct therapeutic strategies would be experimented with on each cohort, with the purpose of identifying the most effective one.[10] Moreover, deeming that it was not easy to find good-quality medicines in Noja and the surrounding province, Cotugno requested that an adequate quantity of drugs of proven effectiveness, prepared in the capital's apothecary shops, should be sent to the plague-ridden town.[11] On 1 February, a counsel of the Magistrate for

[9] For an introduction to the life and works of Cotugno, see Premuda (1984). Among the most recent bibliographical contributions are Iacovelli (1988: 53–61 and passim), Borrelli (2000), and Mansi (2006).

[10] See Archivio di Stato di Napoli, *Magistrato di Salute*, b. 194, *Registro de'Reali dispacci. Anno 1816*, letter of the Minister of the Interior to the Superintendent General of Health of 31 January 1816.

[11] See Archivio di Stato di Bari, *Sanità pubblica – Intendenza*, b. 5, *Cassa de'medicamenti da essere spediti a Noja per servire alla cura degli ammalati affetti di febbre pestilenziale*, and [Bozzelli] (1816: 97).

Health approved the use of the rubbing of camphor oil on the body of the diseased, a new prescription that clearly highlights the disorientation of the medical profession when confronted with a disease whose nature continued to be largely unknown.[12]

That was the situation when, in the middle of February, a new delegation of doctors was sent to Noja, among whom was Arcangelo D'Onofrio, who filled the post of president of the internal medical committee. D'Onofrio, an aggressive individual who was by his own admission guilty, like all the other doctors present in Noja, of having handled the diseased 'aloofly', visited the *lazaretto* only occasionally and prescribed treatments and therapies only based on the symptoms reported to him by nurses busy at the bedside of persons infected with plague. Nevertheless, he had very precise opinions on the disease, which he synthesised doctrinally in a treatise on the plague in Noja.[13] In his opinion, on the basis of its manifested symptoms, the plague should always be considered a typical asthenic disease. The sthenic symptoms, under which forms the plague manifested itself misleadingly at times, were simply apparent types of an irritative condition, resulting in any case from physical prostration (D'Onofrio 1817: 33).[14] On the contrary, in this respect, he observed that the distinction between sthenic and asthenic diathesis introduced by Brown was largely unfounded. There was only one diathesis, the asthenic one, given that every pathological process weakened the body.

From this starting point D'Onofrio inferred that therapeutic criteria for sustaining the diseased with invigorating substances were to be recommended. Wanting to cure the plague with debilitating remedies (or anti-excitants) was totally inappropriate. Hence, also when confronted with severe fevers, remedies such as emetics, cream of tartar, nitre, or James's powder were counter-indicated. Bloodletting itself was to be considered 'the most perfidious of all remedies' (D'Onofrio 1817: 34). The most suitable therapeutic strategy was using invigorators,

[12] See Archivio di Stato di Napoli, *Magistrato di Salute*, b. 194, *Registro del Supremo Magistrato di Sanità*, volume II, f. 2r, resolution of 1 February 1816.

[13] Sebastiano Tagarelli (who should be considered the most reliable among the historians of the Noja plague) writes in this regard that during the entire winter season 'D'Onofrio led a withdrawn life, far from the hospitals, from which he was indeed far at all times, and from any other healthy occupation foreseen by his mandate' (1934: 106). Other evidence of contemporary views of D'Onofrio includes the short anonymous poem 'Verboncaro' that was written in the local dialect, a succession of invectives and of defamatory accusations against his behaviour. The complete text of the composition, which was unpublished for more than a century, was published in Tagarelli (1934: 151–4).

[14] On the medical thinking of D'Onofrio, see Catapano (1990: 147–8).

although D'Onofrio honestly acknowledged that substances to which the traditional pharmacopoeia ascribed such effects had also produced poor results in the case of the plague in Noja. Medicines such as Gloutton tincture, castoreum tincture, musk, camphor, and the ever-present theriac had not produced the expected effects. As for opium and liquid laudanum, they had often caused 'an immediate failure of the brain, with comatose states' (D'Onofrio 1817: 34). Yet these anomalous results could be explained as follows: these remedies excited the body beyond its normal needs. The only medicine with truly healing effects therefore had been the infusion of chinchona bark, whereby the feverish sick had become 'apyretic' and those who were prostrate and moribund had regained their strength.

Having greatly praised the infusion of chinchona bark as a supreme remedy against the plague, D'Onofrio completed his treatise with some further remarks. The suppuration process of the buboes had to be facilitated naturally by using maturing and emollient substances like posca (a mixture of water and vinegar) (D'Onofrio 1817: 46). Moreover, contradicting Smith's optimistic opinion on the vaccine's universal preventive effects, D'Onofrio (1817: 70) asserted that having been vaccinated (or also having had smallpox) did not have immunisation effects with respect to the plague.

6.3 Conclusions

A critical assessment of all the therapeutic interventions described in this chapter (both those developed theoretically and those actually deployed in the field) highlights first of all that they were generally conceived on the basis of the identification of the nature of the disease. In this respect, the nosological categories devised by Brown, which despite their sketchiness still provided an interpretive basis, were universally accepted.

Were all the treatments devised by the doctors harmful for their patients? Actually, no: some empirical observations had indeed led to relatively sound approaches. For example, bloodletting, which had been a universal therapeutic aid for centuries, was included in the list of debilitating remedies, hence contraindicated for plague, by Brown's nosography. The prescription of camphor oil anointments, although totally ineffective for those already infected by the disease, was on the contrary an excellent preventive remedy, given that this substance has an effective repellent action against fleas. Further, infusions of chinchona bark and cold baths, albeit lacking any intrinsic healing power, nevertheless had a good anti-pyretic effect.[15] And the application of cataplasms on buboes, with the purpose of facilitating their suppuration and the expulsion of the pyogenic material through incision, was also effective: a surgical intervention on the bubo was the only treatment that, if completed appropriately and in timely fashion, enabled the infection of the lymph node stations to be relieved, thereby giving some hope of recovery.[16]

However, these positive outcomes were outweighed by the negative ones. If the plague was – in Brunonian terminology – an asthenic disease, as the great majority of the doctors here reviewed seemed to believe, the drugs had to be of the sthenic or invigorating kind. The problem was that the medicines to which such properties were ascribed were at best useless drugs or simple palliatives, and at times highly toxic. For instance, the Gloutton tincture, which a nineteenth-century pharmacopoeia described as 'being used as an excitant' (Cassola 1846: 726–7), was actually a lethal preparation made from sulphuric acid and muriatic acid that is extremely harmful for the body. Mercurial preparations were considered beneficial insofar as they caused hypersalivation, deemed to be a means of expelling infected humours; it was not suspected that an increased salivary secretion was the first symptom of mercury poisoning that, in prolonged therapy, produced even more severe effects.[17] A compound like laudanum was actually a drug whose ingestion, especially in cases of overdose, could lead to serious respiratory and circulatory depression.[18]

On balance, therefore, when confronted with the plague at Noja in 1815, medical science continued to struggle in the interstices between theory and practice, and the doctors' interventions overall had negative effects, both on the course of the disease and on the rate of fatalities that resulted.

[15] On the origins and spread of the infusions of chinchona bark, see, inter alia, Dousset (1987: 195–8).

[16] Not for nothing had the incision of the bubo been carried out on persons affected by plague since the Middle Ages. On the usefulness of this intervention, see Bruzzone (1987: 161–2), Cassiani (1994: 212–13), and Tanturri (2004: 191).

[17] The next symptoms, for the ill-fated patients, were swelling of the gums and tooth loss (Del Lungo 1983: 776–7).

[18] It is not difficult to believe Tagarelli's (1934: 109) assertion, that is, that among the sick who saved themselves there were some who 'pretended to take the normal medicaments, and then they secretly threw them away'.

REFERENCES

Bonnemain, Bruno. 2010. La thériaque à l'époque moderne (XVIIe au XXe siécle). *Revue d'Histoire de la Pharmacie* 367: 301–10.

Borrelli, Antonio. 2000. *Istituzioni scientifiche, medicina e società. Biografia di Domenico Cotugno*. Florence: Olschki.

[Bozzelli, Francesco Paolo]. 1816. *Giornale di tutti gli atti, discussioni e determinazioni della Soprantendenza generale e Supremo magistrato di Sanità del Regno di Napoli. In occasione del morbo contagioso sviluppato nella città di Noja*. Naples: Presso la Stamperia Reale.

Bradley, Richard. 1721. *The plague at Marseilles consider'd: with remarks upon the plague in general, shewing its cause and nature of infection, with necessary precautions to prevent the spreading of that direful distemper, published for the preservation of the people of Great Britain*. London: Mears.

Brown, John. 1803. *The elements of medicine translated from the Latin with comments and illustrations by the author*. Portsmouth: Treadwell.

Bruzzone, Egidio. 1987. *Storia e medicina nella storiografia della peste*. Genoa: ECIG.

Cassiani, Gennaro. 1994. Medici, magistrati e filosofi contro i miasmi della peste. Ricerche in margine ad alcuni documenti sull'epidemia di Roma del 1656–57. *Ricerche di Storia Sociale e Religiosa* 23: 187–215.

Cassola, Filippo. 1846. *Dizionario di farmacia generale*. Naples: Reale Tipografia Militare.

Catapano, Vittorio Donato. 1990. *Medicina a Napoli nella prima metà dell'Ottocento*. Naples: Liguori.

Catellani, Patrizia, & Renzo Console. 2007. The rise and fall of mithridatium and theriac in pharmaceutical texts. *Pharmaceutical Historian* 37(1): 2–9.

Chast, François. 2010. La thériaque à l'époque moderne. Chronique d'une fin annoncée du XVIe au XIX[e]siécle. *Revue d'Histoire de la Pharmacie* 368: 439–510.

Conforti, Maria. 2006. Peste a stampa: trattati, relazioni e cronache a Roma nel 1656. In Irene Fosi (ed.), *La peste a Roma (1656–1657)*. Rome: CROMA-Università Rome Tre. Monographic issue of *Roma Moderna e Contemporanea* 14:135–58.

Cosmacini, Giorgio. 1987. *Storia della medicina e della sanità in Italia dalla peste europea alla Guerra mondiale 1348–1918*. Rome; Bari: Laterza.

D'Onofrio, Arcangelo. 1817. *Dettaglio istorico della peste di Noja in provincia di Bari sviluppatasi a novembre del 1815*. Naples: Garruccio.

Da Molin, Giovanna. 1983. Una crisi di mortalità nell'età della Restaurazione: la carestia e l'epidemia del 1816–17 in Puglia. In *Atti del III Convegno di studi sul Risorgimento in Puglia. L'età della Restaurazione (1815 – 1830)*, 297–346. Bari: Bracciodieta.

Del Lungo, Mariella. 1983. Aspetti dell'organizzazione sanitaria nella Genova del Settecento: la cura delle malattie veneree. *Società e storia* 6: 769–801.

Della Valle, Cesare. 1816. *Ragguaglio istorico della peste sviluppata in Noja nell'anno 1815*. Naples: Trani.

Do Sameiro Barroso, Maria. 2014. The bezoar stone: A princely antidote, the Távora Sequeira Pinto Collection – Oporto. *Acta Medico – historica Adriatica* 12(1): 77–98.

Dousset, Jean-Claude. 1987. *Storia dei medicamenti e dei farmaci. Dalle origini ai giorni nostri*. Genoa: ECIG.

Duffin, Cristopher, J. 2016. Nathaniel Hodges (1629–1688): Plague doctor. *Journal of Medical Biography* 24(1): 30–5.

Espinoza González, Ricardo. 2016. Bezoares gastrointestinales: mitos y realidades. *Revista médica de Chile* 144(8): 1073–7.

Frasca, Elena. 2014. *L'eco di Brown. Teorie mediche e prassi politiche (secoli XVIII–XIX)*. Rome: Carocci.

Giannini, Giuseppe. 1805. *Della natura delle febbri e del miglior metodo di curarle; con alcune deduzioni sulla natura delle convulsioni, e in generale delle malattie di parossismo; sul trattamento e sull'estinzione delle febbri contagiose; sull'uso delle immersioni fredde; sull'esistenza ed indole della complicazion morbosa, e sulla relativa modificazione da introdursi nella indicazion curativa*, vol. I. Milan: Pirotta e Maspero.

Grassi, Francesco. 1843. *Risposta ai sette quesiti concernenti la peste bubonica orientale*. Pistoia: Cino.

Griffin, John P. 2004. Venetian treacle and the foundation of medicines regulation. *British Journal of Clinical Pharmacology* 58(3): 317–25.

Hancock, Thomas. 1821. *Researches into the laws and phenomena of pestilence, including a medical sketch and review of the plague of London in 1665, and remarks on quarantine, with an appendix containing extracts and observations relative to the plagues of Morocco, Malta, Noya and Corfu, being the subject of the anniversary oration delivered before the Medical Society of London in the spring of 1820 and published at their request*. London: Philips.

Iacovelli, Gianni. 1988. *Gli acquedotti di Cotugno. Medici pugliesi a Napoli tra Illuminismo e Restaurazione*. Galatina: Congedo.

Kampmeier, Rudolph H. 1976. Syphilis therapy: An historical perspective. *Journal of the American Venereal Disease Association* 3: 99–108.

Karaberopoulos, Demetrios, Marianna Karamanou, & George Androutsos. 2012. The teriac in antiquity. *The Lancet* 379: 1942–3.

Mansi, Maria Gabriella. 2006. I libri di Cotugno e i documenti della Biblioteca Nazionale di Napoli. *Scrinia* 3: 101–14.

Morea, Vitangelo. 1817. *Storia della peste di Noja*. Naples: Trani.

Nockels-Fabbri, Christiane. 2007. Treating medieval plague: The wonderful virtues of theriac. *Early Science and Medicine* 12(3): 247–83.

O'Shea, John, G. 1990. 'Two minutes with Venus, two years with Mercury'. Mercury as an antisyphilitic chemotherapeutic agent. *Journal of the Royal Society of Medicine* 83: 392–5.

Panvini, Pasquale. 1816. *Chiara dimostrazione de' veri preservativi della peste, e de' rimedj che distruggono il contagio, con l'esposizione delle circostanze che infieriscono la peste e del miglior metodo di curare gli appestati, con l'aggiunta delle più interessanti regole sanitarie*. Naples: De Dominicis.

Petraccone, Claudia. 1977. La difesa contro la peste: prevenzione e controllo dell'epidemia nelle pestilenze in Terra di Bari (1690–1692) e Noja (1815–1816). *Archivio Storico per le Province Napoletane*, 3rd series, 16: 261–80.

Premuda, Loris. 1984. *Cotugno Domenico*. In *Dizionario Biografico degli Italiani*, vol. 30, 480–3. Rome: Istituto della Enciclopedia Italiana.

Romani, Francesco. 1816. *Ricordi su la peste redatti in un sistema teorico – pratico*. Naples: Masi.

Sanders, Michael K. 2004. Bezoars: From mystical charms to medical and nutritional management. *Practical Gastroenterology* 28: 37–50.

Scofield, Samuel. 1803. *An inaugural dissertation on the nature and origin of vaccina or cow-pock, submitted to the public examination of the Faculty of Physic*. New York: T. & J. Swords.

Smith, Luigi. 1817. *Della peste. Trattato completo*, vol. I. Naples: Nella Stamperia della Società Tipografica.

Tagarelli, Sebastiano. 1934. *La peste di Noja (1815–1816)*. Noicattaro: Fiorentino.

Tanturri, Alberto. 2004. Terapie contro la peste nel Mezzogiorno moderno. *Ricerche di Storia Sociale e Religiosa* 33: 181–93.

Tanturri, Alberto. 2014. *'L'infausto dono dell'Arabia'. Vaiolo e vaccinazione nel Mezzogiorno preunitario (1801–1861)*. Milan: Unicopli.

Tilles, Gérard, & Daniel Wallach. 1996. Le traitement de la *syphilis* par le mercure. Une histoire thérapeutique exemplaire. *Histoire des Sciences Médicales* 30(4): 501–10.

Tisci, Caterina. 2015. *Lo scudo contro il vaiolo. Antonio Miglietta e la profilassi nel Regno di Napoli (1801–1826)*. Lecce: Edizioni Grifo.

Valerio, Sebastiano. 2011. Noja, la peste e il Grand Tour: il viaggio 'letterario' di Richard Keppel Kraven. In Patrizia Guida & Giovanna Scianatico (eds.), *Saggi di letteratura italiana. Selected papers of the 2010 AATI Annual Conference, Lecce, May 29–30 2010*, 103–17. Lecce: Pensa Multimedia.

Williams, Randolph S. 1986. The fascinating history of bezoars. *Medical Journal of Australia* 145(11–12): 613–14.

Willis, Thomas. 1691. *A plain and easie method for preserving (by God's blessing) those that are well from the infection of the plague, or any contagious distemper in city, camp, fleet & c. and for curing such as are infected with it*. London: Crook.

[Zocchi, Giuseppe]. 1816. *Pensiere sulla peste*. Naples: Tipografia Chianese.

CHAPTER 7

On Excitability

Jeremy J. Smith

Medical language – like all forms of living language – is subject to change. The 'scientific currency' (de Almeida 1991: 13) of the late eighteenth and early nineteenth centuries differs from our own. One word in English that had special meanings at the time, as identified by Professor Alberto Tanturri, is *excitability*, and the linked terms *excite*, *excitant*, and so on, which in the late eighteenth century came to develop specifically physiological meanings. This usage seems to derive from the writings of John Brown (1735–88), an Edinburgh physician of the Scottish Enlightenment whose biography is conveniently available in the *Oxford Dictionary of National Biography* (Lawrence 2004; see also Beddoes 1795; Bynum & Porter 1988). Brown, the founder of an eponymous innovative nosographic system known as *Brunonianism*, held that *excitability* was the fundamental feature of living bodies, being triggered by interaction with the environment to produce excitement; that is, the life force. Brunonianism thus pointed forward to Vitalist and Romantic notions of the operation of the body, going beyond the dominant earlier eighteenth-century conception that living bodies could be understood as the outcome of mathematical or physical laws alone.

Although Brunonianism's experimental basis was problematic in several ways, its author seems to have become convinced of his system through experimenting on himself. This was an approach regularly adopted by later Romantic scientists such as Humphry Davy (see further Holmes 2009, especially ch. 6). Brown suffered from gout, but reported that abstention from meat and alcohol, as recommended by an anonymous medical adviser, was ineffective. (The adviser was possibly the great William Cullen, who had once been Brown's mentor, but with whom he had quarrelled.) He therefore decided to go to the opposite extreme, ingesting 'liberally' (Lawrence 2004) not only substantial quantities of food and drink but also opium, with, it seems, satisfactory results. His approach to medicine was promulgated through a series of university lectures, and subsequently published as *Elementa Medicinae Brunonis* (1780), and (anonymously) as *Observations on the Principle of the Old System of Physic* (1787). His views achieved considerable acclaim from many contemporaries, including students attracted by his charismatic manner of teaching: '[i]n Edinburgh, espousing Brunonianism was often the choice of young Turks whose medical radicalism might be matched by a socio-political radicalism' (Bynum & Porter 1988: ix). However, the system remained controversial, not least because of Brown's perceived personal faults. Thomas Beddoes (1760–1808), the radical (and teetotal) chemist and physician, who had also attended Cullen's lectures in Edinburgh, offered the following anecdote in his hostile 'Observations on the Character and Writings', prefixed to his posthumous translation of Brown's *Elementa*:

(1) One of his pupils informs me that when he found himself languid, he sometimes placed a bottle of whisky in one hand, and a phial of laudanum on the other; and that, before he began his lecture, he would take forty or fifty drops of laudanum in a glass of whisky; repeating the dose four or five times during the lecture. Between the effects of these stimulants and voluntary exertion, he soon waxed warm, and by degrees his imagination was exalted into phrenzy. (Beddoes 1795: lxxxvii)

Beddoes's considered views on the author of the *Elements* were summed up by the dedication of his translation: 'To the ingenious, the candid, and humane, the following production of unfortunate genius is inscribed by the editor.' Brown's influence was nevertheless widely felt, notably in Germany and – as Professor Tanturri has shown – in Italy.

Brown's *excitability*, and the related form *excitant*, are both derivatives of the verb *excite*, from Latin *excitāre* ('to set in motion'). Other related words include *excitancy*, *excitation*, *excitative*, *excitator*, and *excitatory*. According to the *Oxford English Dictionary* (OED), the earliest specifically medical usage of any of these terms dates from Middle English, where *excite* simply refers to the process whereby a purge is induced. John Trevisa's translation of Bartholomaeus Anglicus's encyclopaedia *De Proprietatibus Rerum* (1398) describes how 'It is generall medycyne to excyte spewinge', and that the form has no special medical significance is confirmed by its usage in the near-contemporary *Three Kings of Cologne*: 'Þe deuyll [...] excited [...] among þe pepil diuers opynyouns of heresy.'

More relevant to the later development of the term is its appearance in Sir Thomas Browne's *Pseudodoxia Epidemica* (1646), where magnetism is referred to: 'If an iron or steele not formerly excited, be held perpendicularly or inclinatorily unto the needle, the lower end thereof will attract the cuspis or southerne point.' Magnetism fascinated contemporary writers; Sir Thomas was said to have been drawn to his wife Dorothy 'by a kind of Natural Magnetism' (Lawrence 2004), and magnetism was a trope for metaphysical poets such as John Donne, used to refer to both profane and sacred love. Indeed, interchange between scientific and religious meanings of these words is characteristic of this early usage. *Excitant*, for instance, is first recorded in the OED in the puritan preacher Richard Crakenthorpe's *A sermon of sanctification* (1608): 'Gods grace in our conversion is not onely an excitant, but a viuificant grace.' Interestingly, the OED classifies the citation from Crakenthorpe, glossing *excitant* as 'That rouses, excites, or stimulates; exciting, stimulating', alongside a 1774 reference to the Royal Society's *Philosophical Transactions*: 'Cushions [. . .] covered with silk [. . .] are much more powerfully excitant.'

The physiological meaning of *excitability* seems to emerge from these earlier usages, both religious and secular, and underpinned Brown's extension of the term's meaning. The OED shows how swiftly the term became current in contemporary scientific discourse, for example in the writings of Brown's contemporary Erasmus Darwin (1731–1802), an Edinburgh-trained physician as well as polymath who, in addition to favouring Brown's 'strong interventions' such as opium (though not alcohol), used 'swinging machines' (Lawrence 2004). Darwin's *Phytologia* (1800) refers to how 'The buds of vegetables [. . .] possess irritability, and sensibility, and voluntarity, and have associations of motion [. . .]. But [. . .] the three latter kinds of excitability are possessed in a so much less degree by vegetable buds.' Darwin was hugely influential on Romantic writers. Mary Shelley, for instance, seems to have been inspired to write *Frankenstein* after a discussion with Lord Byron and her husband Percy about 'the experiments of Dr Darwin' (1831: ix–x).

Fascinatingly, as Romantic thinking developed it seems to have sustained a broad approach to the notion of *excitability*, and here the key figure is the poet and philosopher Samuel Taylor Coleridge (1772–1834). Numerous citations from Coleridge relating to the term and its congeners appear in the OED. Coleridge was clearly aware of the scientific sense of these words, accompanied by a good understanding of Brunonian principles. As Neil Vickers has pointed out, Coleridge is on record – in a letter to his publishers of 1819 – as ranking Brown 'alongside Cicero, Luther, Giordano Bruno, Milton, Dryden, Wolfe, Hunter and Wordsworth, as a "man of great Genius and original Mind"' (1997: 48). It is no surprise to learn that Coleridge was close to Beddoes, who encouraged him to travel to

Germany in 1798–1799 to develop his philosophical education (in 1799 Coleridge was to enrol as a student at Göttingen). An OED quotation from Coleridge's *Table-Talk* (1833), which catches something of the poet's inspired casual conversation, reads as follows: 'The English affect stimulant nourishment—beef and beer. The French excitants [...] alcohol, champagne.' And *excitability* is used in a less flippant way in Coleridge's much more serious, and highly influential, *Aids to reflection in the formation of a manly character on the several grounds of prudence, morality, and religion* (1825): 'Pleasure [...] consists in the harmony between the specific excitability of a living creature, and the exciting causes correspondent thereto.' Coleridge, in truly Romantic fashion, clearly saw the connexion between physical and metaphysical approaches to the world, reminding us incidentally why science used to be referred to as 'natural philosophy'. It is intriguing in this context that *excitability* and *excitant* continue to be current terms in neurology (see for instance Izhikevich 2000, with 1,876 citations to date in Google Scholar).

REFERENCES

de Almeida, Hermione. 1991. *Romantic medicine and John Keats*. Oxford: Oxford University Press.

Beddoes, Thomas (trans.). 1795. *The elements of medicine of John Brown, M.D. Translated from the Latin*. London: Johnson.

Bynum, William F., & Roy Porter (eds.). 1988. *Brunonianism in Britain and Europe*. London: Wellcome Institute.

Holmes, Richard. 2009. *The age of wonder*. London: HarperCollins.

Izhikevich, Eugene. 2000. Neural excitability, spiking and bursting. *International Journal of Bifurcation and Chaos* 10: 1171–266.

Lawrence, Christopher. 2004. Brown, John (*bap.* 1735, *d.* 1788), physician. *Oxford Dictionary of National Biography*. www.oxforddnb.com/view/10.1093/ref:odnb/9780198614128.001.0001/odnb-9780198614128-e-3623 (accessed 3 June 2021).

Shelley, Mary. 1831. *Frankenstein*. 2nd ed. London: Colburn and Bentley.

Vickers, Neil. 1997. Coleridge, Thomas Beddoes and Brunonian medicine. *European Romantic Review* 8: 47–94.

CHAPTER 8

Systems and Centos

Some Eighteenth-Century Dictionaries

Roderick McConchie

What is an encyclopaedic dictionary: a dictionary, an encyclopaedia, or a dictionary with encyclopaedic entries (as medical dictionaries archetypically are)?[1] Are they dictionaries of things or of lexical items and definitions, a distinction all the more urgent in medical compilations? Accounts setting out the approaches adopted in such works of reference are rare, and the historian of dictionaries is normally obliged to trawl the evidence of the dictionary itself, including its forematter, to establish how and on what principles it was constructed. In English, we generally search in vain for extensive accounts such as found in the entries for *encyclopaedia*, *dictionary*, and *definition* by the encyclopaedist Denis Diderot (see Diderot n.d.). Further difficulties are caused by the fact that what we now call an encyclopaedia was frequently entitled a 'universal dictionary' in the eighteenth century. The distinction was clearly blurred.

It is therefore refreshing – and illuminating not only to philologists but also to historians of science – to find extended comments on such works of reference, albeit not penned by mainstream lexicographers and encyclopaedists. This chapter examines comments by three disparate eighteenth-century compilers of such volumes on their nature and function. The hugely successful *Cyclopaedia* by Ephraim Chambers (1680?–1740) appeared in 1728. His insights were subsequently applied to the medical dictionary by Robert James (1703–1776), published 1742–1745, and are also relevant to the dictionaries published or projected by James Keir (1735–1820), who translated one dictionary of chemistry (a subject critical to medicine), and later undertook an abortive one of his own, published in part in 1789.

[1] I am taking *dictionary* here in the extended sense of *Oxford English Dictionary* (OED) 1b: 'a book of information or reference on any subject in which the entries are arranged alphabetically; an alphabetical encyclopedia'. Chambers consistently calls his work and others like it a 'dictionary' throughout his 1728 preface.

Diderot's entry for *encyclopaedia* argues that compiling one would require so much time and effort that it would be desperately out of date once published. Words are coined, become obsolete, and change meaning, sometimes quite abruptly. Definitions can be rendered inaccurate and misleading. Diderot also maintains that insightful cross-referencing 'will give an *encyclopedia* the character which a good dictionary ought to possess [...] of changing the common mode of thinking'. 'An encyclopedia', he argues, 'is a rapid and disinterested exposition of the discoveries of men in all places, all kinds, and all centuries' (Diderot n.d.: s.v. *encyclopedia*).[2] Such a work, according to Diderot, provides general and permanent instruction. Thus the 'dictionarist' or encyclopaedist imposes systems of thought on the reader that may enhance and expand knowledge as well as disseminate it.

8.1 Ephraim Chambers on Dictionaries

Ephraim Chambers, born near Kendal, was apprenticed to a London cartographer and conceived the idea of compiling a compendium of knowledge, inspired by John Harris's *Lexicon Technicum* (1704) and the work of Pierre Bayle and Louis Moreri. First published in 1728, his *Cyclopaedia* ran through three editions before his death.[3] Chambers defines a dictionary as 'a Collection of Definitions of the Words of a Language' (1728 Preface: xxi), a definition that draws attention to the meanings ascribed to the word list but not to its constituents.[4] Within this broader category he identifies three kinds of dictionary: grammatical, philosophical and technical (that is, lexical, scientific and those of 'arts and sciences'), the latter incorporating medicine, seen as both art and science. Nevertheless,

[2] The Diderot quotations are from the University of Michigan Collaborative Translation Project version.

[3] For more on Chambers and his methods, see Bocast (2016).

[4] Joseph Priestley offers a slightly different and later definition according more significance to polysemy: 'a *Dictionary* is that which contains all the words of a language, and an account of all the senses in which they are used'. Priestley also commented on

> (i) That immense and valuable performance of Mr. *Johnson's* [which] contains an account of almost all the senses in which all the words of the English language are used: and [...] from little more than [his] examples [...] from our best writers of the use of every word in every sense, to compose a grammar of all the varieties of manner in which words are used [...] which, together with the dictionary, would be a complete system of our language as now used. (1762: 185–6)

Citations from Chambers and other eighteenth-century writers have been accessed on *Eighteenth Century Collections Online (ECCO).*

in the *Cyclopaedia* text Chambers offers 'a Collection, or Catalogue of all the Words of a Language, or an Art, with their Significations; rang'd in Order of Alphabet', now stressing the list of lemmas rather than their 'significations'. He argues that the lexicographer

(1) was an Analyst; that his View was not to improve or advance Knowledge, but to teach, or convey it; and that he was hence led to unty the Complexions or Bundles of Ideas his Predecessors had made, and reduce 'em to their natural parity: which is all that is essential to a Dictionarist [. . .]. (1728 Preface: xxi)[5]

Thus the dictionarist is to achieve parity among discrete items of knowledge by reducing the individual entries to equivalence, a characteristic of Chambers's work that Diderot disparaged, writing of Chambers's perfect and regular encyclopaedic order that:

(2) since he limited himself to compilation from our dictionaries and the analysis of a small number of works, invented nothing, and stuck strictly to what was known, everything being equally interesting or indifferent to him, [. . .] save that of a migraine or spleen, he was a labourer who plowed his furrow, shallow, but even and straight. (n.d.: 49–50)

But Chambers also understood that he was not merely to record, but to analyse and interpret. He was well aware of the limitations of such a classification, and thus of the nuances of the dictionary as a genre:

(3) Tho we have *Dictionaries* under all these Titles; it would perhaps be hard to find any conformable to this Partition [. . .] Dictionarists are far from considering their Subject so closely, or confining themselves to so narrow, tho direct, a Channel: They must have more room [. . .] to use all kinds of Definitions promiscuously. 'Tis no wonder they should not keep to Views which they had not, and which could only arise from Researches they never made. While the Notions of *Term* and *Art*, remain'd yet in the Rubbish [. . .] left by the Schoolmen; those of *Definition* and *Dictionary* must needs be vague and arbitrary enough; and the Dictionarists and Expositors, profited by an Embarrass it was their Business to have remov'd. (1728: xxi)

[5] The 1738 edition (Chambers 1738: xvi) makes two significant changes here: 'parity' has become 'simplicity', suggesting a change in categorization, and 'Dictionarist' now reads 'lexicographer', a term gaining in frequency at the expense of *dictionarist* in this period.

More generally, Chambers claims, lexicographers had been insufficiently discriminating. Latin–English–Latin dictionaries and Vernacular–English–Vernacular dictionaries, despite greater sophistication, remained largely tied to educational ends in terms of both achievement and marketing. Medical dictionaries repeatedly addressed the medical tyro. For Chambers, principles that remained largely undeclared and unconsidered drove lexicography, and articulating them would help to purge dictionaries of their disorderliness and lexical excesses.

With hindsight, Chambers could hardly have made such an argument without the development of the lexical dictionary (see Lancashire 2002), rather than dictionaries of translation equivalents and/or glosses. However, it is significant that he also expressed this emerging view, albeit succinctly. The dictionary for Chambers is also a historical artefact that provides post hoc explanations for what is already known; his vision of the role of the dictionary is thus far more constrained than Diderot's:

(4) THE *Dictionary* [. . .] supposes the Advances and Discoveries made, and comes to explain or relate 'em. The Dictionarist, like an Historian, comes after the Affair; and gives a Description of what pass'd [. . .]. The Dictionary of an Art, is the proper History of such Art: the Dictionary of a Language, the History of that Language [. . .]. The Dictionarist is not supposed to have any hand in the Things he relates; he is no more concerned to make the Improvements, or establish the Significations, than the Historian to atchieve the Transactions he relates. (1728: xxii)

A medical dictionary might thus have to painstakingly incorporate new words for innovative concepts and procedures with full explanations, whereas relisting old ones was relatively straightforward.

For Chambers, the lexicographer's role is qualitatively different from that of the encyclopaedist. What the encyclopaedist undertakes is 'An Attempt towards a Survey of the Republick of Learning [. . .] the Boundary that circumscribes our present Prospect; and separates the known, from the unknown Parts of the Intelligible World' (1728 Dedication) as contemporaneously understood, a boundary that, despite his expressed limitations, Chambers sees as being pushed far back into the unknown 'other Hemisphere' (1728 Dedication) under the King's patronage, leading to new discoveries and as yet unimagined inventions. A vision fit for a king to be sure, but Chambers is less clear on how exactly the *Cyclopaedia* will conduce to this progress.

The dictionary retains a valuable role, however: 'It may even be said, that if the System be an Improvement upon the Dictionary; the Dictionary is some Advantage to the System; and [...] perhaps, the only Way, wherein the whole circle or body of knowledge can be delivered' (1728 Preface: i). He sees a system as the web or chain of logical deductions and conclusions that constitute a science (1728 Preface: ix). Chambers argues that all the minutiae must be 'swallowed up in the Whole' (1728 Preface: i), rather than being allowed to dominate the whole as a purely alphabetical arrangement would surely demand. Each minor point should assist the reader's imagination to envisage the whole, and vice versa. Thus the use of both systems and alphabetisation offers advantages.

Chambers's preface opens nonetheless by comparing his present effort with the monumental labour that produced the dictionaries of the Italian Accademia della Crusca and the French Academy, rather than encyclopaedic works. He also recognises the inheritance these and other works bequeathed him – so much indeed that digesting and organising it into 'one consistent Whole' (1728 Preface: i) has been his greatest problem. Chambers undertook to impose order and coherence on the multifarious materials obtained from previous dictionaries, his purpose being 'as different from theirs, as a System from a Cento' (1728 Preface: i). Cento, a word with a somewhat negative connotation, means a patchwork, something composed of scraps, a work composed of quotations. It is thus disorganised in terms of the items comprising its internal content, just as a dictionary is distinct in this sense from a thesaurus. Chambers does not consider the dictionary cento as diametrically opposed to the encyclopaedic system, however, but merely as representing a deficiency. His forward-looking view suggests that he envisioned a cline rather than an unambiguous divide between the genres:

(5) Former Lexicographers have not attempted any thing like Structure in their Works; nor seem to have been aware that a Dictionary was in some measure capable of the Advantages of a continued Discourse. (1728 Preface: i)

Chambers's method is to rank data on a given subject along a line of inference and logical subordination and dependence, like links in a chain. Further, he explores the interrelations between subjects, intending to set out the whole of knowledge for the reader, which 'appears indeed with the Face of a Wilderness; but 'tis a Wilderness thro' which the Reader may pursue his Journey as securely, tho not so expeditiously and easily, as thro' a regular Parterre' (1728 Preface: i).[6] His multifarious sources, as Kennedy relates at length, demand this level of curation (Kennedy 2016: 14–21, 36–45).

Chambers is also very aware of polysemy, and that monosemous lexemes are rare, as well as acknowledging complex ideas and collocations, so that, for instance, the very polysemous entry for *composition* includes the pharmaceutical sense. A medical and surgical sense appears under *friction*, and the '*Frixion* of Medicines' is also noted separately. The clearly medical term *fistula* is also noted as a pipe through which early communicants sucked wine, and *hermetical* (1728: s.v. *hermetic*) notes causes in medicine and how medicines work. Chambers claims that the mind will 'bundle up its Ideas, and thus pay or receive 'em in Parcels, [leaving] us very few simple ones [. . .] Names which denote only one Idea' (1728: xviii).

Chambers offers several definitions of a *term*, one being 'a Word which denotes an Assemblage, or System of Ideas, relating to some one Point, which the Mind artfully complicates, or associates together, for the conveniency of its own Operations' (1728 Preface: xix).[7] Terms allow readers to assimilate, contextualise, and communicate knowledge more easily. Chambers is also very aware of what he omits, such as the detailed properties of material substances, derived forms, 'plebeian words', and so on (see 1728 Preface: xxiv–xxv).

Words may also become seriously misleading with scientific advances and discoveries. Chambers cites *attraction*, not a completely new term, but one used by Newton in a new way:

(6) the great Author [. . .] explain'd [. . .] the Sense he fix'd to his *Attraction*; yet Experience verifies how much he was overseen; the chief Objections against his whole System being drawn from a Misapprehension of this very Word, which keeps half the Philosophers in *Europe* still at a distance, afraid to admit a most excellent Doctrine, merely out of distrust of the Vehicle that conveys it [. . .]. (1728 Preface: xxviii)

In short, trying to redefine a word as a term has the practical effect of causing confusion and retarding progress.

6 Always remembering that the early eighteenth-century wilderness was a geometrically designed series of gravel walks between rows of trees, often severely clipped or trained and with some central opening with a built feature such as a pavilion or statue.

7 A sense not recognised by the OED.

Further, Chambers's hesitation about the use of an encyclopaedic dictionary in advancing knowledge was unjustified. Dictionaries were of genuine use to more than simply casual or inquisitive users, as was to be demonstrated later by James Keir in introducing his chemical dictionary, which he had not merely translated but also added to. The eminent 'Mr. Macquer [. . .] acknowledged that my [Keir's] notes to the translation of his Dictionary first excited his attention to the discoveries which had been made in England on the elastic fluids' (Keir 1789 Preface: iv).

8.2 Robert James

Robert James was from a well-to-do Staffordshire family. He attended St John's College, Oxford, and received a mandamus MD from Cambridge in 1728. He became an extra-licentiate of the Royal College of Physicians in the same year, and is best known for Dr James's Fever Powder, a hugely popular antimonial nostrum patented in 1747, which sold well into the twentieth century.[8]

James's *A Medicinal Dictionary*, a massive folio work with about 14,000 entries, is far more both encyclopaedic and lexical as well as glossarial than its contemporary rivals. It silently adopts Chambers's notion of the system within a dictionary structure, but fails to exploit its advantages, since large entries are exhaustive, not selective, and are sandwiched between innumerable minor entries of marginal relevance. Multipage entries are commonplace, *anatome* (anatomy), for example, taking up forty-three pages. As with contemporaneous medical dictionaries, headwords are characteristically in Latin or Greek, forms that do not appear in the text itself. Thus *air*, though mentioned often in the text, appears under AER, which is absent, bar cross-references. What James aims for, however, is exhaustiveness, not a system, which would involve disciplined curation.

Other than disambiguation of older terminology, James's Proposals (1741) pays no attention to the linguistic and lexicographical issues prominent in Chambers and (as we shall see) Keir. He does promise alphabetical order, as well as methods of cure in the post-lemmatic material, treatises on anatomy, surgery, and aliments (1741: [1]), restoration of order to the 'perplexity' of the terminology of the *materia medica* (1741: [1]), and select cases to illustrate particular diseases and treatments. The surgical treatise will contain an alphabetical list of 'subordinate articles' to assist the reader

[8] For recent and upcoming work on James, see Lonati (2017), McConchie (2019: ch. 9), and Wright and McConchie (in press).

with 'a distinct View of the whole Science' (1741: [2]). He also stresses veterinary medicine as a 'System of *Comparative Physic* and the lives of famous physicians', but is inconsistent, also suggesting that physicians should not waste their time on theory and systems (1741: [2]).

Turning to the dictionary itself, long and short entries constitute extremes, the disparity being beyond systematic. Many short entries with only a single signification, no definition, or even a medical sense occur often. Robert James's professional readers would already know much of the neoclassical terminology in his *Medicinal dictionary* (1743–1745), which may explain his frequent neglect of definitions.

To illustrate, *ptissana* (decorticated barley) has a solid, single-column entry. The next long one is *pulmo*, but between these are twenty-one short entries, only one of which, *pulegium* (pennyroyal), has much substance. Simple glosses with no medical relevance ('PULEX. A flea') abound, and some are merely cross-references ('PUBES. See ABDOMEN'). The series *alae* to *alaqueca* mentions many entries for stones, only some of which have medical uses. To take a further series, *amurca*, the dregs of pressed olive oil, is actually entered twice, giving every appearance that these entries were prepared independently and then entered without the duplication being noticed. These are followed by the short entry for *amyche* (superficial laceration of the skin);[9] *amydros*, a Hippocratic word meaning barely visible; *amygdalæ* (almonds, tonsils); *amygdalia* (also almonds), given another Hippocratic reference; *amygdalatum*, almond milk; *amygdaloides* (a species of spurge, euphorbia), for which a number of synonymous cross-references are offered; then *amygdalopersicum*, the almond peach. The medical significance of these varies greatly from obvious (*amyche*) to less obvious but perhaps useful as an ingredient (*amurca*) to none at all (*amygdalopersicum*) to unstated and apparently entered only because they are Hippocratic.[10] James's use of large-scale terms and entries to incorporate information into a 'system' is inconsistent, however, since under *febris* (fever), we find simply a cross-reference to a treatment (*cathartica*), some fever types (*depuratoria, miliaris*), and a main article (*pyretos*). James's own use of *system* is largely confined to 'the nervous system'. Many entries simply provide a Greek term, as in 'PROSCOLLEMA, ϖροσχολλεμα. An Agglutination'. *Agglutinatio* is defined under its own headword. As with earlier English dictionaries, Erasmus's encomiums on copiousness seem

[9] No genuine eighteenth-century use of this word in an English text has been found.

[10] At the same point, Chambers (1728) has *amurca* – *amy* (law term) – *amygdalæ* – *amygdalate* (= amygdalatum), but his main entry is under *almond*.

still to dominate (Erasmus 1512). James's dictionary in this respect could be seen as allowing the minutiae to swallow the systems whole.

Chambers had sought 'extracts and accounts from books of all kinds' as sources and to create a coherent system out of 'a confused Heap of incongruous Parts' (1728 Preface: i). He offers *anatomy* as an example, considered not simply within itself, but also in relation to medicine generally. He starts with a definition and a guide to the related terminology and concludes with a brief history and survey of anatomical writers. By contrast, James begins with a one-word gloss and an extended historical and practical argument for the use and necessity of anatomy. The history of anatomy comes much later. Chambers thus offers a series of fingerposts; James a disquisition beginning with the circulation of the blood, the skin, liver, and so on. James sought to be all-inclusive, not to curate systems, stressing inclusiveness repeatedly in his proposals: 'every particular Muscle [...] all the Glands [...] nothing shall be willingly omitted [...] everything to which a Name has been assigned [...] all the minute Inquiries of the Microscope', and so on. He also saw his dictionary as 'medicinal', not philosophical ('scientific'), and did not want physicians 'mis-spending their most improveable Days in reading Compilers of Theories and Systems' (James 1741: [1]). James does not list *system* at all, merely offering *systema*, the sediment at the bottom of the urinal. His full copiousness remained unrealised, as several of his later publications were medical translations intended for his library-replacing dictionary, but cut by the anxious publisher. 'The following Sheets were intended for the *Medicinal Dictionary*,' James complained, but 'the Impatience of the Bookseller [...] oblig'd me to omit it' (Hoffmann and Ramazzini 1746: ix).

8.3 James Keir

James Keir originally went to Edinburgh to study medicine in 1754 (King-Hele 1977: 32), where he became a life-long friend of Erasmus Darwin, and later moved to Birmingham.[11] His training in the foremost British medical school would have piqued his interest in the two-century tradition of iatrochemistry stemming from Paracelsus and van Helmont. He became a member of the Lunar Society of Birmingham, and worked mainly as an industrialist, including ventures in glassworks and the manufacture of alkali and soap.

[11] For Darwin, see Priestland (1990).

While several English medical dictionaries appeared up to 1800,[12] chemical dictionaries, such as William Johnson's *Lexicon chymicum* of 1652, were infrequent. A close relation between medicine and chemistry subsisted during this period, Keir contributing two such works in later eighteenth-century England.[13]

Keir's lexicographical activities included a translation of the *Dictionnaire de chymie* by Pierre-Joseph Macquer (1718–1784), and his own incomplete dictionary of chemistry. Macquer's successful dictionary was published in French in 1766, and Keir was already working on it by 1769 (Schofield 1963: 79 n.).

Macquer's original preface (Macquer 1766) advances Chambers's argument that alphabetisation would be disadvantageous, since the parts of chemistry are interrelated. This was resolved somewhat by many of his entries being extensive essays about the headword; again, an encyclopaedic dictionary.

Keir's additional notes enhanced the translation considerably.[14] Commenting on *air*, Keir notes that Macquer is apparently unaware of recent findings, including those 'of Dr. Black, from experiments so conducted and related, that his treatise may be considered [showing] the best method of investigating and demonstrating chemical truths' (Macquer 1771: 33).[15]

Keir issued his second edition in 1777. In prefacing his 1789 dictionary, Keir explains that additions to Macquer's work would improve it, specifying 'the valuable discoveries that had been made [...] by Dr. *Black* and Mr. *Cavendish*, on fixed and inflammable airs; a knowledge of which had

[12] The seventeenth- and eighteenth-century English medical dictionaries are Anon. 1657. *A physical dictionary*. London: G. Dawson; Blancard, Steven. 1684. *A physical dictionary*. London: J. D.; Cruso, John. 1701. *Medicamentorum Ευποριστο thesaurus*. Londini: Impensis Sam. Smith & Benj. Walford. (In Latin with English glosses); Quincy, John. 1719. *Lexicon physico-medicum; or, a new physical dictionary*. London: for Andrew Bell, William Taylor and John Osborn; [Duddell, Benedict?]. 1732. *Prosodia chirurgica*. London: for Charles Corbett and Richard Chandler; James, R[obert]. 1742–1745. *A medicinal dictionary*, 3 vols. London: for T. Osborne; Barrow, John. 1749. *Dictionarium medicum universale*. London: for T. Longman, and C. Hitch; and A. Millar; Motherby, G[eorge]. 1775. *A new medical dictionary*. London: for J. Johnson; Lara, Benjamin. 1796. *A dictionary of surgery*. London: for James Ridgway; Turton, William. 1797. *A medical glossary*. London: for J. Johnson.

[13] There was an efflorescence of chemical dictionaries in the early nineteenth century. For more on Keir, see Schofield (1963: 75–82) and Smith and Moilliet (1967).

[14] 'I became acquainted with Mr. Keir, at the time when he was employed in translating Macquer's Dictionary of Chemistry, a work which was rendered doubly valuable by the notes of the translator' (cited in Schofield 1963: 79).

[15] In 1775, however, in a letter to la Rouchfoucault (12 May), Macquer mentions the 'seven kinds of air' that Priestley had discovered. See Smeaton (2000).

not then reached Mr. *Macquer*'.[16] His work was thus positively received – 'more consideration than is due to a mere translation' (Keir 1789 Preface: i).

Keir's forematter to Macquer sets out some of his basic principles, which credit the reader's knowledge and intelligence. He argues for the dictionary arrangement, mentioned in both the translator's preface and the advertisement. Keir argues that chemistry is insufficiently systematic to be considered an independent discipline: 'But the Chemistry [. . .] now known is scarcely entitled to the name of science, so defined. It is at present little more than a collection of facts [. . .] [and] incapable of a more systematical arrangement' (Macquer 1771: ii).[17] In short, a cento. While chemistry does have systematic elements, Keir fears that a systematising work would omit other less connected or unconnected components. Alphabetisation thus implies completeness but undermines interrelations. The advertisement claims that:

(7) The alphabetical arrangement does indeed seem to interrupt and disconcert the regularity of plan and system, with which a science ought to be treated. But [. . .] this apparent want of order allows the readers to form such plans [. . .] as they may judge proper; and they may possibly make a better choice than the author would have done. (Macquer 1771 Advertisement)

Another advantage of alphabetical order is that if all the potential elements of chemistry are there, the reader can decide objectively and independently about internal coherences, and not admit preconceived notions.

Keir also claims that this 'is not a mere vocabulary, or dictionary of definitions; but rather a number of dissertations, generally full and extensive' (Macquer 1771 Advertisement), thus stressing its encyclopaedic nature. It seems clear that Keir ideally wants an internally coherent, systematised encyclopaedic work like that Chambers anticipated, rather than a dictionary, and, while preferring to minimise the essential dictionary functions, cannot see how to achieve this.[18] A little of this preface is

[16] Schofield makes detailed comments on Keir's additions to Macquer (1963: 80–1; 180–2). A very thorough exposition of Macquer's intentions and achievements appears in Anderson (1984).

[17] For a fuller account of the preface in terms of theoretical chemistry, see Schofield (1963: 299–300).

[18] In deference to the systematising skills of his readers and the awareness that chemical vocabulary was in a state of flux, Erasmus Darwin interleaved his copy of Keir's translation, now in the Wren Library at Trinity College, Cambridge, with largely blank pages.

retained verbatim in the introduction to his abortive later dictionary, as well as some of these arguments. Keir also added supplementary material and notes of his own, and promised to publish supplements as necessary.[19] Finally, it is curious that Keir omitted Macquer's long and insightful preface, especially when translating the original author's preface was a common practice. He does however cite it in his own, as well as mentioning Macquer's attempt to overcome the disjointed nature of the subject by providing generous cross-referencing.

In the preface to the second edition, he explains that recent progress superseded his original article on fixable air. As a result, he added an appendix entitled *A Treatise on the various kinds of permanently elastic fluids, or gases,* clearly intended as a report on current research and knowledge. Unusually, Keir indicates his sources very precisely, using letter symbols to distinguish between a borrowing from Macquer, one from Leonhardi's German translation of this work, and his own additions. Keir also explains this brings Macquer up to date, even though the translations into German and Italian had done this to some extent (Macquer 1777 Preface: i).

Keir later returned to lexicography, publishing *The first part of a dictionary of chemistry* (1789), mentioned by Erasmus Darwin to Richard Edgeworth on 20 February 1788: 'And He is now printing a new improved edition of his chemical dictionary.' Darwin also comments puckishly that 'Keir makes soap and dictionaries [. . .] and thrives I dare say' (King-Hele 1977: 179). Keir was probably more seriously engaged, however, since he had anticipated in his first preface that 'some person of eminently perspicuous genius may unfold the laws and causes of chemical analysis, collect and methodize the scattered facts, and form the several parts of Chemistry into one regular, connected science' (Macquer 1771: iii). Keir was presumably now taking his first halting steps in that direction, and adding greatly to what had appeared previously. Keir employs Chambers's distinction between dictionaries and encyclopaedias and between systematic structure and alphabetical order: that encyclopaedias enjoin systematic thought on the reader, but dictionaries allow freer judgement (1789 Preface: iii).[20]

In the event, Keir's own dictionary only reached its first part (A–Acid), apparently because of devastating theoretical and terminological problems, and despite much more being intended.[21] King-Hele attributes this to

[19] The first, resulting from Keir's work on Macquer's second edition, appeared in 1779.

[20] He makes no reference to Chambers here or indeed elsewhere.

[21] A letter of 20 November 1789 in the archives of the Library of Birmingham (MS 3147/3/504) indicates that he was then still at work on it.

Keir's recognition that he was wrong in clinging to the phlogiston theory, a seemingly reasonable supposition (King-Hele 1977: 182, 192). Keir found himself awkwardly placed at a crucial time in chemistry as the ground-breaking discoveries during the 1780s were becoming known, especially that of oxygen. This meant that Keir, a committed phlogistian,[22] seems to have found accepting the new nomenclature for these phenomena demanded by the French chemists overwhelming. The immediate problem seems to have been *air*, part of the meaning of which was to be overtaken by the term *gas* for its various constituents, *air* being still understood as the irreducible element air when Keir was working on his dictionaries. Keir would have had to accept terms like *oxygen*, *hydrogen*, *nitrogen*, and so on without seeing sufficient evidence that these were other than variant kinds of air.

Keir was at pains to position himself theoretically, specifically rejecting the 'antiphlogistic' terminology, since it 'cannot be considered as the general language of Chemistry' (1789 Preface: ii). Keir says much on phlogiston later in his preface (esp. vi–ix), but his friend Darwin joined the winning side by accepting the French innovations. It seems that part of Keir's objection is that antiphlogistic theory required an entirely new nomenclature for chemistry and that his scepticism prevented accepting this. His complex view on terminology may well have arisen from profound doubts about his own theoretical position. By the early nineteenth century, Morveau's and Lavoisier's nomenclature had been largely accepted.[23] Far more was at stake, however, than simply new terms replacing equivalent older ones – a paradigm shift from the Aristotelian notion of air as a single primary element to understanding the gaseous state as a fundamental condition of matter. When Joseph Black discovered carbon dioxide, he called it merely 'fixed air' (Black 1756: 199). Air had been regarded as containing impurities rather than as a mixture of gaseous elements (Crosland 2000: 86–8).

Keir makes several insightful remarks about language, especially that of science, which show his sensitivity to the issue of how facts and theories relate, as well as the words and terminologies that describe them. There are two jobs, the first being to purge chemical terminology of the inappropriate and misleading detritus of the past, while the second is to accommodate the new terms. The first is relatively straightforward, but the second

[22] As did Priestley. For phlogiston theory and why Priestley and others clung to it, see Woodcock (2005).

[23] Louis-Bernard Guyton-Morveau (1737–1816), who first introduced the new nomenclature.

presents considerable difficulties. Keir takes a conservative but even-handed view of the new terminology:

(8) The same philosophers who have introduced the new or antiphlogistic theory, have, with the same laudable zeal for promoting the interest of the science, attempted to reform the language of chemistry, and indeed to introduce an entirely *new Nomenclature* of almost all the substances, and of some of the operations employed by chemists. (Keir 1789 Preface: xiv)

This new theory was jumping the gun for Keir. His sensitivity to this issue seems to have left him too undecided to continue with what could have been a major scientific dictionary. He adumbrates two sources of imprecision and variability in language. These are the vagaries of its users and the attempts by chemists and their predecessors to reform it:

(9) every language being the invention of many different men, and at different times and places, partakes of the irregularity and imperfection of its origin. In chemistry, accordingly, the language is full of improper and absurd names, some [. . .] owing to the general causes of imperfection of all language, and some [. . .] introduced by the Alchemists, who wished to veil alike their knowledge and their ignorance under mysterious words; and lastly, some [. . .] from the false philosophy of the times, supposed then to be true and unalterable. Some of these names are merely barbarous, such as *powder of Algaroth*[24] and *Turbeth Mineral*;[25] and others lead to false ideas of the properties of the substance, as *oil of vitriol* and *butter of arsenic*[26] [. . .]. It is however [. . .] desirable [. . .] to purge the science of these remains of barbarism and alchemical mystery, and to introduce terms more *precise* and *elegant*, and especially such as shall clearly distinguish the objects, either by *proper names*, or by such as indicate some *sensible* and *obvious property*; and above all, which have *no theoretical etymology*, and consequently no tendency to give *false ideas*, or to give stability to such as are *uncertain* and *hypothetical*. (Keir 1789 Preface: xiv)

Keir wants a chemical terminology based on clear and unambiguous reference to the realia of the subject, stripped of the fanciful and obfuscatory as well as terms with no basis in anything other than theory. The essential problem was that Lavoisier and the French chemists, bar

[24] Antimony oxychloride (SbOCl). [25] Mercuric sulphate ($HgSO_4 \cdot 2HgO$).
[26] Arsenic trichloride (AsCl3).

Macquer, by inventing an entirely new terminology, had anticipated and interdicted the English adherents of the phlogiston theory. Different words (*dephlogisticated air*, *phlogisticated air*, etc.) represented different and incompatible conceptual structures (Brock 2008: 73–4).

Keir also used their public acceptance and demonstrable usefulness to defend dictionaries of sciences. He quotes his earlier translation of Macquer in asserting that because the discipline of chemistry is not yet inherently coherent, that is, 'not yet capable either of the synthetic or analytic modes of explanation' (Macquer 1771: ii), that an alphabetical arrangement has its advantages (as Ephraim Chambers, indeed, saw in acknowledging and reproducing such a coherence within his *Cyclopædia*). Reference is rendered easier than in a work that attempts to systematise the subject, and adherence to one theory rather than another is rendered unnecessary.

Change outran Keir's evolutionary approach, however, despite his eminently sensible understanding of how languages change: 'But as language is the common property of all, no authority is equal to any other alteration, however well imagined, but what is effected gradually, and [. . .] by universal consent' (Keir 1789: xiv). He goes on to claim that the effort to change chemical terminology by the French chemists is very difficult – admirable, but doomed.

According to Keir, the proponents of the new French nomenclature

(10) maintain that a science cannot be perfected without, at the same time, perfecting the language; and, that by using words conveying just definitions of the substances represented, we facilitate the attainment and the accurate comprehension of the science. With this intention they have given names expressive of the *constituent parts* and *characteristic properties* of the substances. A language *justly* and *completely* formed on these principles would be a truly philosophical language, and greatly conducive to the ends proposed. (Keir 1789: xv)

Keir fears that this certainty has not yet been achieved, much as he seems to approve. He is still wedded to phlogiston and, while not rejecting the antiphlogistic position out of hand, remains sceptical of its truth and general acceptability. In this genre, the system and consensus on it must prevail:

(11) They are however sensible of the fault of others in giving names founded on theory; such as *phlogisticated* and *dephlogisticated air*, &c. in which I perfectly agree with them, although these names accord

> with my own theory; but, as they imagine, that their own system is only a mere exposition of facts, they perceive no impropriety in giving the permanency of language to their ideas, by the words *oxygene*, *hydrogene*, &c. Accordingly their nomenclature is intirely relative to their peculiar theory. [. . .] we cannot speak the language of the new Nomenclature, without thinking as its authors do. (Keir 1789: xv)

He goes on to discuss *oxide*, *combustion*, *potash*, and other terms. Accepting a word entails general acceptance, as well as a corresponding acceptance that the theory and the facts agree. Competing nomenclatures would only lead to confusion (Keir 1789: xvi).

The subtlety of Keir's discussion shows us the insufficiency of simple generalisations on lexical change. The familiar notion that as new discoveries were made the terminology moved in lockstep with it belies the complexity of the relationship between the words and the system of words and the world of things, and the profound doubt that motivated Keir. This raises a fundamental research problem. Failure to understand the nature of the process of change and how to approach it is an obstacle in itself. The still common notion that naming moves in lockstep with discovery and classification is overly simple. Such a post hoc view obscures the process of making the terminological transitions that Keir saw so clearly. The difficulty with contenting oneself with this oversimplification is that the process of achieving the transition and adjustment is much more interesting and revealing than describing its outcome, and helps to obscure what really needs to be investigated. Likewise, the ultimate success of a chemical experiment for Lavoisier depended primarily on the conceptual language and terminology by which it was conceived, not on its observable outcome, as Anderson points out (1984: 95–8).

As it happened, Keir was quickly superseded in this respect by *A dictionary of chemistry* (1795) by William Nicholson (1753–1815), a work that accepted the new French theories and terminology.[27]

Keir felt the lexicographical dilemma very strongly. Puerperal fever, as conceived in the eighteenth century, provides a case in point. The various names for this condition – childbed fever, milk fever, sepsis puerperalis,

[27] Note that Nicholson claims that 'The man who has been habituated to explain chemical phænomena by the doctrine of phlogiston, will not be an impartial judge in that controversy, until he has acquired a facility in explaining them by the doctrine which rejects that principle' (1795: vi). In spite of also expressing doubts about the French nomenclature, he does still include *hydrogen* (a short entry cross-referenced to air, inflammable) and *oxygene* (simply cross-referenced to *nomenclature*), but does not include *nitrogene* at all, despite using it in the *nomenclature* entry.

postpartum metritis—are based on theories about its cause, including cold, inflammation, putrefaction, nervous spasms, and so on. The way a disease is conceived crucially determines how research is conducted and progress made. Thomas Trotter, discussing the role of names and definitions in medical research in his *Medicine Nautica* (1797–1803), wrote insightfully that:

(12) The name and definition of a disease are perhaps of more importance than is generally thought. They are like a central point to which all converging rays tend: they direct future inquirers how to compare facts, and become the base on which accumulating knowledge is to be heaped [. . .]. (Trotter 1797–1803, iii: 467)[28]

The disjunction between Keir's theory and what he thought should go into the dictionary was noted by Moilliet in 1868:

(13) Mr. Keir [. . .] discontinued this great undertaking when he became convinced that his theory would not fully explain some of the many curious facts which were afterwards discovered during the rapid progress which then occurred in experimental chemistry [. . .] [to] which perhaps his own writings and personal character [. . .] mainly contributed. (Moilliet 1868: 95)[29]

Perhaps we should conclude by citing Erasmus Darwin's terse remark of 12 September 1789 on reading Keir's introduction about this infant system: 'You have successfully combated the new nomenclature, and strangled him in the cradle before he has learnt to speak' (cited in Moilliet 1868: 96).

8.4 Conclusion

The compilers of *A new and complete dictionary of arts and sciences* of 1754 invoke the instability of the scientific lexicon, arguing that authors capriciously coin 'a multiplicity of names for the same object [. . .] subject [ing] lexicographers to the cruel and almost endless task of explaining the various terms [. . .] for one and the same thing' (Society of Gentlemen

[28] Trotter (1760–1832) was a naval physician and medical author, who helped pioneer an effective treatment for scurvy, and became an ardent abolitionist after first-hand experience on a slave ship.

[29] A letter of 15 March 1790 to Darwin shows that at that date he still intended to proceed, since he accepts Darwin's suggestion that the new terms be included, as well as expressing the conviction that Lavoisier's theory, and the new terms with it, would be overturned in time (Moilliet 1868: 110–11).

1754, I: iv), a matter that occupied James as well (James 1741: [ii]). Their answer is essentially Diderot's plan to cross-reference consistently, both to synonyms and to subjects and their subdivisions, in order to create systems. They thus see encyclopaedias as digesting and explaining the compass of human knowledge 'in the form of dictionaries' (s.v. *cyclopaedia*). Chambers's preface ends optimistically in justifying the dictionary as a 'farrago of arts', the cento that forms part of the dictionary, especially for the potential of each datum to spawn new systems: 'the least of 'em may possibly be the Foundation of a new System' (1728 Preface: xxix), but James does not envision or embrace this opportunity.

Both Chambers's and Keir's expansive and insightful theoretical commentaries put James's lack of a theoretical stance, despite the sheer ambition of his dictionary, into perspective. Although utilising a structure apparently like that of Chambers, James gives little thought to the more general principles, concentrating simply on the details of what should be included in his entries and the value of the work. His dictionary nevertheless sufficiently exemplified the enlightenment reference work to induce Diderot to have it translated and published by 1746–1748, but it seems so almost inadvertently, more for its mass than for its adherence to encyclopaedic principles. James has both bloated his systemic entries and overstuffed the dictionary with the intervening ones in the interests of comprehensiveness. Both Chambers and Keir are much more enlightening and 'enlightened', whereas James, far from being an 'analyst' *pace* Chambers, has produced a work of superogation, more cento than system. Keir, caught out by rapid paradigmatic change, found himself stranded, whereas Chambers coped by being fortunate enough to come in the wake of the Newtonian revolution.

REFERENCES

Anderson, Wilda. 1984. *Between the library and the laboratory: The language of chemistry in eighteenth-century France*. Baltimore; London: Johns Hopkins University Press.

Black, Joseph (1756) Experiments upon Magnesia alba, Quicklime, and some other Alcaline Substances. In *Essays and observations, physical and literary. Read before a society in Edinburgh, and published by them*, vol. 2, 157–225.

Blancard, Steven. 1684. *A physical dictionary*. London: J. D.

Bocast, Alexander K. 2016. Definition in Chambers's *Cyclopaedia*: Chambers on definition. Enlightenment Views of Definition 1.1. McLean, VA: Berkeley Bridge Press.

Brock, W. H. 2008. Joseph Priestley, enlightened experimentalist. In Isabel Rivers & David L. Wykes (eds.), *Joseph Priestley, scientist, philosopher, and theologian*, 49–79. Oxford: Oxford University Press.

Chambers, Ephraim. 1728. *Cyclopaedia: or, an universal dictionary of arts and sciences*. London: for James and John Knapton et al.

Chambers, Ephraim. 1738. *Cyclopaedia: or, an universal dictionary of arts and sciences*. London: for James and John Knapton et al.

Crosland, Maurice. 2000. Slippery substances: Some practical and conceptual problems in the understanding of gases in the pre-Lavoisier era. In Frederic L. Holmes & Trevor H. Levere (eds.), *Instruments and experimentation in the history of chemistry*, 79–104. Cambridge, MA: MIT Press.

Diderot, Denis. n.d. *The encyclopedia of Diderot & D'Alambert*. n.p.: Michigan Publishing. http://quod.lib.umich.edu/d/did/index.html (accessed 27 May 2021).

Erasmus, Desiderius. 1512. *De Utraque verborum ac rerum copia* [UT *De copia*]. Paris: Josse Bade.

Harris, John. 1704. *Lexicon technicum*. London: for Daniel Brown et al.

Hoffman, Frederick, & Bernado Ramazzini. 1746. *A dissertation on endemial diseases [. . .] and the diseases of tradesman*. Trans. Dr. James. London: for Thomas Osborne.

James, Robert. [1741]. *Proposals for printing A medicinal dictionary*. [London]: Society of Booksellers for Promoting Learning.

James, R[obert]. 1743–1745. *A medicinal dictionary; including physic, surgery, anatomy, chymistry, and botany, in all their branches relative to medicine. Together with a history of drugs [. . .] With copper plates*, 3 vols. London: for T. Osborne.

Johnson, William. 1652. *Lexicon chymicum: Cum obscuriorum verborum, et rerum hermeticarum, tum phrasium Paracelsicarum inscriptis ejus*. London: William Nealand.

Keir, James. 1789. *The first part of a dictionary of chemistry, &c*. Birmingham: for Elliot and Kay.

Kennedy, Krista. 2016. *Textual curation: Authorship, agency, and technology in* Wikipedia *and Chambers's* Cyclopædia. Columbia: University of South Carolina Press.

King-Hele, Desmond. 1977. *Doctor of revolution: The life and genius of Erasmus Darwin*. London: Faber and Faber.

Lancashire, Ian. 2002. 'Dumb significants' and early modern English definition. In Jens Brockmeier, Min Wang, & David R. Olson (eds.), *Literacy, narrative and culture*, 131–54. London; New York: Routledge.

Lonati, Elisabetta. 2017. *Communicating medicine: British medical discourse in eighteenth-century reference works*. Milan: Ledizioni.

Macquer, P.-J. 1766. *Dictionnaire de chemie*. Paris: Lacombe.

Macquer, Pierre Joseph. 1771. *Dictionnaire de chymie. A dictionary of chemistry. Containing the theory and practice of that science*, 2 vols. London: for T. Cadell, and P. Elmsly; J. Robson.

Macquer, Pierre Joseph. 1777. *A dictionary of chemistry*. London: for T. Cadell, and P. Elmsly.

McConchie, Roderick. 2019. *Discovery in haste: English medical dictionaries and lexicographers 1547 to 1796*. Lexicographica Series Maior 156. Berlin: De Gruyter.

Moilliet, A. 1868. *Sketch of the life of James Keir, Esq., F.R.S.: With a selection from his correspondence*. London: R. E. Taylor.

Nicholson, William. 1795. *A dictionary of chemistry, exhibiting the present state of the theory and practice of that science, its application to natural philosophy, the processes of manufactures, metallurgy, and numerous other arts dependant on the properties and habitudes of bodies, in the mineral, vegetable, and animal kingdoms*. London: G. G. and J. Robinson.

Priestland, Neal. 1990. *Erasmus Darwin: Philosopher, scientist, physician and poet*. Nottingham: Ashbracken.

Priestley, Joseph. 1762. *A course of lectures on the theory of language, and universal grammar*. Warrington: W. Eyres.

Quincy, John. 1719. *Lexicon medico-physicum*. London: Andrew Bell et al.

Schofield, Robert E. 1963. *The Lunar Society of Birmingham: A social history of provincial science and industry in eighteenth-century England*. Oxford: Clarendon Press.

Smeaton, William A. 2000. Platinum and ground glass: Some innovations in chemical apparatus by Guyton de Morveau and others. In Frederic L. Holmes & Trevor H. Levere (eds.), *Instruments and experimentation in the history of chemistry*, 211–37. Cambridge, MA: MIT Press.

Smith, Barbara M. D., & J. L. Moilliet. 1967. James Keir of the Lunar Society. *Notes and Records of the Royal Society of London* 22: 144–54.

Society of Gentlemen. 1754. *A new and complete dictionary of arts and sciences*, 4 vols. London: for W. Owen.

Trotter, Thomas.1797–1803. *Medicina Nautica; An essay on the diseases of seamen*. 3 vols. London: T. Cadell et al.

Woodcock, Leslie V. 2005. Phlogiston theory and chemical revolutions. *Bulletin for the History of Chemistry* 30(2): 63–9.

Wright, Alexander, & R. W. McConchie. In press. *A medicinal dictionary* (1743–45) by Robert James: an Enlightenment reference work. In Jeff Loveland & Stéphane Schmitt (eds.), *Specialized dictionaries and encyclopedias, 1650–1800: A tribute to Frank Kafker*. Oxford Studies in the Enlightenment. London: Liverpool University Press for the Voltaire Foundation for Enlightenment Studies.

CHAPTER 9

Medical Vocabulary in English Romantic Literature

Jeremy J. Smith

9.1 Romantic Medicine

The importance of medical thinking in Romantic poetry is now a commonplace of literary-critical discourse (see e.g. Vickers 2004, or the essays in Roe 2017). However, its presence is sometimes disguised for present-day readers since medical language – like all forms of living language – is subject to change; the 'scientific currency' (de Almeida 1991: 13) of the early nineteenth century differs from our own. As a result, many words that are no longer considered to be primarily medical in denotation or connotation had quite specific medical meanings for Enlightenment and Romantic writers.

New resources have led to new insights into the history of English medical vocabulary. The completion of the *Historical Thesaurus of English* (HTE, https://ht.ac.uk, 2nd ed., 2020), for instance, linked to the ongoing revision of the *Oxford English Dictionary* (OED) and its location online, has enabled the reconstruction of the medical lexicons for particular periods of the history of the language.[1] We are increasingly aware moreover of the importance of the OED not just as a source for the lexicon, but also as an extensive repository of citations, allowing for the enhanced study of intertextuality. In addition, the appearance of large machine-readable corpora has made it possible to contextualise particular idiolectal usages much more comprehensively than was possible until recently, and thus draw robustly evidenced conclusions. Such developments have allowed the better understanding of what might be called authorial invention. That is

I am most grateful to Rod McConchie, Irma Taavitsainen, and two anonymous reviewers for their valuable comments on an earlier version of this chapter, originally delivered as a paper at the Helsinki CHIMED-2 (the second International Conference on Historical Medical Discourse), June 2019. Any remaining flaws are my own responsibility.

[1] See e.g. Smith (2006) for an early harnessing of HTE materials, including a preliminary account of Keats's usage, discussed below.

the focus of the current chapter, which is intended as part of a longer-term project on specialised vocabularies in the history of English.

Imaginative writers do not make their own language; rather, they harness, creatively, the linguistic forms that they encounter in the spoken or written modes of their own times, a process that is basic to the notion of style. Had they lived at other times, they would have expressed themselves in different ways. To use a term that would have been familiar to medieval or early modern readers, they practise *inventio*. According to classical and medieval rhetoricians *inventio* meant 'finding something', distinct from the modern understanding of 'invention', that is, 'creating something new'. *Inventio*, then, the primary activity involved in literary creation, was essentially about discovery. Once the 'matter' was determined through *inventio*, 'poetic art' – in the words of the medieval rhetorician Geoffrey de Vinsauf, Chaucer's 'Gaufred, deere maister soverayn' – 'came forward to clothe the matter with words' in an appropriate manner.[2]

In what follows, *invention* will be examined in texts by three English Romantic writers who were all closely engaged with contemporary scientific (and specifically medical) thinking. They are Samuel Taylor Coleridge (1772–1834), representing the 'first generation' traditionally identified, and John Keats (1795–1821) and Mary Wollstonecraft Shelley (1797–1851), representing the second. Their usages will be compared to that of one of the most significant and influential medical practitioners of the period, William Cullen (1710–1790), whose substantial correspondence has recently become accessible for large-scale searching and analysis, and whose impact, both direct and indirect, can be traced in the outputs of all three writers, offering further insights into their creative – and inventive – practice.

9.2 *Panting* in the Verse of Samuel Taylor Coleridge

Coleridge, like all the Romantics, was intensely interested in his own personal formation and development, and his writings reveal a great deal about his health. The first volume of Richard Holmes's authoritative biography (1989) lists in the index a string of ailments ranging from rheumatic fever through neuralgia, problems with his teeth, influenza,

[2] Reflecting widespread views in antiquity on the subject, the nineteen-year-old Cicero composed *De inventione*, defining the notion as 'the discovery of valid or seemingly valid arguments that render one's thoughts plausible', and this discovery of arguments was to be extended to the broader notion of 'materials'. It is *inventio* to which Thomas Hoccleve was referring when he called Geoffrey Chaucer 'The firste fyndere of our faire langage' (*Regement of Princes*, c. 1412, line 4978).

and gout. In later life, of course, his opium addiction, acquired initially as a medical response to eye infections that gave him insomnia, was notorious. The second volume (1998) of Holmes's biography famously opens with Coleridge, en route to Malta, being given an enema – which Coleridge himself recorded in somewhat gory detail – to address the severe constipation his addiction had caused. His family were also afflicted by illness: his father died young, of a heart attack, as did his sister, of consumption, and his brother Luke – who was training as a doctor at London Hospital – died of 'a fever' (Holmes 1989: 38). Poetry famously became for Coleridge associated 'with sickness, feverish dreams, and isolation, set against the consoling, healing presence of the beloved' (Holmes 1989: 38). More positively, Coleridge was from early in his career profoundly interested in medicine as a scientific discipline, having attended lectures on physiology during his sojourn in Germany in 1798–1799, and assisting his own medical adviser, James Gillman, in writing *An Essay on Scrofula*, to be submitted for the Royal College of Surgeons' Jacksonian Prize in 1816 (Holmes 1998: 432). The material Coleridge developed for the *Essay* prefigured his later metaphysical thinking on biological evolution, *The Theory of Life* (see Jackson 1977).

It is unsurprising therefore that there are many places in Coleridge's verse where we can detect a medical presence, albeit at times somewhat hidden. In 1797, Coleridge wrote one of his best-known poems, inspired it seems by having taken 'two grains of Opium [. . .] to check a dysentery' while on a walking tour in Somerset. Famously the poem is unfinished, the poet having been – as he tells us in his preface (Coleridge 1967: 295–6) – 'unfortunately called out by a person on business from Porlock', causing the rest of the poem to have 'passed away like the images on the surface of a stream into which a stone has been cast, but alas! without the after restoration of the latter!', a trope of interruption that was later to influence writers as different as Sir Arthur Conan Doyle and Stevie Smith (White 2006–2007). Coleridge was to publish the fragment many years later, in 1816, as what he called – intriguingly – a 'psychological curiosity'. This poem was the celebrated *Kubla Khan*, which contains the following lines:

(1) But oh! that deep romantic chasm which slanted
Down the green hill athwart a cedarn cover!
A savage place! as holy and enchanted
As e'er beneath a waning moon was haunted
By woman wailing for her demon-lover!
And from this chasm, with ceaseless turmoil seething,

As if this earth in fast thick pants were breathing,
A mighty fountain momently was forced: [. . .] (Coleridge 1967: 297, lines 12–19)

The passage is usually interpreted as drawing on Coleridge's observation of the scenery in the Quantock Hills in Somerset, transmuted by his imagination. But there is also something more, suggested by citations in the OED from the verse of another Romantic poet, Percy Bysshe Shelley:[3]

(2) 1819 SHELLEY *Cenci* II. ii. 34 Her very name, But spoken by a stranger, makes my heart Sicken and **pant**.
1820 SHELLEY *Prometheus Unbound* III. iii. 109 My spirit Was **panted** forth in anguish whilst thy pain Made my heart mad. (OED s.v. *pant*)

These citations from *The Cenci* and *Prometheus Unbound* explicitly link the word *pant* with poor health (*sicken*, *pain*), and there is some evidence that *pant* – hitherto found primarily in literary works with a more general set of meanings – had been developing a specifically medical connotation from the later eighteenth century onwards. This evidence is supplied by a recently released corpus of medical correspondence; it is to that corpus that we will now turn.

9.3 *Panting* in Enlightenment Medical Discourse

William Cullen (1710–1790) was a major and hugely influential figure in the later Scottish Enlightenment. A friend of Joseph Black, William Hunter, and Adam Smith, he held professorships first at Glasgow and subsequently at Edinburgh. However, he continued to practise medicine, and in that role he undertook the usual custom of receiving consultations and then responding. In accordance with contemporary practice, this process was undertaken by letter, both to and from the doctor, and by good fortune a vast archive of these materials survives. An electronic corpus, derived from the archives of the Royal College of Physicians in Edinburgh and of the University of Glasgow, has been published online as *The Consultation Letters of Dr Cullen* (www.cullenproject.ac.uk).

The following letter from 1782, citing a patient's 'distressful pantings', was written to Cullen by a close colleague and friend, Alexander

[3] Emboldening has been added here and elsewhere to flag the form under discussion in citations.

Stevenson, Professor of the Theory and Practice of Medicine at Glasgow from 1766 and a fellow member of Edinburgh's elite Select Society:

(3) I have visited a patient of yours Mr Neilson. I am afraid his fate is fixed, but am not sure how near. You have his late history, as well as the former part, from Mr Taylor. I found him in that bent posture so usual to those who have an Effusion in the Thorax : at times having sudden & distressful **pantings** - & now & then ritchings to Vomit. I observed a reddish tinge in that which He Coughed up. His Pulse not so quick as might be expected, but the stroke hard. Mr Taylor said it had been much more so & that you had suspected Aneurism. I found the stroke of the temporal Arteries soft & small, those of the Wrist & foot hard & [corded?]. (Stevenson 1782 at www.cullenproject.ac.uk)

Pant and *panting* are terms regularly deployed by Dr Cullen's correspondents, even if not by the good doctor himself. Here is an excerpt from a letter from a Dr James Robertson, dated to 1789:

(4) Mrs. Fraser has had no return of the complaint alluded to, & during the Northern Jubilee held at Inverness she was able to go thro' a weeks fatigue in attending it; When I last wrote you, tho' she at that time complained of no pectoral uneasiness, yet I should have mentioned that she often ailed with in the course of the Spring & Summer before her attack in August; she often used to complain of uneasiness in the chest, arising from a sense of tightness across it; this was attended with some Dyspnœa; to me it seemed rather a kind of nervous **panting**, than arising from any inflammatory tendency of the lungs; [. . .]. (Robertson 1789 at www.cullenproject.ac.uk)

The expression 'nervous panting' is here notable; Cullen was famously on record as stating that '[i]n a certain view, almost the whole of the diseases of the human body might be called NERVOUS' (1827–1828, 2:330), and Robertson seems to have been reflecting this view. Cullen took a holistic view of physiology, connecting his thinking to wider cultural concerns, as flagged by William Bynum: 'Cullen's doctrine of the nervous system was central to his more general beliefs about culture, civilization, improvement, and sensibility' (Bynum 2004b). It seems that 'nervous panting' was being used by Robertson in a technical sense with which he expected Cullen to be familiar.

The medical views of Cullen and his circle were well known to Coleridge. He seems to have encountered them through his close friendship with the distinguished physician Thomas Beddoes (1760–1808), who had been taught at Edinburgh by Cullen's friend Joseph Black (see Vickers 2004: 80–5; see also Vickers 1997). It seems at least possible therefore that Coleridge's lines from *Kubla Khan* are worth revisiting in the light of their medical connotations:

(5) As if this earth in fast thick **pants** were breathing,
A mighty fountain momently was forced: [. . .] (Coleridge 1967: 297, lines 18–19)

The traditional gloss for this image – encouraged by the rise of criticism informed by psychoanalysis – is male ejaculation (see e.g. Logan 1985 and references there cited, especially Bliss and Bliss 1949), but an alternative interpretation is possible. It can be plausibly argued that the earth is clearly struggling for breath, and the mighty fountain is envisaged as a vomiting forth – or as Cullen's correspondent (Stevenson 1782 in www.cullenproject.ac.uk) might have termed it, 'ritchings to Vomit'. The earth is, in such a view, sick, an interpretation aligning with recent 'ecocritical' approaches to literary works from the Romantic period (see famously Bate 1991; for a recent survey, see Rigby 2014). Indeed, it was suggested some time ago – by a critic inspired by a distinct psychoanalytic approach – that there was a link between the explosive force described and Coleridge's unfortunate enema already flagged (Sloane 1972). It might be suggested that the association of *panting* with illness could align with such an interpretation.

9.4 Mary Wollstonecraft Shelley's *Frankenstein; or The Modern Prometheus*

We are on firmer ground with the second text discussed here: Mary Wollstonecraft Shelley's *Frankenstein; or The Modern Prometheus* (1818). The story of the writing of *Frankenstein* is almost as celebrated as the narrative it contains. It is famously the product of competitive ghost-story writing, at Lord Byron's suggestion, during a stormy summer night in 1816, in the Villa Diodati near Lake Geneva in Switzerland. Two seminal Romantic works arose from that event: *The Vampyre* by Byron's personal physician Dr John Polidori (1795–1821), later to inspire Bram Stoker, and *Frankenstein* itself. Polidori's discussions of physiology – as Nigel Leask points out, his doctoral thesis was on somnambulism (Leask 2004) – seem to have influenced Mary, though the imaginative creation was undoubtedly her own, drawing on her attendance, at the age of fourteen, at one of the famous Royal Institution lectures delivered by Humphry Davy (1778–1829). Mary went on to read, precociously, Davy's 'Introductory Discourse', in which he spoke of how in the future man would 'interrogate Nature with Power [. . .] as a master, active, with his own instruments' (cited in Holmes 2009: 326).

Mary Shelley was, remarkably, only eighteen when she composed *Frankenstein*. Her achievement was for some time occluded, overshadowed because of her relationship with Percy Bysshe Shelley, the poet. In recent years, however, the originality and significance of her writings have been given appropriate and independent recognition. In many ways she comes across as a much more sympathetic and attractive figure than her husband. She was brought up by her father, the philosopher William Godwin. Her mother Mary Wollstonecraft, the leading feminist political writer of her generation, had died of puerperal fever a few days after her daughter's birth. Godwin's circle included many of the most prominent thinkers and scientists of the period, and Mary was 'well read and painstakingly educated in the radical tradition' by her father (Holmes 1995: 170). She had attended Coleridge's lectures in 1811, delivered to the newly founded Philosophical Institution. Tickets for these lectures were sold at Godwin's bookshop, among other venues (Holmes 1998: 265).

Mary continued her learning habits into later life, after her elopement with Percy Bysshe Shelley in 1814, and while in Geneva seems in this way to have encountered what she herself described as 'the physiological writers of Germany' (Shelley 1818; see below). Holmes considers that Dr Frankenstein was modelled at least in part on Johann Wilhelm Ritter (1776–1810), originally of Jena and later of Munich, where he is alleged to have attempted to revive dead animals – and even humans – by means of 'electrical action' (2009: 329). Ritter died, insane, at the age of thirty-three.

Mary was also influenced, directly or indirectly, by Erasmus Darwin (1731–1802), and through him by Cullen. Mary explicitly cited Darwin in the preface to the second edition of *Frankenstein*:

(6) [Byron and Shelley] talked of the experiments of Dr. Darwin, (I speak not of what the Doctor really did, or said that he did, but, as more to my purpose, of what was then spoken of as having been done by him,) who preserved a piece of vermicelli in a glass case, till by some extraordinary means it began to move with voluntary motion [. . .]. (Shelley 1831: ix–x)

The last year of Darwin's study at Edinburgh (1753–1756) coincided with Cullen's appointment to a chair at that university. The second volume of his *Zoonomia* (1794), on nosology (i.e. classification of diseases), drew extensively on Cullen's work, although modified by Darwin's engagement with the 'Brunonian' theories of the radical Edinburgh physician John Brown (1735–1788). Brown had also influenced (albeit with severe reservations) Beddoes's – and subsequently Coleridge's – thinking.

9.4.1 *Medical Uses of Passion in Shelley's* Frankenstein

This engagement with current scientific – and specifically medical – thinking may be illustrated from Mary Shelley's use of the word *passion*, which occurs no fewer than fifteen times in *Frankenstein* (see Figure 13 in the Image Gallery). For instance, Mary used the word in the prefatory remarks she placed at the very beginning of the first edition, flagging its centrality to the themes of the book:

(7) The event on which this fiction is founded has been supposed, by Dr. Darwin, and some of the physiological writers of Germany, as not of impossible occurrence. I shall not be supposed as according the remotest degree of serious faith to such an imagination; yet, in assuming it as the basis of a work of fancy, I have not considered myself as merely weaving a series of supernatural terrors. The event on which the interest of the story depends is exempt from the disadvantages of a mere tale of spectres or enchantment. It was recommended by the novelty of the situations which it developes; and, however impossible as a physical fact, affords a point of view to the imagination for the delineating of human **passions** more comprehensive and commanding than any which the ordinary relations of existing events can yield. I have thus endeavoured to preserve the truth of the elementary principles of human nature, while I have not scrupled to innovate upon their combinations. (Shelley 1818: 2)

Mary seems to have used the word *passion* with some quite precise meanings, and in this context the OED's citations are illuminating. The earliest citations, from the Middle and Early Modern English periods, are focused on physical sensation, for example:

(8) *a*1398 J. TREVISA tr. Bartholomaeus Anglicus *De Proprietatibus Rerum* (BL Add.) f.316 Mete..bredeþ þe **passiouns**, colica passio & Iliaca passio.

1547 A. BORDE *Breuiary of Helthe* I. f. xxxix In latyn it is named Ventralis passio. In englyshe..the bely ache or a **passion** in the bely.
1563 T. GALE *Certaine Wks. Chirurg.* IV. II. f. 28ᵛ It is of ryght good effecte in the **passions** of the ioyntes.
1624 W. LAUD *Diary* 7 Aug. in *Hist. Troubles* (1695) 13 My **passion** by Blood, and my fear of a Stone in my Bladder.
1684 tr. T. Bonet *Guide Pract. Physician* XVI. 566 Thirst is a **Passion** of the Mouth of the Stomach. (OED s.v. *passion*)

Later citations, however, seem to focus rather on mental states, for instance:

(9) 1710 J. NORRIS *Treat. Christian Prudence* vii. 323 By the **Passions** I think we are to understand certain Motions of the Mind depending upon and accompanied with an Agitation of the Spirits.
1733 POPE *Of Use of Riches* 9 The ruling **Passion** conquers Reason still.
1791 A. RADCLIFFE *Romance of Forest* I. i. 4 A man whose **passions** often overcame his reason.
1797 *Encycl. Brit.* XIV. 2/1 The common division of the **passions** into *desire* and *aversion, hope* and *fear, joy* and *grief, love* and *hatred*, has been mentioned by every author who has treated of them. (OED s.v. *passion*)

The deployment of 'passions' in Anne Radcliffe's *Romance of the Forest*, a highly influential 'Gothic' bestseller, is perhaps significant. Mary and Percy Shelley were certainly reading Radcliffe in 1814 (Holmes 1995: 274). The term was also widely deployed in other high-profile works with a similar meaning, for example in Joanna Baillie's *Plays of the Passions* (1798–1812), where, as Norma Clarke flags, 'often hidden psychological processes [gave] rise to passionate action' (Clarke 2004).

William Cullen's correspondence again offers numerous interesting parallel usages, demonstrating how medical terminology is at the heart of the word's later deployment by fictional writers (Baillie being the niece of the physicians John and William Hunter; William was, as indicated above, a friend of William Cullen, providing another possible link). Here is an incoming letter of 1755 responding to Cullen's request for advice, signed by a team led by Dr John Stevenson, father of Alexander. We might note the reference to 'passion of the mind':

(10) We have considered your patients case with all due attention, & as we are informed that her present indisposition was initially owing to

passion of the mind, we are of opinion that on that account chiefly the case has proved so obstinate, & the cure so difficult & uncertain, tho' we are not without hopes even of a thorough recovery. (Stevenson 1755 in www.cullenproject.ac.uk)

In this context, the significance of many of the occurrences of the word *passion* in *Frankenstein* becomes more salient. Here, for instance, is the narrator, Dr Frankenstein:

(11) Memory brought madness with it; and when I thought on what had passed, a real insanity possessed me; sometimes I was furious, and **burnt** with **rage**, sometimes low and despondent. I neither spoke nor looked, but sat motionless, bewildered by the multitude of miseries that overcame me. Elizabeth alone had the power to draw me from these fits; her **gentle** voice would soothe me when transported by **passion**, and inspire me when human feelings were sunk in torpor. She wept with me, and for me. When reason returned, she would remonstrate, and endeavour to inspire me with resignation [. . .]. (Shelley 1818: 219)

We might note in this passage not only *passion*, referring to the mental state in quite a precise way, but other words that seem to have developed a specifically medical meaning when Mary Shelley was writing, such as *rage* and *gentle*. Here are some relevant citations in the OED for *gentle*, sense 6d:

(12) Of a medicine: Acting without violence; mild.
1576 A. FLEMING tr. Hippocrates in *Panoplie Epist.* 289 I would therfore, that a stronger remedie be prepared: for this emplaster is too **gentle**.
1790 J. B. MORETON *Manners & Customs West India Islands* 25 If you find yourself costive, take a **gentle** purge.
1835 J. FORBES et al. *Cycl. Pract. Med.* IV. 587/2 By mild and frequently repeated doses of **gentle** aperients. (OED s.v. *gentle*)

It seems that Elizabeth's 'gentle voice' was undertaking a distinctly therapeutic function. Here are some similar citations for *rage*, sense 4b, defined by the OED as 'Madness, insanity; a fit or attack of madness. Now *archaic*'. The citation from Percy Shelley might be noted as a link to Mary's writing:

(13) 1700 J. DRYDEN *Chaucer's Palamon & Arcite*, in *Fables* 20 Museful Mopings, which presage The loss of Reason, and conclude in **Rage**.

1774 S. JOHNSON *Patriot* 21 By the howling violence of patriotic **rage**, the nation was for a time exasperated to such madness.
*a*1822 P. B. SHELLEY *Peter Bell III* VII, in *Poet. Wks.* (?1840) 246/1 To wakeful frenzy's vigil **rages**, As opiates, were the same applied.
1874 *Appleton's Jrnl.* 4 July 30 Saul, in the last paroxysm of royal **rage** and madness, slays himself. (OED s.v. *rage*)

The words *gentle* and *rage* both appear regularly in the Cullen correspondence. *Gentle* is very frequent, commonly in relation to purging (as in the 1790 OED citation). We may recall the 'gentle evacuations' recommended to John Stevenson in 1755, and here is another use of *gentle*, some twenty years later, in the following letter of advice to Lord Charles Cathcart (1776):

(14) I am sorry to find the appetite for dinner not so good as before, but Impute it to the milk which after repetition in such quantity is not so easily digested as at first and I am of opinion that your Lordship must either take a **gentle** vomit, if you vomit with any tolerable ease or if you do not you must diminish for some days the quantity of your milk and I think your noon and afternoon doses are the most fit to be omitted. (Cullen 1776 in www.cullenproject.ac.uk)

'Gentle vomit' seems from the frequency of its occurrence in the corpus to have been a favourite technical expression of Cullen's circle. As for *rage*, here is the unhappy Reverend Henry Elliot of Beadnell and Bamburgh in Northumberland, reporting to Cullen in 1778 how, despite a range of treatments, he is still suffering from the 'rage' of a 'wandering mind':

(15) [...] after all I applied to your prescription and pukes above mentioned, but still the heats, and all these doubts, & wanderings of the mind seem to **rage** as much as ever; [...]. (Elliot 1778 in www.cullenproject.ac.uk)

9.5 On *Burning*: Shelley's Creature and the Case of John Keats

Another word that is linked in *Frankenstein* to *passion* is *burning*. Here speaks Mary Shelley's Creature, who has been brought to life by means of the doctor's infernal craft:

(16) 'For some days I haunted the spot where these scenes had taken place; sometimes wishing to see you, sometimes resolved to quit the world

and its miseries for ever. At length I wandered towards these mountains, and have ranged through their immense recesses, consumed by a **burning passion** which you alone can gratify. We may not part until you have promised to comply with my requisition. I am alone, and miserable; man will not associate with me; but one as deformed and horrible as myself would not deny herself to me. My companion must be of the same species, and have the same defects. This being you must create.' (Shelley 1818: 158)

In both the cases of the unfortunate Reverend Elliot and the Creature, it is clear that the 'passion' is 'of the mind', but in this latter instance the 'passion' is *burning.*

The Cullen correspondence interestingly links *burning* with *rage*, as in this passage from an enquiry of 1783, concerning an unfortunate schoolmaster, Mr David Watson:

(17) The Conflict begins about the Neck of the Bladder where the Patient feels a severe **burning** Pain that passes along the Urethra & from that sometimes to the Glans. But the forcible strainings communicate to the neighbouring parts very violent pains which not only adds greatly to the Patients agony during the time of passing the Urine but continue to afflict him for a long time after. [. . .] The Pains will sometimes **rage** both in the Lumbar Region & in the Thighs at the same time but not in equal degree so that when very severe in one part they are less so in the other and they will sometimes seem to shift from the low parts of the Back to the Thighs & vice versa. (Cullen 1783 in www.cullenproject.ac.uk)

Burning here was evidently the result of gonorrhoea, and the term seems to have become used both for the effect of the disease and the disease itself; the connexion with tormented sexuality is one that may be relevant for Mary Shelley's Creature as well. The OED defines the term as 'Heat attendant upon disease or a serpent's bite; the disease itself; *esp.* erysipelas or St. Anthony's fire, and venereal disease', and offers several relevant citations from the late medieval period to the middle of the nineteenth century, for example:

(18) 1728 E. CHAMBERS *Cycl.* **Burning**,..an infectious Disease, got in the Stews.
1753 *Chambers's Cycl.* Suppl. **Burning** is more particularly used for.. erysipelas.
1860 R. G. MAYNE *Expos. Lexicon Med. Sci.* **Burning**, an old English name for Gonorrhœa. (OED s.v. *burning*)

The medical denotation of *burning* seems therefore to be established, and in this instance the final figure under review, John Keats (1795–1821), is relevant, both for his deployment of the word in his poetry and also his personal experience, as a professional medical practitioner and as a sufferer from that unfortunate condition.

Keats is best known to present-day readers now as a poet, but by professional training he was an 'apothecary', a medically trained practitioner who had studied at one of the premier London teaching hospitals of the period, Guy's, under a leading surgeon, Astley Cooper (1768–1841). Cooper had himself studied not only at another major institution, St Thomas's, but also in Edinburgh, where, as William Bynum describes, he had attended Cullen's lectures (Bynum 2004a). Cullen's medical taxonomy was a standard part of Keats's curriculum (Curran 2017: 1709). And this fact has implications for his poetry, since, as Robert Gittings put it many years ago,

> [Keats] could, and did, transmute almost any experience into poetry [...] This is why no part of Keats's life should be neglected, and every incident, once truly recorded, may have immense value in interpreting his poetry. (Gittings 1968: 627–8)

Indeed, there is good evidence that Keats saw his poetry as not distinct from his medical practice, something that contemporaries understood and has been emphasised by recent research, ranging from Hermione de Almeida's foundational *Romantic medicine and John Keats* (1991) through Nicholas Roe's recent important edited collection *John Keats and the medical imagination* (2017). Cooper and his associates always emphasised that 'the practitioner of "first rank" must know "more than Medicine"' (de Almeida 1991: 36), and this axiom seems to have underpinned Keats's thinking:

> While we read his work and notice its consoling luxuries, its healthy and unhealthy airs, its medicinal flowers, its systems of nervous sensibilities, its working brains, its ethereal flights, its emphasis on 'sensation', its fluctuating temperatures, its marvellous chemical transformations, and its restorative sleeps, we realise that these things are not just incidental details, but the components of a selfless and moral imagination [...]. (Motion 1997: 131)

Medical situations are found, for instance, throughout Keats's first major poem, *Endymion*. Sporadic metaphors and similes hint at a medical context, such as 'nature's lives and wonders pulsed tenfold' (Barnard 1988: book I, line 105); Peona, Endymion's sister and confidante, has healing powers 'like some midnight spirit-nurse' (book I, line 413), which allow Endymion's 'brain' to become 'healthier' (book I, line 465); 'atomies' 'buzz about our slumbers, like brain-flies,/Leaving us fancy-sick' (book I, lines 851–3; see also 'brain-sick', book II, line 43). The speech of the aged Glaucus in book III plays with images of mortality ('remorseless as an infant's bier', book III, line 520), describing Circe as a kind of anti-physician inflicting sickness: 'soon these limbs became/Gaunt, withered, sapless, feeble, cramped, and lame' (book III, lines 637–8). The subsequent resuscitation of the nymph Scylla clearly has a medical parallel. Furthermore, in a discussion of the poem in his letters Keats refers, perhaps significantly, to 'Pleasure's Thermometer' (cf. Barnard 1988: 567–8), demonstrating his engagement with cutting-edge science. However, it should be noted that medical use of the thermometer was not current in Keats's day, possibly because the instrument had not become appropriately refined for clinical use (Porter 1997: 344–6).

Keats uses the word *burning* a good deal in his poetry. In his posthumously published *The fall of Hyperion*, for instance, the word appears in the Dreamer's narrative as follows, with a generalised medical connotation:

(19) For by my **burning** brain I measured sure
Her silver seasons shedded on the night,
And every day by day methought I grew
More gaunt and ghostly. (cited from Barnard 1988: part I, lines 393–6)

Such usages correspond with the widespread use of *burning* in the Cullen correspondence, referring to a range of symptoms in various parts of the anatomy.[4]

However, Keats also seems to have used *burning* in a more specific sense, for personal reasons. As is now generally accepted by scholars, Keats suffered from gonorrhoea, contracted most probably during his visit to Oxford in 1817 (Gittings 1968: 236; Motion 1997: 196–7). Keats seems – in accordance with contemporary, entirely erroneous medical views on the

[4] The rarer technical term deployed by some other contemporary medical writers, viz. *adustion*, does not occur in the Cullen corpus. *Adustion* rarely occurs outside medical contexts, and a perhaps-significant humorous deployment of the related verb, clearly drawing on medical usage on the basis of the other terms used in the reference, is cited in OED from *Bubble and squeak: a gallimaufry of British beef with the chopp'd cabbage of Gallic philosophy and radical reform* by the satirical poet George Huddesford (d. 1809). Huddesford, interestingly, refers to a 'reeking hot' poet's brain:

(i) 1799 G. Huddesford *Bubble & Squeak* I. 55 Frícando of verse From brain of poet reeking hot, is Likely to parch the epiglottis Of patient readers, who neglect Red Lane adusted to humect. (OED s.v. *adustion*)

connexion between the diseases – to have been worried that an ulcerated throat (contracted during his visit to Scotland in the summer of 1818) may have been a sign that his gonorrhoea was developing into the much more serious disease of syphilis.

The reference to how Hyperion's 'ample palate' (cited from Barnard 1988: part II, line 32) tasted 'poisonous brass and metals sick' (Barnard 1988: part II, line 33) may be connected to this unhappy and humiliating experience. Contemporary medical opinion required, as a remedy for this condition, the sparing use of mercury (quicksilver), usually administered either by rubbing on the skin or in pill form. In 1780, for instance, Dr Cullen wrote to a certain Lachlan Campbell, with reference to a decently anonymous 'Mr —', as follows:

(20) He suspect [sic] relics of a venereal disorder, but his symptoms are slight & I think his suspicions groundless. But to quiet his mind give a course for two or three weeks of Corrosive sublimate with Decoction of Sarsaparilla & Mezereon avoiding letting the Mercury touch his mouth on account of the scorbutic taint there. Milk & vegetables diet. (Cullen 1780 in www.cullenproject.ac.uk)

'Corrosive sublimate' or mercuric chloride, the chemical compound of mercury and chlorine, was the notorious 'common blue pill' that, according to an OED citation from 1861, had 'literally bec[o]me a part of the national diet' (s.v. *blue pill* n.). Keats would have been able to self-prescribe, which he did, taking fairly heavy doses of mercury. However, the therapy had dangers, as Cullen flagged, in terms of inducing a general debility: thus the reference to 'scorbutic taint' – that is, scurvy, a diagnosis used rather generally in the eighteenth century. Combined with the hardships Keats underwent during a rain-soaked tour to the highlands and islands of Scotland, this dosage seems to have made him especially susceptible to catching tuberculosis from his brother Tom, a condition from which he eventually died (Gittings 1968: 343).

9.6 Keats on the *Sympathetic Touch*

Another term Cullen used in his letter to Campbell (1780) was *touch*: 'avoiding letting the Mercury **touch** his mouth'. *Touch* was one of Keats's favourite words, often cited by literary critics as linked to his 'tendency [. . .] to ally his other sensory images more closely with the sense of touch and consequently render them stronger and more concrete' (Bate 1945: 3). *Touch* occurs no fewer than twenty-one times in Keats's *Endymion*, and undoubtedly contributes to the perception that that poem is particularly concerned with sensuality. As the philosopher John Locke put it, *touch* is 'a sense spread over the whole body, tho' it be most eminently placed in the ends of the fingers' (*Elements of natural philosophy* xi.50; cited in the OED s.v. *touch* n.).

However, according to the OED citations, *touch* had primary and specific medical meanings during the eighteenth and nineteenth centuries. Several citations in the OED confirm Cullen's usage, flagging that the usage was long established and linked to mercury:

(21) 1569 R. ANDROSE tr. G. Ruscelli *4th Pt. Secretes Alexis of Piemont* II. 52 Take Plantine water and mixe it with oyle of Brimstone, and **touch** [It. *toccarai*] therwith the gummes.
1659 *Secrets Phioravante* II. xxix. 73 in tr. L. Fioravanti *Exact Coll. Exper. Physick & Chyrurg.* (new ed.) Ulcers that are caused of *Morbo Gallico*, if you will cure them, you must first remove the cause..and **touch** them with our *Castick*.[5]
1713 W. COCKBURN *Symptoms Gonorrhoea* v. 165 The Crystallin is to be **touched** with this Tincture Five Times, at most, after it is first humbled with sublimate or precipitate Mercury.
1793 T. BEDDOES *Observ. Nature & Cure Calculus* 142 Some persons whose skin is no sooner **touched** with quicksilver ointment than it is felt in the salivary glands.
1888 W. R. GOWERS *Man. Dis. Nerv. Syst.* II. IV. 326 The patient should be brought slightly..under its [*i.e.* mercury's] influence, so as just to '**touch** the gums', as the phrase is. (OED s.v. *touch* n.)

In medical parlance *touch* had further meanings, and the word was also associated with early gynaecology, for example:

(22) 1655 N. CULPEPER et al. tr. L. Rivière *Pract. Physick* XV. ii. 404 If a wise Midwife **touch** the inward Mouth of the Womb, it will not be so close shut as in women with Child, but rather hard, and contracted, and full of pain.
1734 E. HODY *Giffard's Cases Midwifry* lxxxi. 192 I thought it proper to **touch** her.

[5] *Morbus Gallicus*, 'the French disease', was syphilis. The expression was first used in Ulrich von Hutten's treatise *De morbo Gallico* (1519); von Hutten's portrait by Holbein the Younger is the first known representation of a sufferer from the disease (Riccomi & Giuffra 2018). Girolamo Fracastero's epic poem *Syphilis sive morbus gallicus* (1530) encouraged the usage.

*a*1763 W. SMELLIE *Treat. Midwifery* (1764) III. 424 Upon touching I found the *Os Uteri* a little more dilated. (OED s.v. *touch* n.)

This last meaning of *touch* is especially relevant to Keats's usage in *Endymion*. In book I of the poem, Endymion, in conversation with his sister Peona, develops an argument about the human aspiration for the spiritual life:

(23) Behold
The clear religion of heaven! Fold
A rose leaf round thy finger's taperness,
And soothe thy lips; hist, when the airy stress
Of music's kiss impregnates the free winds,
And with a sympathetic **touch** unbinds
Aeolian magic from their lucid wombs;
Then old songs waken from enclouded tombs;
Old ditties sigh above their father's grave;
Ghosts of melodious prophesyings rave
Round every spot where trod Apollo's foot [. . .].
(cited from Barnard 1988: book I, lines 780–90)

The gynaecological reference point is obviously relevant to the image Keats is developing (cf. 'impregnates', 'wombs').

Further complexities may be distinguished in the use of *touch* in this passage. It seems that the phrase 'sympathetic touch' seems to have had a quite specific – and quite complex – meaning for Keats, the interpretation of which depends in part on understanding contemporary physiological language. 'Sympathetic' had both physiological/pathological and anatomical meanings, with two relevant definitions offered by the OED. The first, 'applied to a condition, action, or disorder induced in a person, or in an organ or part of the body, by a similar or corresponding one in another', is supported by citations such as the following:

(24) 1728 E. CHAMBERS *Cycl.* ***Sympathetic***, is particularly applied to all Diseases which have two Causes; the one remote, the other near. In which Sense, the Word is opposed to Idiopathetic.
1774 O. GOLDSMITH *Hist. Earth* III. 92 He had only to gape or yawn, and the professor instantly caught the **sympathetic** affection.
1804 J. ABERNETHY *Surg. Observ.* 22 Perhaps these vessels undergo a kind of **sympathetic** enlargement.
1849 H. M. NOAD *Lect. Electr.* (ed. 3) 486 The action of Electricity on the muscles and nerves produces two distinct kinds of contractions; the first, which he [*sc.* Marianini] calls *idiopathic*, are the result

> of the immediate action of the current on the muscles; and the second, which he calls ***sympathetic***, arise from the action of Electricity on the nerves which preside over the motions of the muscles. (OED s.v. *sympathetic*)

This usage is found in a note of 1780 within the Cullen materials, about a gentleman of sixty-nine simply referred to as 'A.B.':

(25) At present he is free of Acidity of stomach the **sympathetic** headache it usually occasiond, & as he says the flatulence, yet he has a pain of the left side which, very tolerable in any other position, won't suffer him to lie on it. (Cullen 1780 in www.cullenproject.ac.uk)

The second OED definition of *sympathetic* describes the term as 'designating one of the two great nerve-systems in vertebrates [. . .], consisting of a double chain of ganglia, with connecting fibres, along the vertebral column, giving off branches and plexuses which supply the viscera and blood-vessels and maintain relations between their various activities; belonging to or forming part of this system.' Citations include:

(26) 1771 J. JOHNSTONE in *Philos. Trans. 1770* (Royal Soc.) **60** 35 The intercostal, or as they are otherwise called, the great **sympathetic** nerves.
1830 R. KNOX tr. P. A. Béclard *Elements Gen. Anat.* 337 The particular action of the heart..is directly under the influence of the **sympathetic** nerve;..digestion, under the combined influence of the par vagum and **sympathetic** nerve. (OED s.v. *sympathetic*)

In the light of these definitions and citations of *sympathetic* and *touch*, the collocation of the two words in

(27) [. . .] when the airy stress
Of music's kiss impregnates the free winds,
And with a **sympathetic touch** unbinds
Aeolian magic from their lucid wombs; [. . .].
(cited from Barnard 1988: book I)

becomes explicable. For Keats, music has become the midwife, whereby human invention harnesses natural sounds.

This interpretation is supported by a contemporary meaning of *touch* recorded in the OED: 'The action or an act of touching a musical instrument, its strings, keys, etc., in order to produce music; the manner in which an instrument (esp. a keyboard instrument) is touched or handled so as to produce particular tones or effects' (OED s.v. *touch*). Relevant OED citations include for the noun:

(28) 1673 J. MILTON *At Vacation Exercise* in *Poems* (new ed.) 65 Listening to what unshorn Apollo sings To th' **touch** of golden wires.
1828 W. SCOTT *Fair Maid of Perth* x, in *Chron. Canongate* 2nd Ser. I. 264 I hear no unpleasing **touch** of minstrelsy.
1879 A. J. HIPKINS in G. Grove *Dict. Music* I. 647 A sensitive instrument of **touch**, instead of one of mere percussion. (OED s.v. *touch*)

For the verb:

(29) 1580 J. LYLY *Euphues & his Eng.* (new ed.) f. 130 Instruments sound sweetest, when they be **touched** softest.
*a*1640 P. MASSINGER *Guardian* II. iv. 60 in *3 New Playes* (1655) I'll **touch** my horn (Severino blows his horn), they know my call.
1697 J. DRYDEN *Alexander's Feast* ii. 2 Timotheus..With flying Fingers **touch'd** the Lyre.
1779 *Mirror* No. 43. □6 The organ was **touched** with a hand less firm.
1799 E. S. GOOCH *Fancied Events* I. i. 9 She sat down at some distance, and again **touched** the strings of her lute.
1827 J. BARRINGTON *Personal Sketches Own Times* II. 164 I recollect Moore..one night..**touching** the piano-forte, in his own unique way.
1888 J. W. BURGON *Lives Twelve Good Men* II. ix. 214 Having **touched** the piano, [he] was requested to sing. (OED s.v. *touch*)

Keats himself collocates *touch* and *sound* in

(30) [. . .] or ye, whose precious charge
Nibble their fill at ocean's very marge,
Whose mellow reeds are **touched** with **sounds** forlorn
By the dim echoes of old Triton's horn.
(cited from Barnard 1988: book I, lines 203–6)

The link also accounts for yet further elements in the passage under analysis, as when 'the airy stress [. . .] with a sympathetic touch'

(31) [. . .] unbinds
Aeolian magic from their lucid wombs;
Then old songs waken from enclouded tombs;
Old ditties sigh above their father's grave;

Ghosts of melodious prophesyings rave
Round every spot where trod Apollo's foot [. . .].
(cited from Barnard 1988: book I, lines 785–90)

The culminating reference to Apollo – the god of music, as well as of poetry and medicine – is surely significant.

9.7 Romantic Invention

The reference to an Aeolian harp is a characteristically Romantic gesture, which Keats had already used in his early *Ode to Apollo* of 1815 (see also, for instance, Coleridge's *Effusion XXXV: The Eolian harp* and *Dejection: an ode*). Aeolian harps are string instruments designed to be played by the wind, Aeolus being the relevant Greek god. It is surely also significant that the Aeolian harp functioned as a model for the operation of the human nervous system in the eighteenth and early nineteenth centuries.[6]

Such examples demonstrate Keats's astonishing ability to harness polysemy in complex ways. They also demonstrate a traditional artistic activity, as flagged at the beginning of this chapter: *inventio*. A parallel may be drawn with 'found art', as demonstrated for example by Picasso's famous – notorious? – linking of a bicycle saddle and handlebars to create a bull's head. Coleridge, Mary Shelley, and Keats are all drawing on available materials to deliver remarkable creative outcomes.

But what perhaps comes across more strongly in all the literary case studies discussed in this chapter is something rather strikingly of the period: they are all profoundly impacted by medical practice, but on Romantic terms. Until comparatively recently, Romanticism was seen as hostile to science, 'its ideal of subjectivity eternally opposed to that of scientific objectivity' (Holmes 2009: xvi). Examples like those cited here demonstrate that such a view is, as Richard Holmes has eloquently argued, simplistic: Romanticism drew profoundly on its scientific inheritance, but transformed this inheritance through 'imaginative intensity' (2009: xvi). The result was a breaking-down – through shared 'wonder' – of the boundary between sciences and the humanities, developing a holistic conception of the body and the psyche in a way that, at the beginning of the twenty-first century, we are only gradually rediscovering. Analyses of the kind presented here, drawing on both established resources such as the OED and new electronic corpora, are increasingly confirming the correctness of Holmes's claim.

6 See further Trower (2009) for a fascinating discussion.

REFERENCES

de Almeida, Hermione. 1991. *Romantic medicine and John Keats*. New York: Oxford University Press.

Barnard, John (ed.). 1988. *John Keats: The poems*, 3rd ed. Harmondsworth: Penguin.

Bate, Jonathan. 1991. *Romantic ecology: Wordsworth and the environmental tradition*. London: Routledge.

Bate, Walter. 1945. *The stylistic development of Keats*. New York: Modern Language Association of America.

Bliss, Hilde, & Donald Bliss. 1949. Coleridge's *Kubla Khan*. *American Imago* 6: 261–73.

Bynum, W. F. 2004a. Cooper, Sir Astley Paston, first baronet (1768–1841), surgeon. *Oxford Dictionary of National Biography*. https://doi.org/10.1093/ref:odnb/6211.

Bynum, W. F. 2004b. Cullen, William (1710–1790), chemist and physician. *Oxford Dictionary of National Biography*. https://doi.org/10.1093/ref:odnb/6874.

Clarke, Norma. 2004. Baillie, Joanna (1762–1851), playwright and poet. *Oxford Dictionary of National Biography*. https://doi.org/10.1093/ref:odnb/1062.

Coleridge, Ernest (ed.). 1967. *Coleridge: Poetical works*. Oxford: Oxford University Press.

Cullen, William. 1827–1828. *The Works of William Cullen*, ed. John Thomson (Edinburgh: Blackwood).

Curran, Stuart. 2017. 'The Feel of Not to Feel It': The life of non-sensation in Keats. In Nicholas Roe (ed.), *John Keats and the medical imagination*, 153–72. Basingstoke: Palgrave.

Gittings, Robert. 1968. *John Keats*. Harmondsworth: Penguin.

Holmes, Richard. 1989. *Coleridge: Early visions*. London: HarperCollins.

Holmes, Richard. 1995. *Shelley: The pursuit*, 2nd ed. London: HarperCollins.

Holmes, Richard. 1998. *Coleridge: Darker reflections*. London: HarperCollins.

Holmes, Richard. 2009. *The age of wonder*. London: HarperCollins.

Jackson, H. J. 1977. Coleridge on the King's Evil. *Studies in Romanticism* 16: 337–47.

Leask, Nigel. 2004. Polidori, John William (1795–1821), physician and writer. *Oxford Dictionary of National Biography*. https://doi.org/10.1093/ref:odnb/22466.

Logan, Richard. 1985. From Eros to Thanatos: Condensation and repetition compulsion in Coleridge's *Kubla Khan*. *Psychoanalytic Review* 72: 657–63.

Motion, Andrew. 1997. *John Keats*. London: Faber.

Porter, Roy. 1997. *The greatest benefit to mankind: A medical history of humanity from antiquity to the present*. London: HarperCollins.

Riccomi, Giulia, & Valentina Giuffra. 2018. First portrait of a syphilitic patient: Ulrich von Hutten. *American Journal of Medicine* 131: 714–15.

Rigby, Kate. 2014. Romanticism and ecocriticism. In Greg Garrard (ed.), *The Oxford handbook of ecocriticism* (online publication). Oxford: Oxford University Press. https://doi,org/10.1093/oxfordhb/9780199742929.001.0001.

Roe, Nicholas (ed.). 2017. *John Keats and the medical imagination*. Basingstoke: Palgrave.

Shelley, Mary. 1818. *Frankenstein; or The Modern Prometheus*. London: Lackington et al.

Shelley, Mary. 1831. *Frankenstein; or The Modern Prometheus*, 2nd ed. London: Colburn & Bentley.

Sloane, Eugene. 1972. Coleridge's *Kubla Khan*: The living catacombs of the mind. *American Imago* 29: 97–122.

Smith, Jeremy J. 2006. Notes on the medical vocabulary of John Keats. In Graham D. Caie, Carole Hough, & Irene Wotherspoon (eds.), *The power of words: Essays in lexicography, lexicology and semantics in honour of Christian J. Kay*, 150–70. Leiden: Rodopi.

Trower, Shelley. 2009. Nerves, vibration, and the Aeolian Harp. *Romanticism and Victorianism on the Net* 54 (online publication). https://ronjournal.org.

Vickers, Neil. 1997. Coleridge, Thomas Beddoes and Brunonian medicine. *European Romantic Review* 8: 47–94.

Vickers, Neil. 2004. *Coleridge and the doctors 1795–1806*. Oxford: Oxford University Press.

White, Laura. 2006–2007. The person from Porlock in *Kubla Khan* and later texts: Inspiration, agency, and interruption. *Connotations* 16: 172–93.

CHAPTER 10

Foreign Ingredients in Early and Late Modern English Recipes

Isabel De la Cruz-Cabanillas

During the Early and Late Modern English periods[1] medical writing experienced an increasing growth of interest as a result of different factors: the position of English as the language of science and medicine, the adoption of unknown products from the New World, the proliferation of old and new diseases, and a fast-developing print culture, among others (Pahta & Taavitsanen 2011; see also Taavitsainen, Jones, & Hiltunen 2019). Likewise, recipe compilations witnessed a dramatic increase in their production and publication during the sixteenth and seventeenth centuries. Cabré (2011: 170) claims that 'vernacular genres compiling practical knowledge flourished in Western Europe in the sixteenth and seventeenth centuries from the so-called books of secrets to commonplace books, conduct books, manuals of healthcare and, especially, collections of medicinal receipts'. Furthermore, even if the printing press made the recipe collections available to a wider audience, the manuscript tradition continued being an important source of transmission. Thus, 'the printed handbooks, designed to appeal to a broad range of people as aides to ordinary life, coexisted with manuscript domestic guides in the form of recipe collections and compilations, notebooks and so on' (Cabré 2011: 170).

The focus of this chapter is on manuscript medical recipes in early and late modern England as a reflection of the time period, to learn about the novelties introduced in terms of ingredients. From a long-standing tradition inherited from Antiquity and preserved in the Middle Ages, recipes retain their prototypical features over the centuries, but will also incorporate innovations, especially in the ingredients section. Since recipes often tell us 'about the cultural expectations and parameters of any given society'

The author would like to thank here the University of Glasgow Library Visiting Research Fellowship for the year 2019, which made the consultation of the manuscripts held in Glasgow University Library possible. My gratitude goes also to the staff of Special Collections for their kind assistance.

[1] The Early Modern English period is understood to cover the years from 1500 to 1700 and Late Modern English from 1700 to 1800.

(Pennell 2009: 15), changes in society will be mirrored in recipe collections. Probably no other genre is so permeable to alterations in the cultural and social spheres, reflecting fashion, traditions, and conceptions of their time of writing. The food and medicine culture of modern Europe was revolutionised in the wake of the 1492 encounter with America.[2] Thus, the importation of substances from the New World would have an impact not only on European diet and medicine, but also on social, economic and cultural history (López-Piñero et al. 1992: 13).

Regarding the structure of the present chapter, after the introduction to the topic the methodology is explained, followed by a section on the new commodities from America and other products incorporated mainly from Europe. The newly introduced substances are examined in medical terms and illustrated with passages extracted from the corpus of manuscript recipes compiled for the research. Finally, the conclusions drawn from the analysis are presented in the final section.

10.1 Methodology

The methodology followed here has been refined through a series of processes: first, through reading a wide range of relevant works by historians and contemporary authors; second, by the selection of representative recipe collections ranging from the sixteenth to the eighteenth centuries kept in Glasgow University Library (henceforth GUL). The corpus has been balanced to include *receptaria* from the three centuries, even though the number of recipes in each manuscript varies. Thus, Hunter MS 93 and Hunter MS 95 are sixteenth-century texts, whereas Hunter MS 64, General MS 831, and Ferguson MS 61 are seventeenth-century collections. Finally, samples of eighteenth-century manuscripts, Hunter MS 43, Ferguson MS 15, and Ferguson MS 43, have been included in the present study.

Before analysing the material, it is worth mentioning that the contents of the manuscripts under consideration have not been examined thus far, with the exception of Hunter MS 93 (Ortega-Barrera 2014) and the present author's studies based on three of them (De la Cruz-Cabanillas 2016, 2017, 2020). This explains why the material of this study is

[2] I follow Barrera-Osorio's use of the word *America* to refer to the American continent. According to him, 'this usage was already in place in the sixteenth century and is still current in many American countries, with the exception of the United States, where "America" means only the United States' (2006: 12).

remarkably valuable. Additionally, no images are available on the University of Glasgow website, which made the visit to the Library Special Collections Reading Room essential. In addition, the transcription of the texts was necessary to process the information contained in the manuscripts.[3] After this, the ingredients were identified manually by reading the manuscripts. Finally, the products were classified according to their origin: whether they came from America, Asia, or continental Europe.

The provenance of the ingredients, as well as the dates of their introduction into the English language, relies on the information provided by the *Oxford English Dictionary* (henceforth OED). Nevertheless, other lexicographic references have also been taken into consideration, such as the *Lexicons of Early Modern English* (https://leme.library.utoronto.ca), the *Middle English Dictionary* (https://quod.lib.umich.edu/m/middle-english-dictionary/dictionary), and the *Dictionary of Medical Vocabulary* by Norri (2016), to check whether the word had already appeared in the Middle Ages, even if the OED dated the first occurrence in the Renaissance period.

10.2 New Commodities in the Early Modern Period

10.2.1 From the New World

The encounter with the New World from the fifteenth century onwards made possible the regular movement of people, plants, diseases, products, and cultural practices back and forth across the Atlantic Ocean (Canny & Morgan 2012: 1). This exchange between the Old and the New Worlds was intense. On the one hand, Spaniards carried food from Spain with them. Thus, grains and pulses – such as lentils and chickpeas – were transported from Europe, as well as vegetables like 'lettuce, escarole, edible thistles, chard, cabbage, cauliflower, artichoke, spinach, eggplant, turnips, radishes, beets, and carrots; fruits such as quince, peaches, cherries, pomegranates, melons, mangos, and, especially, citrus fruits including oranges, lemons, and grapefruit' (Pérez-Samper 2014: 19).

On the other hand, Spain also benefited from the new goods found in the Americas, which made available a whole new range of products to be employed both in the kitchen and in household medicine. Most recipe

[3] In the transcriptions of the texts, the original spelling has been maintained, whereas the abbreviations have been silently expanded.

collections in early modern England were compiled to be used in the author's domestic environment and relied upon easily accessible ingredients (Leong & Pennell 2007: 136). However, remedies prepared in the period also made use of new substances, especially from America, as shown in the *receptaria* analysed below.

Furthermore, European nobles and middle classes were keen on using new products as a sign of identity to show their status. New foodstuffs percolated into Britain, through a well-established trade with continental countries that brought spices, fruits, and herbs from all over the world. Several products had already shown their efficacy in their places of origin. Nonetheless, the employment of plants from the New World for medicinal purposes was not always obvious. As Barrera-Osorio notes, there were insufficient references to their properties according to humoral theory, which was still prevalent in Europe:

> Perhaps the single most important difference between the development of natural history in the Atlantic world and in the Old World was that the natural products of the Atlantic world lacked a reference in classical traditions. Not a single classical or religious text could provide information on an avocado or cochineal (an organic red dye). Sometimes the texts did provide a clue, but it was never specific enough. (Barrera-Osorio 2006: 102)

European physicians sometimes disagreed on the classification of American plants (Estes 1995: 12). Thus, having no proof of their real qualities, the products were used because American Indian people had proven their efficacy in the treatment of some diseases, but often also because they were considered sophisticated, being new to the market. In addition, the outbreak of unknown diseases in the Old World made it necessary for physicians to resort to new remedies. This could be the case for ailments such as syphilis, or new episodes of the plague, to which several medical preparations were applied. Many of these included newly introduced American commodities.

Several of the substances coming from America may have had a direct medical use, but others, like tobacco, were definitely employed for other purposes. First of all, Stewart (1967: 229) and López-Piñero et al. (1992: 45) mention the fact that tobacco was not the name of the plant, but referred to the instrument used by indigenous Americans to inhale it. Secondly, 'Monardes reported that the Spanish had brought tobacco to the Old World as an ornamental flower' (Estes 1995: 9). Nonetheless, it had also entered medical practice by 1570s, and it became the focus of learned pamphlet controversies arguing both for and against its medicinal uses (see Ratia 2011). Matthee claims that

> tobacco was considered to be a disinfectant in a time in which frequent outbreaks of the plague left people desperate for preventive medicine. Praised as such during the 1635–6 epidemic in Holland, tobacco maintained that reputation during the 1665 plague of London and the epidemic that afflicted Vienna in 1679. (1995: 29–30)

De la Cruz-Cabanillas (2020: 51) records 'A Receipt for Buggs' in Wellcome MS 1322, where tobacco is used as a disinfectant:

(1) Take a pail of Water and put to it some unslaked Lime and let it stand all Night then pour of the Water clear and Boyle in it Tobacco stalks and Coloquintida, boyl them well and strain it wash the floor of the room & all the wainscott and Jester & Bedstead let it dig on & do it 3 times or more together it was never known to fail [. . .]. (Wellcome MS 1322, f. 50v)

In addition to preventive use for sanitary purposes, tobacco could be used together with other herbs to treat a quartene fever, as said in General MS 831 (2) and diseases, such as asthma (3) and gout (4), as mentioned in Hunter MS 93:

(2) Take Currants and bruse them and strew uppon it the pouder of Tobaco; and it to the wrest of the handes, and lett it remaine till the Medcine be drie.//. (GUL, General MS 831, f. 55)

(3) This is excellent for Asthmaticall and Consumptive distempers for ye Lungs in case of arSthysis for any sore cough and difficulty of breathing the best time to make it is in Aprill./ Take two twenty shilings of apaned hould waight of Bitteny, and ye same quantity of Sweet Margerum, dryed bery green in a fier shobell or Ouen, then pound it in a Woden Morter and Sarce them through Tiffeny or Leume then take 15 gould waight of Spanish tobacco dryed and Sarced likewise; then you may put thervnto twenty graines of Muskell, let them all be well mixed togeather and put up in boxes. This being used to be snufft up once or twice a day morning & euening into ye Llostwitt that is most stopt soe much at a time as wilbe held betweene ye Thumbe and ye finger end, is a rare experienct remedy against ye Gout [. . .]. (GUL, Hunter MS 93, ff. 269–70)

(4) The Tobacco must bee bruised to a fine powder, ye Cloves dryed and beaten and soe sifted through Tistiney, then mixe ye muske and Ambergreece with the Cloves and beate them and then bruise them with a knife together and then after that mixe both Cloves & Tobacco

powder, and soe reserve it a close boxe for your use but first wrapt vp in paper. you must take above ye quantity of a greate pins head in each nostril. [. . .]. (GUL, Hunter MS 93, f. 270)

American substances were also employed to heal several rampant diseases in the period, one of which was the French pox or syphilis, which was known to Europe since the end of the fifteenth century. The first outbreak took place in Italy in 1495 and its origin is often linked to the return of Christopher Columbus two years earlier with ten natives of the West Indies and a crew of forty-four men, some of whom are said 'to have joined the troops of Gonzalo de Cordoba who marched with Charles VIII to Naples' (Cartwright & Biddiss 2000: 44).

In modern Europe several procedures were used to treat the French pox, especially mercury and guaiac, a resin obtained from *Guaiacum officinale* and *Guaiacum sanctum*, indigenous trees to South America and the West Indies. The guaiac was the usual remedy among Indian people (López-Piñero et al. 1992: 16). The product became very popular in Europe, even though it was expensive, due to the fact that 'the monopoly in its trade was sold by the Spanish Crown to the Fuggers, the wealthiest bankers in Europe' (Wear 2000: 70) and, therefore, it was available only to patients who could afford the treatment. Estes refers to the cost of guaiac, which 'seems to have been prescribed chiefly by physicians whose clientele included those who could pay most for the new drug, while the cheaper mercurials were more likely to be prescribed by barber-surgeons, whose patients were less affluent' (1995: 7).

The popularity of guaiac is evidenced due to the fact that several treatments recorded in the corpus refer to using it for the French pox. One of them is included in Hunter MS 43, whereby not only guaiac but also sarsaparilla,[4] 'the most popular remedy from the New World in the sixteenth century' (Estes 1995: 7), are mixed with other ingredients:

(5) A Wonderfull good Diet for ye French Pox. Take Coloquintida drachm ij. The bark of Guajacum, Sarsaparilla, Liquerishe ana. ounce semisse [. . .]. (GUL, Hunter MS 43, f. 3)

In turn, in Hunter MS 95 there are several similar remedies for the same disease. In the next example, apart from guaiac and sarsaparilla, sassafras, another American plant, is prescribed. The demand for sassafras was so

[4] These ingredients were not only used for the treatment of the French pox, but also for the different episodes of the plague in the modern period. Tanturri, in Chapter 6 in this volume, also reports on their use in Italy in the nineteenth century.

great that 'expeditions were sent to New England in 1602 and 1603 to collect it for English entrepreneurs, who hoped to sell it for fifty pounds a ton' (Estes 1995: 8). Hunter MS 95 has the following recipes:

(6) Recipe. ligni guiaci libra ij, Cortexe ounce ij, sarsaperilla libra semis. sarsafras Cardus benedictus.manipulus. 4. Camamell flowers melelott flowres ana manipulus ij pollipodi libra semis liquerish ounce .6. sene libra .j. hermodacteles ounce 6. turbit ounce 8. blacke helebor ounce .6: pulp Colloquinted a ounce iiij aneseedes ounce iij ginger. ounce: v semis. Cinamon. ounce ij put all these beinge prepared in aglasse boddye and Couer them ij fingers on with speritt of wine or distilled vineger. (GUL, Hunter MS 95, f. 2r)

(7) Recipe guiaci libra. semis. sarsaparilla ounce iij. China. ounce. j. seep these in :8: libra of faire water. 20: houres then ad ounce. ij of the rootes of vipers grasse, of Cardus benedictus, ffumitory, ana. manipulus. j. then boyle these till the halfe be spente & when it is almost enough boyled ad: ounce ij of sarsaphras & ounce j. of liquerish & when it is cold strayne it for. vse [. . .]. (GUL, Hunter MS 95, f. 9v)

In (7), along with other herbs, one finds China root or China-grass, which is 'a small shrubby plant with broadly cordate leaves, native to China and Sumatra' (OED). China root is included in recipes to prepare restorative broths. Albala claims that these kinds of recipes 'verge on the medicinal' (2012: 326). Thus, the mixture of cooking and medical recipes is common in the period, and diet and medicine are clearly interconnected. Furthermore, Thirsk claims that plants served two purposes, as food and as medicine, and 'these two separate interests mingled instinctively in the minds of contemporaries whenever they sat down to eat' (2007: 287). In fact, a medical recipe collection, such as the one in Ferguson MS 61, also includes what could be considered culinary instructions for a strengthening broth:

(8) Take halfe An ounce of prepared woormes A spoonefull of shaveings of harts horne and halfe a spoonefull of Ivory, ty those up in A Cloth and boyle them with A Chickening and A suffitient quantity of water ading a spoonefull of ffrench Barly nine or ten prums and a halfe A handfull of Raysons of the sun stooned A Crust of manchet one spoonefull of Currants A Sprig of Rousemary and time, Sucory Sparrowgrasd fennell Rootes of each one ounce steepe these in whitte wine thet night beefore and halfe a Spoone full of Capers well wayshed from the Salt Drinke A Draught of this Brath every morneing worme by seaven of the Clocke [. . .]. (GUL, Ferguson MS 61, f. 3)

Often the newly introduced herbs were used to treat new diseases, but they were also employed to treat several already well-known ones. *Crab-tree* or *eryngo* is first attested in 1769 in the OED meaning 'a South American tree, *Carapa guianensis*'. Despite this dating, *crab-tree* is already documented in Hunter MS 64, a seventeenth-century text, in a recipe for healing a canker or any other wound:

(9) Take the barke of a crabtre that groweth in a wood & seath it in ale till it hath sodd to the third parte then cast away the barke & straine it well & then put to it a pinte of milke then sethe them together till it be as thicke as honey & ever more washe the canker with womans milke & make a playster and change it twise in a daye . [. . .] (GUL, Hunter MS 64, f. 10r)

These several products are among the most widely used introduced from America, but they were not the only ones. The corpus records other gums and resins, such as tacamahaca. This is mentioned by Monardes, a Spanish botanist and physician, whose main work was *IOYFVLL NEWES out of the newfound world, wherein are declared the rare and singular vertues of diuers and sundrie Herbs, Trees, Oyles, Plants, & Stones.*[5] Similarly, a resin known as carana, obtained from a West Indian tree, *Bursera acuminata*, has medical applications. Both are present in Ferguson MS 43 in a description of a plaster for an ache:

(10) Take of ij Gummes ye one called Tackame-hacka & ye other Carana ye one being a hard Gumme must be first spread on with a hot knyfe vpon a peece of leather, and then you must spread on ye other Gume and lay it to ye place where ye paine is, and lett it remaine till ye paine be quite gone [. . .]. (GUL, Ferguson MS 43, f. 4v)

In turn, in Hunter MS 64 carana is used in a recipe for sciatica:

(11) Take caranna iiij ounce & put to it of the strongest sacke you can get put in almost halfe a pinte melt them together in a peuter bason & so sone as it is molten strenie it then boyle it till the sacke be wasted then tak fine shepes lether & spread this thereon making your plaister fit for the plane. [. . .] (GUL Hunter MS 64, f. 54v)

Likewise, several GUL manuscripts document the use of *Benjamin*, whose name refers to three different trees. According to the OED, they are '*(a) Styrax benzoin*, the tree from which benzoin is obtained; a native of

[5] For an analysis of Monardes, see Taavitsainen (2009).

Sumatra, Borneo, etc.; *(b)* the *Benzoin odoriferum* or *Lindera Benzoin*, a North American shrub, which has an aromatic stimulant tonic bark, and berries yielding an oil of similar properties; called also Benjamin-bush and in U.S. Benjamin; *(c)* sometimes applied to *Ficus Benjamina*'. We cannot know for certain which one the recipe compiler meant. The plant could serve diverse purposes: in Hunter MS 64 it is used to make a pomander (12), for washing the teeth (13), and for a perfume for the head (14), whereas in Ferguson MS 43 (15) it appears only once in a recipe for a perfume:

(12) To make a very Excellent Pomander

> Take halfe an ounce of gum dragagant & infuse it in Rosewater till it becum all a musklage this done heate your morter very hote pestell & all then take this receite as followeth storax calamite halfe an ounce beniamin ij drames labdanum one ounce cloves yealow sanders of each one dram musk xv graines sevet tene graines first take your gumes & beate them in your hote morter then take the cloves & sanders beinge in fine powder & beate it all together with the muske and sevet then take of the foresaid gum infused to a musculage & put therto as muche as you thinke shall suffice then beate all together and Rowle them vp as you woulde have them [. . .]. (GUL, Hunter MS 64, f. 1r)

(13) A decoction to washe & scoure the mouthe to fasten lose tethe to consolidate, & make sounde the gummes & to make the fleshe to growe agayne beinge decayed./

> Take halfe a glasse full of vineger with as muche water of lettis of Rosemary mirre masticke boule-armoniacke, the moysture that distilleth put of dragons bloud roche allom burned of eache of them an ounce fine sina mon halfe an ounce well, Ryver, or fountaine water three glasse full mingle all well together, & let it boyle with a small fier addinge to it halfe a pounde of honey scuminge it then put in a little beniamyn, when it hath boyled a quarter of an hower cole yt & put it in a clene viall & washe your tethe often therewith as well before as after meate & houldinge it a while in your mouthe yt is very good for the heade & maketh a sweet breath bringe a thinge of greate excellencye . [. . .] (GUL, Hunter MS 64, f. 8r)

(14) A perfume for the heade./

> Take olibanum, veruxxe, beniamin & storax of eyther on once beate them together grosley to perfume the head & soe imbast A pece of

graye paper with flax & hould it over the perfume beinge burnt vpon coles & then soe lay it to the fore parte of the heade . [. . .] (GUL, Hunter MS 64, f. 16v)

(15) A Receipt of ye Rose perfume.

Take three ounces and a halfe of Beniamine and lay it a night in Rose water, then beate it fine and take halfe a pound of Dammaske Roses ye whites being taken away, beate them fine, then take ye beniamine and put them to ye Roses, and beate them together vntill it come to a past, then mingle with it half a quarter of an ounce of Muske finely beaten, then put to it halfe a quarter of an ounce of Ciuett finely beaten, and an ounce and halfe of sugar finely searsed, then make them vp in little Cakes betwixt Rose leaues on both sides, and dry them on sheetes of paper where no Ayre comes. [. . .] (GUL, Ferguson MS, 43 ff. 15r–15v)

Other products, such as cochineal, found in 'several species of cactus in Mexico and elsewhere' (OED), were prescribed along with other medical ingredients in recipes:

(16) To make Tincture of Carroways

Tis good for ye Cholick or Gripes
Take a quart of spirit's of wine & put it in to ½ a pound of sugard carroway's & shake it every day for a week then put in a quarter of a pound of powder sugar & shake it well together & put in 6 grains of cochenele & keep it close stop't [. . .]. (GUL, Ferguson MS 15, f. 119)

10.2.2 From Europe

By the end of the fifteenth century, England had an established trade not only from the Netherlands and France, but also from the Mediterranean (Thirsk 2007: 10). Apart from figs, raisins, oranges, dates, and pomegranates, not to mention all the currently familiar spices like turmeric, cinnamon, and cumin, several other products that are present in the recipe collections of the period came from the Mediterranean area. Among those was, for instance, alkermes, 'the dried bodies of scale insects (females of *Kermes ilicis* and *K. vermilio*, family Kermesidae), found in the Mediterranean region on the kermes oak (*Quercus coccifera*) and formerly used medicinally and as a source of red dye; a medicinal preparation containing these insects' (OED).

In Hunter MS 93 it is recorded along with other substances as ingredients for a surfeit water:

(17) Put three quarts of Anniseeds water into a new earthen glased pot or pipkin with soe many red feild poppies as can be wett in it when they grow pale straine away the water and if it be high Coulored as Alligant put into it 3 ounces of browne sugar candie and a quarter of a Ounce of Alcarmes afterwards keep it close stopt in a Glasse if the first poppies doe not sufficiently staine ye water put in more before you add ye two last Ingredients
Giue one or two or three spoonfull of it as ye degree of ye surfeit requiers and ye age and strength of ye patient permitts. [. . .] (GUL, Hunter MS 93, f. 260)

Likewise, in an extensive recipe of a mixture that was thought to prevent miscarriage, alkermes is listed along with other ingredients:

(18) Take 2: ounces of Barley water, Cinaman water 2 ounces, Juce of Citrons ½ an ounce on dram of Confect Alkermes without muske, & 2 ounces Cordiall frigida Saxoniae, mix all well together [. . .]. (GUL, Ferguson MS 61, f. 62)

Also from the Mediterranean area is angelica, the 'angelic herb' or 'root of the Holy Ghost', so named on account of its reputation against poison and pestilence, probably from the fragrant smell and aromatic taste of its root. The plague was particularly pestilent, and several recipes against the smell can be found in different manuscripts of the corpus. One of them is *To make a perfume to smell vnto against ye Plague*:

(19) ffirst take halfe a pinte of red Rosewater and putt thereto the quantitie of a hasellnutt of Venice Treacle or Metredate stirring them together vntill they be well infused, then putt therto a grain of an ounce of Synnamon broken into small peeces and bruised, in a Morter, xij Cloues bruised, ye quantitie of a good hasell nutt of Angelica Roote slyced very thyn, as much of Zedoarie rotte slyced, 3 or 4 spoonfulls of white wyne Vinigar, so putt them altogeather into a glasse, and stop it verie close, and shake it two or three tymes a day for two or three dayes [. . .]. (GUL, Ferguson MS 43, f. 10r)

Apart from angelica root, a new ingredient in the period mentioned in (19) is *Venice treacle*, which is 'an electuary composed of many ingredients and supposed to possess universal alexipharmic and preservative properties', according to the OED. The term was first attested in 1617.

Unlike the previously mentioned plants, the origin of scurvy grass is unknown. As can be deduced from its name, scurvy grass, 'a cruciferous plant, *Cochlearia officinalis*, believed to possess anti-scorbutic properties' (OED), was the most widely used herb to treat the scurvy. The disease had been known for centuries, but its prevalence was probably higher in the sixteenth and seventeenth centuries, especially in sailors. In fact, according to Elmer's estimations, 'on long voyages a ship could lose between a quarter and a third of its crew to the disease, not to mention those who were temporarily incapacitated' (2004: 276). The high mortality rate among navy personnel inspired James Lind, a Scottish surgeon in the Royal Navy, to carry out a dietary experiment on those sailors who fell ill with scurvy. The experiment is described by Porter:

> Twelve scurvy patients were chosen. Lind gave two of them a quart of cider a day; two had oil of vitriol; two vinegar; two sea-water; two had oranges and lemons; and two an electuary of garlic, radish, Peru balsam and myrrh. The pair on oranges and lemons were fit for duty in six days, and put to nurse the other, who remained sick. (1997: 295)

Finally, Lind published his results in *Treatise of the Scurvy*, in 1753. No immediate action was taken after Lind's findings, but his proposals for preventing the illness were eventually adopted in 1795, when measures were taken to provide lemon juice to 'crews who had been on salted provisions for six weeks' (Elmer 2004: 276). Nonetheless, the fact that citrus fruits were good for the scurvy was already known in the sixteenth century, as recorded in Dr John Feckenham's *Book of Medical Receipts*, extant in Hunter MS 93:

(20) The Cofernes of skiruie grasse, roman wormod and of ginger of each two ounces. Of the flowers of rosemary, ye pulpe of Cyterne, cofernes of roses woodsorrell, succory; gilliflowers, of each one ounce [...]. (GUL, Hunter MS 93, f. 259)

Even if some panaceas, such as *Aqua Vitae*, were also used to treat the illness, as in 'any disease where any gross humour aboundeth, as in ye Gout, dropsie, french poxe, scurvey & þe like' (GUL, Hunter MS 43, f. 25), scurvy grass was the most widely used herb. A sample of this is in *An approved drink for ye scurvy*:

(21) Take of water cresses brookcyme of scurvey grass as much as will yeild 3 pints or 2 quarts of juice let your scurvy grass be ye greatest quaintity then take of saxifrage & sarsaparilla of each a good hand full thin shave'd & sew them in a bag of lawn. or some thin cloth but

bruise ye woods be fore you put them into the bag & then have a small firkin of ale of 8 gallons after it hath worke'd put into it ye juice of those herbs befor name'd & ye bagg of saxifrage then stick an orange full of cloves & hang it by a thred in ye firkin it will be fitt' te drink after one day it must be drunk. in ye morning tasting & fast 2 hours after it drink it again at 4 in ye afternoon [...]. (GUL, Ferguson MS 15, f. 124)

Another ailment that was thoroughly described in the British medicine of the period was rickets. It was not defined as a specific medical condition until 1645, when an English physician, Daniel Whistler, provided the earliest known description of the disease in his *De Morbo puerili Anglorum, quem patrio idiomate indigenae vocant 'the Rickets'*. However, it is Glisson who is credited with having discovered the illness when he published a treatise, *De Rachitide sive morbo puerili*, in 1650. An English edition by Nicholas Culpeper appeared a year later with the title *A treatise of the rickets, being a disease common to children.*

Remedies for rickets appear in the corpus in Hunter MS 93, but especially in Ferguson MS 61. The latter is a compilation by a woman, Mary Harrison, who was married and pregnant, as she claims in her recipe 318, where she states 'at Aston 1710 I was with child'. Subsequently, her concern about a disease that affected children seems to be a natural one. Recipes for rickets are documented five times in her book: in recipe 36, *A Dyet Drinke for the Rockettes*; recipe 181, *A Drink for ye Rickets*; recipe 189, *An Ointment for ye Rickets*; recipe 232, *Lady Sharlowes receipt for the Ricketts*; and recipe 272, *for ye Ricketts*. One of these, Lady Sharlowe's recipe, reads as follows:

(22) Recipe of speedwell Liver wort, dandelyon, heart Tongue, of each one handfull, penyroyle ½ a handfull, strawberrye Leaves, & vilet Leaves of each a handfull, of Liqurish & anniseed a ¼ of a pond of Each: 2 or 3 Leaves of Lovage bojle al these in 3 pintes of strong ale tell a pint be consumed, so sweeten it with browne suger & give ye child 2 or 3 spoonfulls [...]. (GUL, Ferguson MS 61, f. 97)

Except for *speedwell*, which was first attested in 1578 according to the OED, none of the ingredients in (22) is new. Liverwort, dandelion, hart's tongue, pennyroyal, strawberry, violet, liquorice, aniseed, and lovage are all herbs used extensively in medieval English recipes.

Other ingredients are also mentioned in the corpus. Venice turpentine is well documented for different purposes. Turpentine, 'the semifluid resin of the terebinth tree', was known in the Middle Ages, but for this specific variety the first record in the OED is from 1744. In General MS 831, a seventeenth-century text, it is used *for an ague*:

(23) Take venice Turpentine. Bole armanick and Mastick spread thes upon sheepes lether and soe apply it to the wrest 2 or three times before the fitt comes [. . .]. (GUL, General MS 831, f. 63)

The ingredients mentioned thus far seem to have been common currency in the period, since they appear in most manuscripts, whereas others not so widespread are recorded in at least one of the chosen manuscripts, such as *coccus indi*, mechoacham, and tetter-berry. The latter is a perennial climbing vine indigenous to Central and Southern Europe, which is known in Britain as *white bryony*, also as *English mandrake* or *ladies' seal.* It is documented for the first time in Gerard's *Herball* (1597). In the GUL corpus it appears in Hunter MS 64 in a recipe for the colic and the stone in the kidneys:

(24) Take a pinte of Saxifrage water & an ounce of titerbery kerneles one ounce of gromewell seed one ounce of alisander seed & ij or iij ackhornes make all these in pouder & put the pouder into the Saxifrage water drinke it every day three morninges conty minge you per may heate it soe hott as you can abyde it [. . .]. (GUL, Hunter MS 64, f. 43r)

Our main topic of interest has been herbs, but other products are also found in medical recipes. *Sack*, a term used for French dry wine (included in Example 11), and Spanish Canary wine both rank high in the frequency of items recorded in the corpus. They provide evidence of the intense trade that took place during Britain and other European nations during the modern period and of how the new products were introduced into medical recipes.

10.3 Conclusions

In this chapter we have explored early and late modern English recipes as a reflection of their time period. In order to do so, a representative compilation of recipe manuscripts was selected from GUL. Since most of them are unexplored texts, the examination of the recipe collections from the sixteenth to the eighteenth centuries contributes to research on what remains largely uncharted territory. The analysis of the manuscript contents reveals several conclusions. The *receptaria* held at GUL are a good example of how recipes reflect the period in which they were written. They deal with the contemporary society's concerns: the outbreak of new diseases, such as syphilis, and other old illnesses that were particularly rampant in the period, such as the plague, rickets, and scurvy.

The remedies used to treat these ailments make use of age-old ingredients known from Antiquity, and also of new products imported from America. It is uncertain whether some of these substances have a specific positive effect, but they seem to be fashionable among and particularly embraced by the better-off population, since these substances were considered exotic. One of the most common goods was guaiac, whose monopoly was granted to the Fuggers, a family of bankers. Tobacco, in our day a major health problem, was used as a disinfectant or even for the treatment of some specific diseases, like asthma, gout, or quartene fever. Of American origin are also sarsaparilla, sassafras, and crab-tree, along with cochineal, among others. Other goods came from Asia or from a territory nearer to Europe, as in the case of angelica and alkermes that grew in the Mediterranean area, or from an unknown origin, like scurvy grass.

Regarding the appearance of new terms in the English language, the focus here was on terms for herbs adopted from the sixteenth century onwards. The OED was taken as the main reference, but some antedatings have been identified, such as the use of *crab-tree*.

The adoption of new ingredient terms has proven significant in a medical context. The exploration of other product words not recorded in the corpus, such as chocolate, could be a topic for further research. It would be intriguing to find out how these commodities were accepted among the European population and how they were introduced as food and medicine into the British diet.

REFERENCES

Albala, Ken. 2012. Food for healing: Convalescent cookery in the early modern era. *Studies in History and Philosophy of Biological and Biomedical Sciences* 43: 323–8.

Barrera-Osorio, Antonio. 2006. *Experiencing nature. The Spanish American empire and the early scientific revolution*. Austin: University of Texas Press.

Cabré, Montserrat. 2011. Keeping beauty secrets in Early Modern Iberia. In Elaine Leong & Alisha Rankin (eds.), *Secrets and knowledge in medicine and science, 1500–1800*, 167–90. Aldershot: Ashgate.

Canny, Nicholas, & Philip Morgan. 2012. Introduction: The making and unmaking of an Atlantic world. In Nicholas Canny & Philip Morgan (eds.), *The Oxford handbook of the Atlantic World: 1450–1850*, 1–18.

Oxford: Oxford University Press. Online edition available at www.oxfordhandbooks.com/view/10.1093/oxfordhb/9780199210879.001.0001/oxfordhb-9780199210879 (accessed 25 April 2022).

Cartwright, Frederick F., & Michael Biddiss. 2000. *Disease and history*. 2nd ed. Stroud: Sutton Publishing.

De la Cruz-Cabanillas, Isabel. 2016. Mary Harrison's book of recipes. Women and household medicine in late 17th century. *Revista Canaria de Estudios Ingleses* 72(1): 79–95.

De la Cruz-Cabanillas, Isabel. 2017. Genre and text-type conventions in Early Modern English women's recipe books. *Revista de Lingüística y Lenguas Aplicadas* 12: 13–21.

De la Cruz-Cabanillas, Isabel. 2020. Early Modern English recipes as a mirror of the time period. *Neophilological Studies* 16: 47–60.

Elmer, Peter (ed.). 2004. *The healing arts. Health, disease and society in Europe, 1500–1800*. Manchester: Manchester University Press/The Open University.

Estes, J. Worth. 1995. The European reception of the first drugs from the New World. *Pharmacy in History* 37: 3–23.

Gerard, John. 1597. *The Herball, or Generall Historie of Plantes*. 1597. Online. 1633 edition. https://quod.lib.umich.edu/e/eebo/A01622.0001.001?rgn=main;%20view=fulltext (accessed 21 May 2022).

Leong, Elaine, & Sara Pennell. 2007. Recipe collections and the currency of medical knowledge in the Early Modern 'medical marketplace'. In Mark S. R. Jenner & Patrick Wallis (eds.), *Medicine and the market in England and its colonies, c. 1450 – c. 1850*, 133–52. Chippenham: Palgrave Macmillan.

López-Piñero, José M., José Luis Fresquet-Febrer, M. Luz López-Terrada, & José Pardo-Tomás. 1992. *Medicinas, Drogas y Alimentos vegetales del Nuevo Mundo*. Madrid: Ministerio de Sanidad y Consumo.

Matthee, Rudi. 1995. Exotic substances: The introduction and global spread of tobacco, coffee, cocoa, tea, and distilled liquor, sixteenth to eighteenth centuries. In Roy Porter & Mikulás Teich (eds.), *Drugs and narcotics in history*, 24–51. Cambridge: Cambridge University Press.

Norri, Juhani. 2016. *Dictionary of medical vocabulary in English, 1375–1550*. 2 vols. London: Routledge.

Ortega-Barrera, Ivalla. 2014. *Un recetario inédito del s. XVI en la Biblioteca Hunteriana de Glasgow: edición y estudio*. Saarbrücken: Editorial Académica.

Pahta, Päivi, & Irma Taavitsainen. 2011. An interdisciplinary approach to medical writing in Early Modern English. In Irma Taavitsainen & Päivi Pahta (eds.), *Medical writing in Early Modern English*, 1–8. Cambridge: Cambridge University Press.

Pennell, Sara. 2009. Recipe and reception: Tracking 'New World' foodstuffs in early modern British culinary texts, c. 1650–1750. *Food & History* 7(1): 11–34.

Pérez-Samper, María de los Ángeles. 2014. The early modern food revolution: A perspective from the Iberian Atlantic. In Bethany Aram & Bartolomé Yun-Casalilla (eds.), *Global goods and the Spanish Empire, 1492–1824: Circulation, resistance and diversity*, 17–36. Basingstoke: Palgrave Macmillan.

Porter, Roy. 1997. *The greatest benefit to mankind: A medical history of humanity from Antiquity to the present.* London: Harper Collins.

Ratia, Maura. 2011. *Texts 'con and pro': The early modern medical controversy over tobacco.* Helsinki: Société Néophilologique de Helsinki.

Stewart, Grace G. 1967. A history of the medicinal use of tobacco, 1492–1860. *Medical History* 11(3): 228–68.

Taavitsainen, Irma. 2009. 'Joyful News out of the Newfound World': Medical and scientific news reports in Early Modern England. In Andreas H. Jucker (ed.), *Early Modern English news discourse: Newspapers, pamphlets and scientific news discourse*, 189–204. Amsterdam; New York: Benjamins.

Taavitsainen, Irma, Peter Jones, & Turo Hiltunen. 2019. Sociohistorical and cultural context of Late Modern English medical texts. In Irma Taavitsainen & Turo Hiltunen (eds.), *Late Modern English medical texts: Writing medicine in the eighteenth century*, 17–30. Amsterdam: Benjamins.

Thirsk, Joan. 2007. *Food in early modern England: Phases, fads, fashion 1500–1760.* London: Continuum.

Wear, Andrew. 2000. *Knowledge and practice in English medicine, 1550–1680.* Cambridge: Cambridge University Press.

CHAPTER 11

Walter Bailey's (1529–1593) Medical Genres

Irma Taavitsainen

> The marvellous effects done by those wels in Warwickshire, not only heard, but also seene by my selfe [. . .] I spent more time in triall and examination of them, [. . .], and so did wholy put mine endeuors for the discouerie of their minerals, natures, and properties [. . .].
>
> (Bailey 1587: A4)

The above early example gives evidence of the new way of thinking in the early modern period, as it places observation above hearsay of old inherited wisdom and enhances empirical evidence as the source of knowledge. Traditionally it was believed that Adam had possessed uncorrupt and pure knowledge; it had become corrupted by the Fall, but could be revived by studying old books and restoring the original meanings of Ancient Philosophers (Shapin 1996: 74–5). This was the idea behind the older thought style of scholasticism that continued as an undercurrent throughout the early modern period and beyond.[1] The discovery of the New World (1492) had opened up new horizons, and keen observers of nature pointed out erroneous descriptions of plants and animals, or, as Bailey put it, 'hath made manifest to vs, how greatly the old authors [. . .] were deceiued' (1588: A5r). Similar conclusions were made, for example, by the Spanish missionary José de Acosta (1540–1600), who describes observations by eye-witnesses as 'difficult' because they were 'contrarie to the ancient and received Philosophy'.[2] Such comments paved the way for changes that were explicitly expressed by Francis Bacon (1561–1626), who advocated the inductive method based on first-hand observation of the 'Book of Nature' instead of musty books by ancient authorities (Porter 2000: 56). This changing worldview corresponded in date to the profound

[1] Thought styles can be defined as underlying intellectual and moral principles as manifested in scientific concepts, objects of inquiry, methods, and evaluations, mediated to us through language (Crombie 1994; see also Taavitsainen & Pahta 1998: 161).

[2] De Acosta travelled in Peru after 1571. The quotations are from the English translation of his book, *The naturall and morall historie of the East and West Indies* (1604: 3), published in Spanish in 1590.

changes taking place in religion in England; Bailey's texts include passages aligned with the new Protestant religion, reflecting the prevailing attitude to old Catholic 'superstitions of our forefathers' (Bailey 1587: A3v).

My point of departure is the variationist theory of language change that describes language as an ever-changing entity with some old varieties dying out and new varieties springing up, with the old and the new forms co-occurring at any one time, and innovative features only gradually taking over.[3] Social history describes the situation at any period in similar terms: 'There is always an overlap of the old and the new continuing side by side in the same country for generations and even for centuries' (Trevelyan 1967 [1942]: 108). But the same view can well be applied to the ideological level of thought styles on the discourse level, as old and new ideas are current in society at the same time but in different discourses. Changes take place at different rates and are more fine-grained than earlier assumed, and features of the new style emerge sporadically in the latter half and turn of the sixteenth century (Taavitsainen & Schneider 2019; Taavitsainen 2009: 56, 2002: 215). They are first introduced into the learned layers of writing and spread only slowly to more widely circulated texts. As a result, older patterns and ways of thinking can be retained for centuries.

The present empirical study is based on medical texts with passages pertaining to several different genres, written by Walter Bailey (1529–1593), an eminent medical doctor who received the highest possible education at Oxford.[4] His earliest text *Mithridatium* (1585)[5] deals with a medical concoction by that name. *A brief treatise touching the preservation of the eyesight* (1586; *Eyesight* hereafter) is a preventive treatise. *A brief discourse of certain bathes of medicinal waters* (1587; *Waters* hereafter) discusses the health-giving effects of Warwickshire wells. *A short discourse of the three kinds of pepper* (1588; *Peppers* hereafter) discusses the question of whether different kinds of pepper grow on one tree or on different trees.

[3] '[. . .] pronunciations are changing, new words and constructions are being adopted and old ones are adapted to new uses. Sometimes change is rapid, and sometimes it is slow, and at any given time some linguistic structures are changing while others remain stable' (Milroy 1972: 1). I am not aware of earlier applications to the ideological level.

[4] Walter Bailey (1529–1593) was born in Dorset, and attended Winchester College and then New College, Oxford. He had a successful medical and academic career as professor at Oxford, was a Fellow of the College of Physicians, and he was one of Queen Elizabeth's medical doctors (Bakewell 2004).

[5] Bailey published his works privately and anonymously; that may be the reason why *Mithridiatum* is not listed among his works in the *Oxford Dictionary of National Biography* (ODNB; Bakewell 2004), although *Early English Books Online* (EEBO; http://eebo.chadwyck.com/home) identifies it as belonging to his canon.

In historical pragmatics, linguistic and stylistic features are assessed in relation to contemporary sociocultural developments (see chapter 1). To contextualise Bailey's genres, we need to know their target audience. In accordance with the old genre conventions, the metatext in *Mithridiatum* refers to a wide and heterogeneous audience, enhancing humility in serving the poor and the needful. The actual audience must, however, have been Bailey's educated peers. Also, the origins of *Peppers* as a New Year's gift applied to the upper classes only and give evidence of a literate audience.[6] Indirect evidence is also provided by the learned style; the specification of diet also points in this direction (see Example 4).[7]

Learned texts by classical authors in their original languages must have been familiar to university-educated doctors; they served as models for vernacular medical and scientific writing.[8] The vernacularisation process of medicine had started already two hundred years before the time in focus, and we can assume that Bailey's discourse community had late medieval texts at their disposal.

After explaining my purpose and method of study, I shall go into detail about his genres and text types, with special attention to features that pertain, on the one hand, to the old scholastic thought style and, on the other hand, to those of empirical science.

11.1 Aim and Method of the Study

This study illustrates ongoing processes of change in learned vernacular medical writing. The present data gives first-hand evidence of the early phases of the transition period. I shall probe deeper into the variationist pattern of change on the discourse level, where both the macrolevel structural composition of genres and the microlevel of linguistic features are of interest. Bailey's medical output is fairly large, with several different genres and text types. *Genres* are related to the speaker's or writer's purpose of communication rather than the form, whereas *text types* are defined according to the text-internal linguistic features, irrespective of genre

6 He wrote to an unknown recipient 'to shew my special affection [. . .] by offering som present, appertaining to the preseruatio*n* of your health: [. . .] in token of a good and prosperous newe yeere, (God grant you many)' (Bailey 1588: unnumbered page).

7 The edition of *Eyesight* has the publisher's preface from 1616. *Waters* is called a 'pamphlet for public benefit' in its original preface.

8 Latin prevailed as the main language of science in England for about a century after Bailey's time (about the changing situation, see Wear 2000: 41).

(Biber 1988: 70, 170; Taavitsainen 2001, 1997: 187–90; Werlich 1982: 38–41). Genres and text types are both abstractions, based on individual texts, and it is useful to keep the terms apart. The advantage of this two-tier model is that it brings out genre dynamics and genre changes. Genres build on conventions and continue with variation and change. Several processes are involved, including genre mutation and innovation that may be initiated by contact with other genres, leading to hybrid forms and eventually to change (Fowler 1982: passim). Genres with their own developing patterns provide a useful tool for my analysis.

Some genres like recipes have received scholarly attention from medieval times to later periods, but learned genres that originate from the prime of scholasticism have not been studied to the same extent.

The approach based on 'family resemblances' sees genres without clear-cut categories and obligatory components, but with fuzzy boundaries and overlapping memberships.[9] A useful analytical tool is also provided by *genre scripts*; that is, typical patterns of language use and sequences in macrolevel structures, with old authorities' knowledge and experience presented first and the text concluded with the author's own opinion. This script is related to both *cultural scripts*, defined as sets of assumptions that relate to particular situations or activity types in a culture (Spencer-Oatey 2000: 61–2), and the *schema theory* that contributes to the meaning-making processes in both authors' and readers' minds, creating expectations of how various situations develop (McIntyre & Busse 2010: 113; cf. Paltridge 1997: 18–19). Texts of a genre may exhibit genre features to different extents, and multiple memberships are also possible. Genre labels give us an ethnographic view indicating social practices with genres as cultural products, linking forms of communication with their sociocultural contexts in regard to their users. The discursive turn in linguistics sees genres, like politeness, discursively constructed and not tied to individual linguistic items (see Jucker & Taavitsainen 2013: 9).

My study relies on a previous exploratory data-driven assessment based on selections from *Middle English Medical Texts* (MEMT) 1375–1500 (Taavitsainen, Pahta, & Mäkinen 2005) and *Early Modern English Medical Texts* (EMEMT) 1500–1700 (Taavitsainen et al. 2010; see Taavitsainen 2018, Taavitsainen & Schneider 2019). Our research questions focused on the distribution of stylistic features of scholasticism versus empiricism.

[9] Fowler (1982: 5) was the first to point out the advantages of the prototype approach (Rosch & Mervis 1975) to genre studies with Wittgenstein's terminology.

In order to define their most salient characteristics, we started by dividing our data into the medieval and the early modern groups according to external criteria of time and text participants' sociolinguistic parameters. The assessment of linguistic features was conducted using a Digital Humanities statistical method of Document Classification that sorts the linguistic features into two groups according to the above division and ranks them in order of importance.

This process indicates an array of positive (and negative) keywords in scholastic texts. Argumentation with *because*, *therefore*, and *wherefore* proved most important,[10] and next came deontic modality with the auxiliary *must* and phrasal verb (*take*) *heed*. Typically scholastic texts mention old authorities like Galen and Avicenna, and use logocentric verbs like *say* and *call*.[11] Topic words of the early period include *humour*, *sickness*, and *medicine*, and moral concerns occur with the dichotomy *evil* vs. *good*, *better*, and *best*. Early modern 'new-style' texts employ different devices with a more tentative mode of knowing, expressed using the auxiliaries *would* and *could*, the verb *seem*, and expressions like *perhaps* and *yet*. Keywords in empirical texts include *observation*, *account*, *found*, and *notice*. The qualitative analysis below is based on the results of this study.

Two of Bailey's books under scrutiny are basically regimen texts, one being a history of a drug, and another a herbal; all four volumes incorporate other genres like recipes and case studies, and features inherited from the commentary genre are present in each. All texts may be classified as 'learned professional writing'[12] and are written in the vernacular within the genre repertoire that was currently available. The commentary had been developed for research at medieval universities in examining old texts in search of the original meanings of ancient authors. The genre was well established in the thirteenth century in Latin, but it took centuries for it to become fully integrated into the vernacular. Earlier studies have shown that its genre features persisted long after the heyday of scholasticism (Taavitsainen & Schneider 2019). Commentary elements occur throughout Bailey's texts, and the first full commentary in English, to my knowledge, is among his achievements. The new thought style characteristic of empiricism is generally considered an innovation regulated from above

[10] This was a new discovery that had gone unnoticed before (Taavitsainen & Schneider 2019: 204–5). Among individual medieval texts, the highest frequency of *for whi* ('because') was found in the newly discovered late medieval Hippocratic commentary (Tavormina 2006).

[11] In an earlier qualitative study (Taavitsainen & Pahta 1998), it was the most conspicuous feature.

[12] In opposition to lay texts for heterogeneous audiences.

almost a century later by the Royal Society (RS), to accord with the declaration of the new, simpler style of writing science without scholastic 'amplifications, digressions, and swellings', with 'positive expressions', 'clear senses', and 'a native easiness'.[13] Seeds can be found in Bailey's text from 1587 (see below).

11.2 Walter Bailey's Medical Works, Their Genres and Text Types

Bailey's medical works were published within four years (1585–1588) and exhibit combinations of several genres. The superordinate term 'medical tract' applies to all, as it describes the main topic, whether medicine, healing method, medical herbs, or other health issues.[14] Bailey's texts use several genres in various combinations, starting from the top of the medieval genre hierarchy. Commentary texts are argumentative with a script that is recognisable by its sequence of sections (Minnis 1979: 397; Taavitsainen 2004: 40–2). In principle, a commentary could be imposed on any text. All texts in the present corpus of Bailey's works contain some elements of the classical pattern: the author shows his learnedness, but is keen to express his own opinion as well.[15] Recipes occur in three of the four texts, with instructions on how to make and use a medicine. The prototypical opening of a *recipe*, 'Take', or R [for Latin *recipe*] in Middle English, triggers expectations of a text belonging to a genre whose function is to instruct in preparing medicine, ink, or something else. Text type features include imperative forms of verbs, measurements, and an optional efficacy part realised in various ways. *Case reports* (also called *case studies* or *case histories*) narrate a patient's illness, treatment, and outcome. Other genres that rely on the narrative text type are *anecdotes* – that is, concise stories allegedly based on actual events – and there is also a passage with a *report* on Bailey's *experiments* with water that can be regarded as an early predecessor of a later RS genre. *Herbals* deal with plants and contain both descriptions according to humoral theory and instructions on how to use their healing power. *Regimen* texts give advice on diet, exercise, and healthy

[13] The lists come from Sprat (2003 [1667]) and the interpretation from Atkinson (1999: 16, 49 n. 3). Besides the *Philosophical Transactions*, the new style occurred in other contemporary medical and scientific writing by the members of the RS community.

[14] In addition, *Waters* overlaps in part with philosophical tracts that deal with issues of human existence.

[15] This is a distinguishing feature; the other typical scholastic genres of compilations, questions and answers, and didactic dialogues do not occur in Bailey's texts.

Table 11.1 *The composition of Bailey's texts of various genres*

Genre	*Mithridiatum*	*Eyesight*	*Waters*	*Peppers*
Anecdote	x			
Case report		x	x	
Commentary	x			x
Report on experiment			x	
Herbal	x			x
Recipes	x	x		x
Regimen		x	x	

Table 11.2 *The composition of Bailey's texts according to text types*

Text types[a]	*Mithridiatum*	*Eyesight*	*Waters*	*Peppers*
Argumentation	x	x		
Description				x
Instruction			x	
Narrative	x	x	x	x

[a]I did not detect expository passages.

living. Descriptive, narrative, argumentative, and instructive text types prevail in these texts. Tables 11.1 and 11.2 summarise Bailey's genres and text types with a model based on keeping the two apart.

These tables show how Bailey both makes use of old genres with long traditions and innovated a new style of reporting. He also combines two or more text types in all his works.

11.2.1 Mithridatium

The text relates an anecdote about an ancient antidote, but the main genre is a herbal 'declaring the firste beginning, the temperament, the noble virtues, and the true use of the same' (title line). The story line contains elements of a romance and overlaps with the literary genre, describing distant events happening to protagonists of high social standing. It follows natural narratives as defined on the basis of oral narratives of life-threatening events (see Labov & Waletsky 1967). Typically such narratives contain an abstract, a statement of orientation, followed by complications in action-recording sentences (in bold) and evaluation of why the story is interesting:[16]

(1) WEe doe read in ye Romaine histories, that Mithridates a Puisante king [. . .] **was assaulted** by Silla, **discomfited by** Lucullus, and **lastly vtterly vanquished** by Pompey the great: and when **this valiaunte king perceiued himselfe to be ouercome**, [. . .] : **first he destroyde his wyfe & daughters with poyson, and then tooke the same poyson,** desiring rather so to dye, then as a captiue to fal into ye hands of his enemyes: **But hauing dronken much of the poyson, could not dye therewith**, and then **caused his seruant** Bistocus [. . .] **to kill him** with a sword.

For **this noble king was** [. . .] also in phisicall matters **very expert, had the knowledg of many hearbes**, and **making tryall of sundry simples** that doe resist poyson in men condemned to dye, **as Galen writeth in his first booke de Antidotis**, [. . .] a mixture of diuerse simples, hoping thereby to haue **a ready remedy against all kindes of poison,** & the same was **termed after his name Mithridatium**: [. . .]. (Bailey 1585: f. A2r–2v; all emphases in the examples are mine)

The coda marks a transfer to the main medical topic. The text unfolds in sequences organised according to the commentary script. The author summarises earlier texts and concludes with his own opinion, according to the commentary tradition, with deontic modality and absolute certainty:

(2) And *it is to be noted*, that where **all writers doe greately co~mend** it, yet *certayne it is*, that they do not in one sorte describe the makinge of the same. But almost **euery authore hath a seuerall description, differinge** in the number of the simples, and also in y^e^ proportions and quantities. [. . .]**In time past** y=e= Apothecaries in making of Mithridatium, folowed most the description of **Nicolaus Prepositus, of Auicenna, and of Nicolaus Mirepsicus, some of Ætius**, **some of Paulus**. [. . .] Wherefore **in these our later daies**, in which learned men haue examined euery thing perfitly, the most part haue commended one of ye three [. . .] **by Galen in 2. de Antid**. of the which, two were taken (**as Galen wryteth**) out of the bookes of Andromachus. [. . .] **Wherefore we may reasonably conclude, that**

[16] See Toolan (2001) and Fludernik (1996); for an analysis of narratives in medical texts between 1375 and 1700, see Taavitsainen (2011).

the first recept transcribed by Galen in 2. de Antid. out of Andromachus workes, is *in truth* **the selfe same that Mithridates vsed, and in mine opinion, in that respect the better to be liked, and the rather to be followed**. (Bailey 1585: f. B1r–v).

Recipes are embedded in a concise and learned form with a long list of ingredients and measures in Latin abbreviations, giving further evidence of the intended target group of professional readers: 'Rec. glicirrizæ +Q vij. ob. iiij. Spicæ nardi +Q vij. ob. iij.' (Bailey 1585: f. B2v). However, the efficacy of the antidote is assured in terms of universal truths.[17]

11.2.2 Eyesight

The full title 'the preservation of the eye-sight' reveals that the text belongs to the regimen genre focusing on preventive medicine, 'partly in good order of diet, partly in vse of Medicines' (titlepage). Food is divided into favourable or harmful, often with further specifications and more precise information. Advice for choosing healthy sites for habitation is given in regard to air and winds, as was customary in regimen texts (see Wear 2000: 157–209):

(3) Concerning diet: some **things hurtfull are to be eschued**, and some **things comfortable to the sight** are **to be vsed**: wherefore they, which may chose their habitations [. . .]: cold and moyst **aire**, and thicke, misty, and rainy weather is **hurtfull: it is best therefore** to abide in dry places, [. . .]: Southerne **windes** doe hurt the sight: [. . .]. (Bailey 1616 [1586]: 1–2)

Advice for diet is otherwise traditional, except for specifications according to the social classes: 'the better sort' has its own diet, while common people may not choose:

(4) [. . .] a young Henne **is greatly commended**: so is Partridge and Pheasant: **Rasis praiseth** the young starne, and the quaile: [. . .] (as **Zoar writeth**). Of small birdes, [. . .] are noted very hurtfull to the sight: and **albeit these birds are seldome, or not at all vsed of the better sort, yet common people happily may be compelled to eate them**. (Bailey 1616 [1586]: 2)

[17] '[. . .] from **all the world in all ages and times'** (f. A 3v), 'for **all men doe know** [. . .]' (f. 3v), 'It is of **all men of our age** co*n*fessed, and taken for a truth [. . .]' (f. B 4v). Such comments are more frequent in texts for heterogeneous audiences. Anecdotes had a wide appeal as well.

Once the author inserts an ironical comment: 'our authors herein are very ingenious, some addressing drinkes with one thing, and some with another' (Bailey 1616 [1586]: 6).[18]

It was customary to add efficacy statements of varying scope to case reports and recipes to convince the readers. The author explains that he has witnessed that '**many** [. . .] **haue found** great good for their sight, not onely to continue in good estate, but also [. . .] **remedie against the dimnes and other impediments**' (Bailey 1616 [1586]: 10), thus expanding the cure to apply to several cases. Short narratives assure the efficacy, for instance '**One** (saith he) which was **blind**, and did see nothing in long time, **by vsing this wine** one yeare, **was restored to his sight**' (Bailey 1616 [1586]: 6–7). A longer passage with multiple cases of efficacy begins with a typical story-telling opening. The first enhances its credibility by orientation with facts, including the location and the name and age of the protagonist, the second uses a list of dignitaries to convince the readers; this device is also used in *Philosophical Transactions* (1665–) experimental reports:

(5) *In truth* **once I met an old man in Shropshire, called M. Hoorde, aboue the age of 84. yeares**, who had at that time perfit sight, and did read small letters very well without spectacles: **hee told me** that about the age of 40. yeares, finding his sight to decay, **he did vse Eiebright** in ale for his drinke, and did also eate the powder thereof **in an egge** three daies in a weeke, being so taught of his father, who by the like order **continued his sight in good integrity to a very long age. I haue heard the same confirmed by many old men.** [. . .]

Rowland Sherlooke an Irish man, **Phisition to Queene Marie**, **did affirme for truth**, that **a Bishop in Ireland perceiuing his sight to wax dimme**, about his age of fifty yeare, by **the vse of eiebright take~ in powder in an egge**, did liue to the age of 80 yeares, **with good integrity of sight**. (Bailey 1616 [1586]: 11–12)

Recipes are included in the traditional form with the imperative as the genre signal (Bailey 1616 [1586]: 22), or more indirectly with a paraphrase and infinitive forms that render the tone prescriptive: 'Montagnana doth mention certaine kind of preparation [. . .] **to take** the iuce of fennell [. . .] and **to put** it [. . .]'. A reward is promised at the end: 'hold this for a secret as miraculous to preserue the sight' (Bailey 1616 [1586]: 19).

[18] This is unusual. A sixteenth-century master of irony was William Bullein (c. 1515–1576), but otherwise this feature becomes common only later in eighteenth-century texts (e.g. Taavitsainen 2020: 143, 145).

11.2.3 Waters

This regimen text instructs on how to use the waters of local wells. The approach is analytical, with the geographical focus on the English climate and soil:

(6) For we find that where **many writers in ancient time** haue largely discoursed of sundrie **bathes in Italie**, [. . .] but that **in this our time later writers do disallow of many positions of the former authors**, and brag of better explanations [. . .] **Therefore** let it not be accounted strange if **learned men do differ in** opinion in consideration of these Warwickshire so late knowen bathes [. . .]. (Bailey 1587: 9)

The text develops into a philosophical tract dealing with human existence and probing into old authorities' sayings with appreciation in places: 'It is well and trulie said, and vpon very sufficient ground & reason, by Aristotle, the *chiefest* learned of the heathen Philosophers [. . .]' (Bailey 1587: 1; emphasis original). But elsewhere, criticism of authorities, in line with the empirical thought style of the text, generally prevails.

Interestingly, this text also contains discourse that predates the advent of the new science in *Philosophical Transactions* by three-quarters of a century, resembling experimental reports with their first-person narration in the past tense and a tentative mode of knowing (see Gotti 2011). The quotation at the beginning of this chapter precedes the following passage that exhibits such features. The author is the acting agent and records his observations considering various possibilities:

(7) [. . .] For the better discouerie of the secret faculties of these waters, **I have taken** certaine quantities of them, and **distilled** them: **I have** likewise **examined** them by filterings and euaporations, and haue alwaie **obserued and found,** in the end after perfect separation of all the waterish parts, that there remaineth a certaine residence [. . .] (*Waters*: 10)

I haue also farther probabilitie heereof, [. . .] **for it is ordinarily obserued** [. . .] **But bicause** it is the propertie of salt **in colour whitish**, and in **taste** somewhat salt **which being put upon a glowing hot iron, doth foorthwith become clearer and whiter** [. . .] **I would thinke it more probable** to refer it vnto Niter, than vnto salt, for that **I haue often noted** it to haue greater acrimonie [. . .]. (Bailey 1587: 11)

But besides all these probabilities I am the rather induced to credite, that this mettall hath place in these waters, for that the vse of them **is daily seene** to be very profitable in affects of the Splene, Reines, and Bladder; **for I myselfe being there present, am an eie witnes** [. . .]. (Bailey 1587: 12)

The old prescriptive mode of writing surfaces again a couple of pages later. Bailey returns to the scholastic mode and, after pondering the matter in a lengthy passage, gives his own opinion:

(8) Therefore it shal not be amisse to mention som conuenient **rules and orders** for the vse of these Bathes, **according to the precepts of our ancient writers, set down to be observed** [. . .] First therfore that we may better knowe [. . .] **as *Fallop*[19] noteth in his booke** *de aquis medicalis* [. . .] **are to be obserued** [. . .]. (Bailey 1587: 16)

I am not ignorant that [. . .] **the learned do dispute** whether [. . .] for that **our authors heerin haue written diuersly, and pronounced contrary opinions**, it seemeth to me not necessaie by long discourse heerof, to detaine the reader: **onely this I say, as I do not thinke** but medicinall waters may be vsed in leape yeares [. . .] **It is an olde obseruation** [. . .] **whereby we are to think for my part I would not rashly cousel** [. . .] Much more then, **we ought to be carefull heereof** [. . .]. (Bailey 1587: 20–1)

The precise location of the fountain is recorded in a case report. The protagonist is introduced as 'a certaine husbandman' and the events follow in chronological order, as in natural narratives. At the end, the significance of the miraculous healings is pointed out:

(9) For it hapned not long since **in Warwickshire, neer vnto a Village called *Newnam Regis*,** that **a certaine husbandman** occupied in lopping of trees, **chaunced to receiue a greeuous would** in his hand, wherupon he repaired presently to a **fountain** which was not far off: **after he had washed and clensed the wound very well** with the water, **he** presently **found all pains of his hurt aswaged, and** in short time **the wounde thoroughly closed & healed**, [. . .] after **another hauing a deepe wound** [. . .] **came to the same fountaine & recouered & was made hole onely with the lotion of the same water**. These and such rare cures [. . .] **many received helpe** of their infirmities, **as is verefied by the testimonies of the worshipfull** [. . .] the same heerof **confirmed now by** often **experience** [. . .]. (Bailey 1587: 3–4).

[19] Gabriel Fallopius (1523–1562) was an Italian anatomist who collaborated with Vesalius in Padova.

11.2.4 Peppers

This text showcases ongoing changes in worldview and thought styles, with emphasis on the contrast between eye-witness testimonies and book wisdom. The text is composed of multiple genres in an unusual combination. The base text is a herbal. Definition of the subject matter is given in terms of language by naming the plant in different languages, in Greek, Latin, and Arabic, as was customary in scholastic texts (Taavitsainen 2002: 209; cf. McConchie & Curzan 2011: 83). The contents of the tract deal mostly with properties of the plants under scrutiny according to the humoral theory with its traditional attributes. Accurate qualities and precise source references are applied throughout:

(10) **DIoscorides and Galen** do yeeld to all the kinds of pepper a faculty to heat and to drie, but neither of them do declare in **what degree they do heate and drie**. After that **Auerrhois in lib. Simplic.** had pronounced long pepper to be moister than the other: And that white pepper was not come to his ripenes, and that black pepper was full ripe: **He concludeth both kinds to be hot in the third degree**, and as **some say in the fourth degree. Auicen in lib. 2. tract. 2.** intreating of white and blacke pepper generally, affirmeth pepper to be **hot and drie tending toward the fourth degree**. [. . .] of long pepper, he writeth that it is **hot in the third degree, and drie in the second**. [. . .] (Bailey 1588: f. B2v–3r)

In line with the empirical thought style, sensory observations by taste are also mentioned (see Example 7). At some places instruction takes over, with guidance by prescriptive phrases and imperative forms of verbs:

(11) [. . .] some do not like of sweet things, and do abhor honie, to such **you must put** the lesse honie, [. . .] **it is good to boile** good store of honie, **so you boile it well**, for then the medicine will not be ouersweet, [. . .] And **you may vse** this medicine [. . .], and **you may put** of it in a Ptisane in steede of pepper. (Bailey 1588: f. C6r)

The genre script of recipes is present in a very concise but well-developed form. It adheres to the genre script with the imperative *Take*, followed by ingredients and measurements:

(12) **Take** of calamints organie, seselios blacke pepper petroselini of ech +Q .iij. +q .ij. leuistici. +Q .ij. +q .j. persley seede +q .j. ammy seede thime, annise seede cinnamon, ginger. of ech +q .ij. (Bailey 1588: f. C1r)

An account of earlier authors' different versions of the ingredients and measures follows with the author's own comments:

(13) In this composition, persley seeds, ammy, annise seedes, ginger, are mo then are set in the description of **Galen**. Some learned men of our time do commend this receit of **Nicolaus** before that of **Galen**, **bicause** it hath mo simples: **but for my part, I do rather allow of that receit of Galen**, [...], it receiueth a sufficient number of simples, so that they which are inserted by **Nicolaus** seeme superfluous. (Bailey 1588: f. C1r)

At the end the author summarises the views and expresses his own opinion, making the text into a fully fledged commentary. The reader is addressed by the inclusive *we*, the deictic pronoun *you*, and the time deixis *our time*. An announcement of where the medicine can be purchased follows:

(14) And where **our authors do differ in opinion,** what is the right Amomum, **and all writers do agree,** that *we* have the right ammi: **I adiuge it better** in these daies to put in this receipt the seeds of ammi, according **as Galen prescribeth**, than amomum, **as Mesue counselleth**. So *you* haue both medicines in vse *in our time* made of three peppers, and are to be sold in the Apothecaries shope, vnder the name of Diatrion pipereon. (Bailey 1588: ff. B7v–8r)

Argumentation is the main text type in *Peppers*, but technical descriptions according to humoral theory are comprehensive. In addition, there is a descriptive passage explaining what these foreign plants look like with reference to the domestic realm:

(15) [...] are not trees of any bignes, but **weake shrubs**, which do **clime vp by other trees, as an Iuie doth in this our countrie**. And haue **leaues like to the apple tree** called Malum Assyrium, and do carrie their **fruit in clusters, like** the clusters of **grapes of vine trees** [...]. (Bailey 1588: f. A5v–6r)

11.3 Summary of Linguistic Features

The co-existence of old and new stylistic features in the above texts gives firm evidence in support of my hypothesis. The variationist approach can fruitfully be applied to discourse features in medical and scientific texts as well as to their underlying thought styles.

11.3.1 Scholastic Features in Bailey's Texts

According to the hierarchy of scholastic features, the most salient pattern of argumentation used is the complementiser *because*. This feature occurs in all four texts, but most clearly in *Mithridatium:*

(16) It followeth, that if [. . .], it **must** remedy such as haue taken poison into the body. And **because** co~mon persons haue not like oportunity to make **this experiment** in men co~demned, as princes haue: **therefore we may** in other beasts (as in dogs, in cokes and hennes, being domesticall creatures) experience the same, geuing to these beasts some poison, and after Mithridatium: **and if** the beast doe take no harme by the poison, **we may be assured** of the goodnesse of the medicine. (Bailey 1585: f. C4v)

Instances of the pattern in other texts include '**because the visible vertue being** coacted and [. . .] but **bicause** the heate of his biting [. . .], **therefore it seemeth** not so hot' (Bailey 1588: f. B3v–4r). Certainty as the mode of knowing was next in importance. It is expressed by verbs like *must* and *shall*, phrasal verbs like *take heed*, and other prescriptive expressions, and commonly emphasised with adverbs like *needs*, *truly*, *forsoth*, and *sothely*, and adjectives like *certain.*[20] Again, the classical pattern is found in *Mithridatium*: 'So **it must needes follow**' (Bailey 1585: f. B4v), 'But *certaine it is*, that' (Bailey 1585: f. B5v), '[. . .] it **must be remembred**, that *it is certayn*' (Bailey 1585: f. A7v), but also in *Eyesight*: 'And he that will continue his sight good, **must be carefull** of ouer-plentifull feeding, and **therefore must end** his meales with appetite' (Bailey 1616 [1586]: 15). *Peppers* abounds in authoritative commands as well: 'Here **it is to be noted** [. . .]' (Bailey 1588: f. A 4r), '[. . .] **it is to be understood**' (Bailey 1588: f. 4v), '**we must** undertand [. . .]' (Bailey 1588: f. A 5r), '**it must be taken** often' (Bailey 1588: f. C5v); '*it is certaine* [. . .]' (Bailey 1588: f. A6r).

Interestingly, *Waters* (Bailey 1587: 27–8) combines the scholastic way of arguing with the new source of knowledge, observation: '[. . .] but **because** I haue **obserued** [. . .] my advice is [. . .]' and prescriptive phrases like '**we must** imagine' (Bailey 1587: 5) and 'we **are to observe** [. . .]' (Bailey 1587: 18). The tone is, however, somewhat different, showing a cautious attitude to knowledge and leaving implicit room for doubt, for instance 'It is well and **trulie said vpon very sufficient ground and reason**, [. . .]' (Bailey

[20] This feature was ranked lower, after moral concerns, and another feature that surfaces only in herbals in this assessment, i.e. humoral theory.

1587: 1) and the first-person expression with a mental verb, 'I **do not doubt** [. . .]' (Bailey 1587: 16).

A very conspicuous feature of scholasticism is the reliance on wisdom inherited from ancient authorities like Galen, Avicenna, Hippocrates, Aristotle, and others. The references are usually precise in Bailey's texts with the original location; this is a distinguishing feature of learned texts, in contrast to general statements in writings for heterogeneous audiences (Taavitsainen & Pahta 1998), for example '**Galen in his first booke de Antidot**. writeth [. . .] The same **Galen in 2. de Antidot.**' (Bailey 1585: f. A5v–6r) and '**The precept of Plato in Charmide**' (Bailey 1616 [1586]: 34). Logocentric verbs like *say* and *call* are often present, emphasising the hearsay aspects, and other reporting verbs occur as well.

In addition to ancient authorities, Bailey refers to contemporary learned doctors. He gives tribute to ancient authors in *Waters*, but cites a sixteenth-century German scholar as the source of the reference: 'It is well and trulie said, and vpon very sufficient ground & reason, by ***Aristotle*** the **chiefest learned of all heathen Philosophers** [. . .] as ***Schegkius***[21] reporteth [. . .]' (Bailey 1587: 1–2), showing his knowledge of recent continental literature.

11.3.2 Predecessors of the Empirical Thought Style of Writing Science

Observation is advocated as the source of knowledge in *Peppers*, where utmost authority is granted to a contemporary Portuguese botanist, 'Garcia, who liued in these parts' and whose writings proved that Dioscorides had been wrong (Bailey 1588: f. A6r).[22] The new style of writing uses first-person narration in reporting the process of experimentation, but in a very different way from its old use, for instance by John Arderne who boasts with his own knowledge, skill, and experience.[23] In contrast, the early modern experimental reports show low modality in first-person narratives. Typical expressions include modal verbs *would* and *could*, and hedges like *seemed*, *perhaps*, and *maybe*, and the author does not claim that his results are conclusive.[24] The new stance is mediated, for example in a modesty claim that almost counts as an apology:

[21] Jacobus Schegkius (Jacob Shegh; 1511–1589) was a German natural philosopher and medical doctor.

[22] Garcia d'Orta (or da Orta) 1501?–1568 was a Portuguese physician and botanist, best known as a pioneer of tropical medicine.

[23] John Arderne's late fourteenth-century *Surgery* contains several case studies with first-person narration, praising the fame and honour that he received throughout the country.

[24] Bailey also mentions probabilities, which is rare in medical texts before the eighteenth century.

(17) **I trust** men in this our time will not take occasion to carpe and reprehend my labors, **if I now in this discourse hap to pronounce** of these late inuented fountains, **assertions contrary to some others opinions, or** if I shall not now in this little pamphlet **sufficiently explane the true minerals of these bathes, or** else shall with some shew of **probabilitie** establish some thing **which herafter may be fou*n*d otherwise.** (Bailey 1587: 8–9)

11.4 Conclusions

The aim of this chapter has been to provide a detailed qualitative assessment with glimpses of changing thought styles in Walter Bailey's medical texts. As a highly educated medical doctor, Bailey was a keen observer and was familiar with pioneering continental authors, like de Acosta and Garcia. He was an exceptionally skilled stylistic virtuoso who could promote his goals by innovation and by applying old models. A special point of interest dealt with features derived from scholastic patterns of argumentation. These features are present in abundance in all his texts, and he brought the old genre script of the commentary to a new perfection in the vernacular as late as in 1588. This is somewhat surprising, as at the same time he expresses doubt about inherited wisdom. A new way of writing emerges in his report on empirical experiments in *Waters*.

Bailey gives us convincing evidence of the onset of the transition period by juxtaposing old and new ideas, combining the old with the new ways of thinking. He demonstrates his skill both in following the genre script of top scholasticism and in relying on experimentation instead of hearsay; for him the anecdotes about the healing power of Warwickshire wells served as a trigger for probing into the causes, showing qualities of curiosity and inquisitiveness that are typically attributed to seventeenth-century scientists. *Waters* is by far the most innovative text in the present data: first-hand evidence by observation is enhanced, and the results are presented as tentative. Furthermore, this innovative report is written in a new style, anticipating the RS way of doing and writing science. The new mode of knowing surfaces at places where observation of nature is preferred to book wisdom. Throughout his literary output, the author includes precise sources to his references. In all, this combination provides a demonstration of the variationist hypothesis of change in action. Even small details work in the same direction: a logocentric definition lists names in various languages, whereas specifying leaf forms and ways of growing belong to the new thought style.

It is obvious that Bailey was conscious of the changing premises of knowledge. He belonged to the learned elite of his medical profession and followed the writings of his peers on the European continent. He was not alone in showing doubt and breaking away from reliance on inherited wisdom (cf. de Acosta and Garcia). In addition, he discussed empirical experimentation in *Waters* as the way of achieving new knowledge and he relied on observation for his conclusions. From the variationist viewpoint, the combination is significant, and shows the mechanism of change on the ideological level in action.

REFERENCES

de Acosta, Joseph. 1604. *The naturall and morall historie of the East and West Indies*. Translated into English by E. G. London. Retrieved from EEBO.

Atkinson, Dwight. 1999. *Scientific discourse in sociohistorical context: The* Philosophical Transactions of the Royal Society of London, *1675–1975*. Mahwah, NJ: Lawrence Erlbaum.

Bailey, Walter. 1585. *A discovrse of the medicine called Mithridatium*. EMEMT.

Bailey, Walter. 1616 [1586]. *A brief treatise touching the preservation of the eyesight*. EMEMT.

Bailey [Baley], Walter. 1587. *A brief discourse of certain bathes of medicinal waters*. London: no publisher. Retrieved from EEBO.

Bailey, Walter. 1588. *Account on the three kinds of pepper, a short discourse of the three kindes of peppers*. EMEMT.

Bakewell, Sarah. 2004. Bayley, Walter (1529–1593). *Oxford Dictionary of National Biography*. https://doi.org/10.1093/ref:odnb/1757.

Biber, Douglas. 1988. *Variation across speech and writing*. Cambridge: Cambridge University Press.

Crombie, Alistair Cameron. 1994. *Styles of scientific thinking in the European tradition*. 3 vols. London: Duckworth.

Fludernik, Monika. 1996. *Towards a 'natural' narratology*. London: Routledge.

Fowler, Alastair. 1982. *Kinds of literature: An introduction to the theory of genres and modes*. Oxford: Clarendon Press.

Gotti, Maurizio. 2011. The development of specialized discourse in the Philosophical Transactions. In Irma Taavitsainen & Päivi Pahta (eds.), *Medical writing in Early Modern English*, 204–20. Cambridge: Cambridge University Press.

Jucker, Andreas H., & Irma Taavitsainen. 2013. *English historical pragmatics*. Edinburgh: Edinburgh University Press.

Labov, William, & Joshua Waletsky. 1967. Narrative analysis: Oral versions of personal experience. In June Helm (ed.), *Essays on the verbal and visual arts: Proceedings of the annual 1966 spring meeting of the American Ethnological Society*, 12–44. Seattle: American Ethnological Society. Rpt. in *Journal of Narrative and Life History* 7(1–4): 3–38.

McConchie, Rod, & Anne Curzan. 2011. Defining in Early Modern English medical texts. In Irma Taavitsainen & Päivi Pahta (eds.), *Medical writing in Early Modern English*, 74–93. Cambridge: Cambridge University Press.

McIntyre, Dan, & Beatrix Busse. 2010. *Language and style*. Basingstoke: Palgrave Macmillan.

Milroy, James. 1972. Linguistic variation and change. Oxford: Blackwell.

Minnis, Alastair. 1979. Late medieval discussions of *compilation* and the role of the *compilator*. *Beiträge zur Geschichte der Deutschen Sprache und Literatur* 101: 385–421.

Paltridge, Brian. 1997. *Genre, frames and writing in research settings*. Amsterdam: Benjamins.

Porter, Roy. 2000. *Enlightenment*. London: Penguin.

Rosch, Eleanor, & Carolyn B. Mervis. 1975. Family resemblances: Studies in the internal structure of categories. *Cognitive Psychology* 7(4): 573– 605.

Shapin, Simon. 1996. *The scientific revolution*. Chicago: University of Chicago Press.

Spencer-Oatey, Helen. 2000. *Culturally speaking*. London: Continuum.

Sprat, Thomas. 2003 [1667]. *The history of the Royal Society of London, for the improving of natural knowledge*. Whitefish, MT: Kessinger.

Taavitsainen, Irma. 2001. Changing conventions of writing: The dynamics of genres, text types, and text traditions. *European Journal of English Studies* (special issue, ed. Lilo Moessner), 5(2): 139–50.

Taavitsainen, Irma. 2002. Historical discourse analysis: Scientific language and changing thought-styles. In Teresa Fanego, Bélén Méndez-Naya, & Elena Seone, *Sounds, words, texts and change*, 201–26. Amsterdam: Benjamins.

Taavitsainen, Irma. 2004. Transferring classical discourse conventions into the vernacular. In Irma Taavitsainen & Päivi Pahta (eds.), *Medical and scientific writing in Late Medieval English*, 37–72. Cambridge: Cambridge University Press.

Taavitsainen, Irma. 2009. *The pragmatics of knowledge and meaning: Corpus linguistic approaches to changing thought-styles in early modern medical discourse.* In Andreas H. Jucker, Danny Schreier, & Marianne Hundt (eds.), *Corpora: Pragmatics and discourse*, 37–62. Amsterdam: Rodopi.

Taavitsainen, Irma. 2011. Narratives as literary commonplaces in late medieval and early modern medical writing. In Greta Olson (ed.), *Current trends in narratology*, 254–73. Berlin; New York: Mouton de Gruyter.

Taavitsainen, Irma. 2018. Scholastic genre scripts in English medical writing 1375–1800. In Richard J. Whitt (ed.), *Diachronic corpora, genre, and language change*, 95–115. Amsterdam: Benjamins.

Taavitsainen, Irma. 2020. A medical debate of 'heated pamphleteering' in the early eighteenth century. In Andreas H. Jucker & Irma Taavitsainen (eds.), *Manners, norms and transgressions in the history of English: Literary and linguistic approaches*, 141–63. Amsterdam: Benjamins.

Taavitsainen, Irma, & Päivi Pahta. 1998. Vernacularisation of medical writing in English: A corpus-based study of scholasticism. *Early Science and Medicine* 3 (2): 157–85.

Taavitsainen, Irma, Päivi Pahta, Turo Hiltunen, Martti Mäkinen, Ville Marttila, Maura Ratia, Carla Suhr, & Jukka Tyrkkö (eds.). *Early Modern English Medical Texts 1500–1700* (EMEMT). 2010. CD-Rom. Amsterdam: Benjamins.

Taavitsainen, Irma, Päivi Pahta, & Martti Mäkinen (eds.). *Middle English Medical Texts 1375–1500* (MEMT). 2005. CD-Rom. Amsterdam: Benjamins.

Taavitsainen, Irma, & Gerold Schneider. 2019. Scholastic argumentation in early English medical writing and its afterlife: New corpus evidence. In Carla Suhr, Terttu Nevalainen, & Irma Taavitsainen (eds.), *From data to evidence in English language research*, 191–221. Leiden: Brill.

Tavormina, M. Teresa (ed.). 2006. *MS Trinity College Cambridge R.14.52: A medieval medical manuscript, its language and scribe*. Tempe: Arizona Center for Medieval and Renaissance Studies.

Toolan, Michael. 2001 [1988]. *Narrative: A critical linguistic approach*. London: Routledge.

Trevelyan, G. M. 1967 [1942]. *English social history*. Harmondsworth: Pelican.

Wear, Andrew. 2000. *Knowledge and practice in English medicine, 1550–1680*. Cambridge: Cambridge University Press.

Werlich, Egon. 1976. *A text grammar of English*. Heidelberg: Quelle and Meyer.

Werlich, Egon. 1982. *A text grammar of English*. 2nd ed. Heidelberg: Quelle & Meyer.

CHAPTER 12

London Bills of Mortality of the Seventeenth Century

Maura Ratia

The significance of the early modern bills of mortality for the development of demographic studies and for the earliest English vital statistics has long been acknowledged. For contemporaries, bills of mortality had a variety of uses and functions: originally printed as reports for government use, they quickly began to interest citizens as well, and turned into commercial publications. Slauter (2011: 1) argues that these bills of mortality gave rise to a new type of 'news consciousness', as the earliest known periodicals in England providing current and potentially life-saving information for their readers. They were meticulously studied by the rich to decide whether to leave the city, stay, or perhaps return. If a given parish had even one plague burial during that week, obtaining health certificates for travel was not possible. Financial concerns were also evident as, for instance, playhouses could be reopened only after the weekly number of plague victims had decreased to under 30 (Munkhoff 1999: 4). This is not, however, the whole picture, and the genre had other functions as well, such as giving religious guidance and even medical advice.

Jenner argues that bills of mortality have been neglected by historians possibly because of their focus on numerical data, although as an inexpensive and maybe even the most common type of plague writing during the 'visitations', they were very influential (2012: 255; see also Sullivan 2011: 76). Some of their functions have been identified in previous studies, but systematic analysis of the genre combining both textual and visual features has been lacking.

In this chapter, I focus on a description of the bills of mortality genre and the changes it underwent in the seventeenth century. In addition to providing statistical data, the genre shared similarities with other genres of plague writing by including remedies and prayers on the page, which was typical of plague treatises of the time (see Ratia 2013). Figures of angels or a *memento mori* could also be found in the margins of tabulated data. The format and typographical conventions of the bills require further scrutiny, as they differ greatly from other genres of plague writing and medical writing in general. The broadsheet as a mode of communication was often reserved for ephemeral topics, and the idea was to give the readers as much up-to-date information in a nutshell as possible. This study will try to account for these numerous and, at times, conflicting functions to give an overview of the genre. The analysis of discourse is accompanied by an analysis of layout and typographical features, showing that in the seventeenth century the genre developed and became more complex in order to accommodate to the changing environment caused by the frequent and severe outbreaks of the plague.

12.1 Background

As a genre, the bill of mortality is a difficult one to tackle. For the present-day reader, what catches the eye is the amount of information barely fitting on a sheet of paper. The printed text and the numbers on the page are so small that they need to be perused closely. The contemporary reader might have also struggled with the use of Roman type instead of blackletter, which suggests that although the contents would surely interest everyone, the readership excluded those with only rudimentary reading skills (Jenner 2012: 261). Later these bills of mortality were compiled together to create a more easily digestible product: a work where the larger trends and developments in the prevalence of certain diseases could be assessed and predicted.[1] For the authorities, bills of mortality were valuable tools in deciding what measures should be taken to respond (Munkhoff 1999: 4). For the public, the contents could mean the difference between life and death.

The role of the plague in the birth and development of the genre is important (Sullivan 2011: 77–8). Contemporary references exist to record-keeping already from the first half of the sixteenth century (Sullivan 2011: 77). Munkhoff (1999: 4–6) claims that the first bills of mortality proper were compiled under the reign of Henry VIII during the years of great mortality, and the main function then was to separate the numbers of plague victims from other deaths. Later, during the 1593 epidemic, London bills of mortality began to be published weekly.

By 1603, bills of mortality were 'subsidized by the city government, printed in considerable numbers by an official printer, and sold for a penny

[1] The recurring outbreaks of the plague in the course of the seventeenth century created the need for the compilations of bills of mortality.

at the bookstalls in the churchyard of the old St. Paul's Cathedral as elsewhere in London' (Greenberg 2004: 510; see also Slauter 2011: 6). It has been claimed that the first surviving printed bills are from this year (Greenberg 2004; Sullivan 2011; Jenner 2012). This probably refers to the more familiar single-sheet format as, for example, *Early English Books Online* (EEBO; http://eebo.chadwyck.com) has a copy from as early as 1582 of a text titled 'The number of all those that hath dyed in the Citie of London & the liberties of the same . . .', containing alphabetical lists of parishes with their diseased and plague victims (Anon. 1582). The numerical data stretches loosely over eight pages, followed by a brief justification of the importance of the data and the total numbers for the earlier epidemic of 1562–1563.[2] The later bills did not have to justify themselves and the weekly numbers of the diseased were printed with a much tighter layout, spread on one sheet, which essentially changed the nature of the text.

Jenner (2012: 262) argues that these official bills by the Company of Parish Clerks were transformed into something else in the hands of anonymous authors coming 'from the literary demi-monde of hack writers'. The statistical data was supplemented by other content derived from more serious works, such as medical treatises, and prayers were taken from contemporary sermons. The whole visual of the broadsheets including woodcuts and death-related imagery was equally important, as Jenner (2012) has shown.

The best-known publication among bills of mortality is John Graunt's compilation work *Observations Made upon the Bills of Mortality* of 1662, which has been claimed to signal the beginning for modern-day vital statistics (see Buck 1977; Greenberg 2004, 1997; Slauter 2011: 2). Compiling together annual bills and data from different parishes, Graunt tried to find patterns to see how the structure of the population developed.

The bills provided a wealth of information to Londoners to know which areas to avoid or whether to flee the city, if they could afford it, by performing 'an anatomy of London' (Stage 2011: 59). Whether the numbers contained in the bills factually reflected the reality is another issue. The information was gathered by employing so-called searchers, often older women, who inspected bodies for signs of plague in order to

[2] The bibliographic information provided by EEBO states that 'This is not an official bill, and the work of which it is a section has not been identified. It is probably based on information gathered by John Stow–STC.'

determine the cause of death (Munkhoff 1999).[3] The numbers were related orally or on paper to parish clerks, registered, and finally compiled by city clerks and published into bills of mortality (Slauter 2011: 10).

The content of these bills was, for reasons of life and death, of the highest importance for readers. However, the visual features, the layout, were also crucial in directing the readers' attention. In the study of seventeenth-century title pages, the first half of the century regarded visual aspects as primary and verbal secondary (Suhr 2011: 126). This meant that creating a certain visual effect, such as a triangle shape in the title or the running text, could even break up words in the middle (Claridge 2013). Only in the latter half of the seventeenth century did titles become more descriptive, and authors become more involved in the process of naming their texts, which had previously often been the responsibility of the editor (Shevlin 1999; McConchie 2013; see Suhr 2011: 125). In my study of title pages of plague treatises, the emphasis on the visual instead of the verbal was still retained during the period of 1603–1666 (Ratia 2013; Ratia & Suhr 2017; see also Shevlin 1999).

Bills of mortality reflect both single-sheet medical adverts and prayer broadsheets (Jenner 2012: 261; see also Watt 1991: 227–9). Medical adverts of the time have been dubbed 'early modern infomercials', as they were read aloud on street corners and thus even reached the uneducated masses (Fissell 2007: 120, 126; see also Chapter 13 in this volume). The bills of mortality also contained medical recipes, prayers, and religious guidance. Ritual healing, where prayers or charms and spells were used to accompany the medicine, was based in the medieval belief of the healing power of the Church. The idea that it was wrong to solely rely on the power of natural remedies, ignoring the role of God, entailed that 'a prayer was always appropriate' (Thomas 1973: 210, 227; see Pahta & Ratia 2010: 99).

Many of these texts have a strong religious undertone, as the outbreaks of the plague epidemic were seen as a punishment for sin. The idea of divine providence advocated by the clergy and theologians was, in general, readily accepted when it came to epidemics and venereal diseases up until the late seventeenth century:

> But howsoeuer God striketh whom he will unmodiatly, yet the Plague being contagious in it owne nature, it cannot be denied, but that one man may be infected by another, except Gods prouidence be to the contrary? (Balmford 1603: 66)

[3] Evidence of employing searchers dates back to at least 1574. Refusing to accept the job, if appointed, resulted in losing one's pension (Munkhoff 1999: 1–2; Slauter 2011: 9).

The plague, especially when affecting whole communities, was seen as a punishment for the sins of the community (see the discussion in Thomas 1973: 90–132). Furthermore, the epidemics in England in 1603 and 1625 coincided with a change of monarch and, at the time, were interpreted as 'a need for the population to be purged of the sins of the previous reign' (Porter 2009: 11). The numbers of the diseased from the plague, therefore, created what was called God's 'Arithmetick', a term used by Dekker in *A rod for run-awayes* (1625: B4r; see Munkhoff 1999: 8).

12.2 Materials and Method

The material, London bills of mortality covering plague epidemics, printed from 1603 to 1666, was selected based on the availability of the texts on EEBO. The bills, listed in Table 12.1, cover the plague years of 1592, 1603, 1625, 1636, and 1665, after which the epidemic in England waned (Greenberg 1997: 392). Minor epidemics of 1591, 1630, 1637, and 1638 are also included in some of the texts, which, except for 1630, are the years surrounding, or coming after, the greater visitations. In addition to specific years, certain months are more prevalent in the material because the numbers of inflicted grew during the warm summer months and dropped in the cold of the winter (see e.g. Porter 2009: 28).

Three types of bills are represented in the material (see Munkhoff 1999: 6):[4]

1) *weekly bills* printed during the outbreaks listing the numbers of deaths in each parish;
2) *yearly bills* compiling the information from these weekly bills;
3) *comparative bills*, often with decorations, which allowed for the comparison of the current situation to earlier, severe plague years.

The official bills by the Company of Parish Clerks of London were excluded because my main interest lies in the development of the genre and the new functions these texts acquired in the course of the seventeenth century, with a focus on layout. The official bills had little decoration; they only contained numerical data of the buried and separate numbers for 'Buried in all' and 'Of the plague' separated by parishes in London, 'within the Walls' and 'Without the Walls', sometimes including numbers from other parishes such as Middlesex (see Greenberg 2004: 508).

[4] An additional subgenre, *collection of bills*, includes John Grant's well-known text, but analysing it here is beyond the scope of this study.

Table 12.1 *Material for analysis*[a]

	Title[b]	Year	Author	Printer/ publisher	Period covered	Subgenre	Layout, additional elements	
1	*A true bill* [. . .]	1603	Anon.	I. R. for Iohn Trundle	14 Jul.– 6 Oct. 14 Jul.– 20 Oct.	Weekly bill	Decorative repetitive pattern flanks the sides of two columns; origin and history of the disease written in blackletter	
2	*The Red-Crosse:* [. . .]	1625	Anon.	Iohn Trundle	23 Jun.– 4 Aug.	Weekly bill	Wide decorated margins; recipe paraphrase, prayer	Two small religious illustrations at the top
	The Red-Crosse: [. . .]	1636	Anon.	H. Gosson	31 Mar.– 26 May			Two small religious illustrations at the bottom
3	*LORD haue mercy vpon vs.*	1636	Anon.	M. S. Junior	*Per week*: 1603, 1625, 1636	Comparative bill	Decorative, short, and catchy title; illustrations of saints in the margins, skeletons, shovels; recipes, verse	
4	*LONDONS* LORD HAVE MERCY VPON VS [. . .]	1637	H. C.	Richard Harper	*Per week*: 1592, 1603, 1625, 1630, 1636	Comparative bill	Verse	Illustration of London; margins decorated with skeletons, bones, shovels; recipe, prayer
	LONDON'S Lord have mercy upon us [. . .]	1665	Anon.	—	*Per week*: 1592, 1603, 1625, 1630, 1636, 1637, 1665 (-> Oct. 31) *Per year*: 1638, 1646, 1647, 1648			No decoration; recipes, recipe paraphrases

	LONDONS LORD HAVE MERCY UPON US [. . .]	1665	Anon.	Francis Coles, Thomas Vere, John Wright	*Per week*: 1592, 1603, 1625, 1630, 1636, 1637, 1665 (-> Nov. 7) *Per year*: 1638, 1646, 1647, 1648		Illustration of London; margins decorated with skeletons, bones, shovels; recipes, recipe paraphrases
5	*The Four Great Years of the Plague* [. . .]	1665	Anon.	Peter Cole	*Per week*: 1593, 1603, 1625, 1636	Comparative bill	Top and bottom margins: illustrations of an angel and crossed bones; new parishes added to the bills
6	*The Mourning-Cross* [. . .]	1665	Anon.	Tho. Milbourn	*Per week*: 1591, 1603, 1625, 1630, 1636, 1637, 1665 (-> Aug. 29) *Per year*: 1638	Comparative bill	Illustration of a thick, black cross in the middle; prayer
7	*Londons Loud Cryes to the Lord by Prayer* [. . .]	1665	Anon.	T. Mabb, R. Burton, R. Gilberson	*Per week*: 1592, 1603, 1625, 1630, 1636, 1637, 1665 (-> Aug. 8) *Per year*: 1638, 1646, 1647, 1648	Comparative bill	Illustration of London; margins elaborately decorated with skeletons, bones, people; long prayer (half of the text)

Table 12.1 (*cont.*)

	Title[b]	Year	Author	Printer/ publisher	Period covered	Subgenre	Layout, additional elements
8	*The General Bill of Mortallity* [...]	1666	Anon.	Francis Coles, Thomas Vere, John Wright	*Per week*: 1592, 1603, 1625, 1630, 1636, 1637, 1665, 1666 (-> Jan. 23) *Per year*: 1638, 1646, 1647, 1648	Comparative bill	Illustration of London; margins decorated with skeletons, bones, shovels; recipe, verse

[a]In addition to the texts available in EEBO, the Guildhall Library copy of *The Red-Crosse* (Anon. 1625, text 2), discussed in Jenner (2012), was also examined.
[b]Full titles are provided in the references.

The method in the analysis of these texts has been influenced by a pragma-philological approach to language study. My understanding of the concept of *genre* is from Swales (1990), referring to a class of communicative events having a shared set of communicative purposes. Genre, therefore, emphasises function and use (see also Biber 1988: 68, 170). Over time, a genre or a group of texts develops similar language-external features, such as layout, headings, organisation of content, and so on. The term *text type*, in contrast, is used to refer to the internal features of a text (for a similar distinction between *genre* and *text type*, see Paltridge 1996; Taavitsainen 2001: 88–90). A well-known typology by Werlich (1976: 39–41) distinguishes five different text types: *description*, *narration*, *instruction*, *exposition*, and *argumentation*. This concept is employed in the analysis as it helps to differentiate between various components present in the text, principally the descriptive passages explaining the history and origin of the plague epidemics as well as the instructive language used to give remedies.

The analysis is based on a close reading of the material in the wider sociohistorical context. The texts were examined on multiple levels including content, text type, and language-external genre features. The content was contrasted to contemporary plague writing as it provided material for these London plague bills. The text type used for different sections of the broadsheet was considered, as were genre features, such as layout, illustrations and decorations, the formulation of titles and headings, and the organisation of content on the page. The right-hand column in Table 12.1 collects together prominent visual features as well as additional textual content, such as remedies and prayers, highlighting the varied nature of these texts.

In the analysis, the earlier texts as the first exemplars of the genre are analysed in more detail, whereas with later broadsheets the focus is on new content and generic functions, including changes in the use of visual features.

12.3 Analysis and Discussion

The changes in the genre across the time period are apparent. The earlier weekly bills (1603 and 1625) display the information in two columns, while comparative bills use a varied layout to include more information on the page. This demand for additional information, especially religious guidance and medical advice, was due to the recurrent outbreaks of the plague epidemic. In 1625 alone, 39,428 people died of the plague in London (H. C. 1637). Weekly bills of mortality had the capacity to reach a wide audience, and new content was added to cater to the needs of a concerned public.

The analysis of *A true bill* (Anon. 1603b), the earliest text in the material, underlines the difference to the official bills containing only numerical data (see Figure 12.1). The first line of the title is in a large font, which speaks of a visual emphasis instead of a verbal one as the line break occurs in the middle of the phrase. The first half of the text, written in the more accessible blackletter and taking almost all of the left-hand column of the broadsheet, relates the origin and the history of the disease. This component was also common in contemporary medical treatises representing the medieval *practica* or compendia tradition (Wear 2000: 117; Taavitsainen 2004; Pahta & Ratia 2010: 75, 79). Other components commonly discussed in these medical treatises on specific diseases are *signs, causes, treatments, names,* and *kinds of disease,* and of these, *causes* are also discussed in the early bills of mortality:

(1) IT is no doubt that the corruption of the ayre, together with vncleanly and vnwholsome keeping of dwelling, where many are pestered together, as also the not obseruing to haue fiers priuate & publiquely made as well within houses, as without in the streets, at times when the ayre is infected, are great occasions to increase corrupt and pestilent diseases. (Anon. 1603b: *A true bill*)

This discussion is followed by other causes of the disease: 'our-boldnesse of many preasing into infected places'. Plague is also compared to other diseases, to 'Leprosie, the Pocks, and sundry such vncleane diseases'. These comparisons were common in early modern medical texts on specific diseases (Pahta & Ratia 2010: 79). The third cause of the disease listed, plague being a punishment sent by God, is ubiquitous in contemporary medical texts (see also Munkhoff 1999: 9).

After the causes, the history of the disease is discussed in detail. Starting from biblical times, the history is presented as a chronology of successive events, with reference either to a specific year or to the reign of a ruler. The descriptive passage lists altogether thirteen such historical events, organised into separate paragraphs such as the following:

(2) In the yeeres 1576. and 77. in Millan, Padua, and Uenice, there fell a hundred thousand in euery Citty: and in Bohemia (beeing but a small Kingdome) there died three hundred thousand the same time. (Anon. 1603b: *A true bill*)

The historical overview ends with a reference to the 'last great visitation, from the 20. December 1592. to the 23. of the same month in the yeere

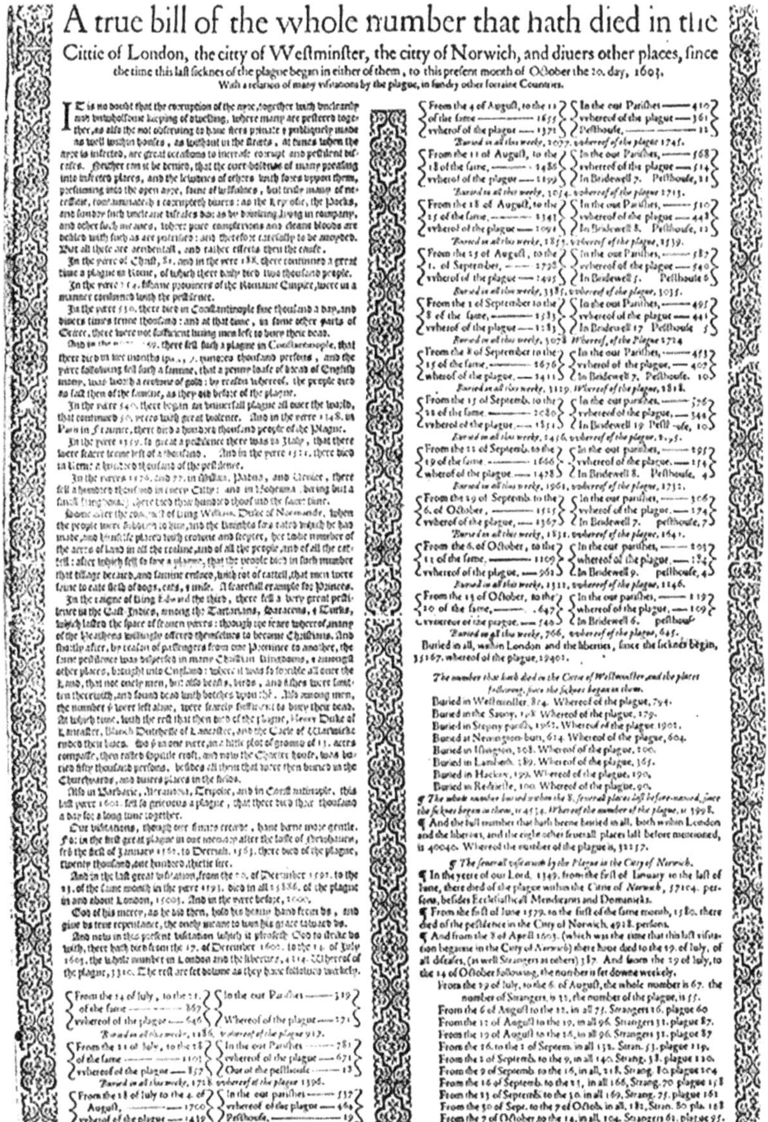

A true bill of the whole number that hath died in the Cittie of London, the citty of Weſtminſter, the citty of Norwich, and diuers other places, ſince the time this laſt ſicknes of the plague began in either of them, to this preſent moneth of October the 20. day, 1603.

With a relation of many viſitations by the plague, in ſundry other forraine Countries.

From the 14 of Iuly, to the 21. of the ſame —— 367, whereof of the plague —— 646. In the out Pariſhes —— 319. Whereof of the plague —— 171.
Buried in all this weeke, 1186, whereof of the plague 917.

From the 21 of Iuly, to the 28 of the ſame —— 1101, whereof of the plague —— 857. In the out Pariſhes —— 781, whereof of the plague —— 671. Out of the peſthouſe —— 13.
Buried in all this weeke, 1728. whereof of the plague 1396.

From the 28 of Iuly to the 4. of Auguſt, —— 1700, whereof of the plague —— 1439. In the out pariſhes —— 537, whereof of the plague —— 464. Peſthouſe, —— 19.
Buried in all this weeke, 2256. whereof of the plague 1922.

From the 4 of Auguſt, to the 11 of the ſame —— 1655, whereof of the plague —— 1371. In the out Pariſhes —— 410, whereof of the plague —— 361. Peſthouſe, —— 11.
Buried in all this weeke, 2077. whereof of the plague 1745.

From the 11 of Auguſt, to the 18 of the ſame, —— 1486, whereof of the plague —— 1199. In the out Pariſhes, —— 568, whereof of the plague —— 514. In Bridewell 7. Peſthouſe, 11.
Buried in all this weeke, 3054. whereof of the plague 1713.

From the 18 of Auguſt, to the 25 of the ſame, —— 1341, whereof of the plague —— 1091. In the out Pariſhes, —— 510, whereof of the plague —— 443. In Bridewell 8. Peſthouſe, 12.
Buried in all this weeke, 1855. whereof of the plague, 1539.

From the 25 of Auguſt, to the 1. of September, —— 2775, whereof of the plague —— 1495. In the out Pariſhes, —— 587, whereof of the plague —— 540. In Bridewell 5. Peſthouſe 6.
Buried in all this weeke, 3385. whereof of the plague, 3035.

From the 1 of September to the 8 of the ſame, —— 2533, whereof of the plague —— 1283. In the out Pariſhes, —— 495, whereof of the plague —— 441. In Bridewell 17 Peſthouſe 5.
Buried in all this weeke, 3078 Whereof, of the Plague 2724.

From the 8 of September to the 15 of the ſame, —— 2676, whereof of the plague. —— 2411. In the out Pariſhes, —— 453, whereof of the plague. —— 407. In Bridewell 7. Peſthouſe. 10.
Buried in all this weeke, 3129. Whereof of the plague, 2818.

From the 15 of Septemb. to the 22 of the ſame. —— 2080, whereof of the plague. —— 1851. In the out pariſhes. —— 376, whereof of the plague. —— 344. In Bridewell 19 Peſthouſe, 10.
Buried in all this weeke, 2456. whereof of the plague, 2195.

From the 22 of Septemb. to the 29 of the ſame. —— 1666, whereof of the plague. —— 1478. In the out pariſhes, —— 295, whereof of the plague. —— 254. In Bridewell 8. Peſthouſe, 4.
Buried in all this weeke, 1961, whereof of the plague, 1732.

From the 29 of Septemb. to the 6. of October, —— 1525, whereof of the plague, —— 1367. In the out pariſhes, —— 306, whereof of the plague. —— 274. In Bridewell 7. peſthouſe, 7.
Buried in all this weeke, 1831. whereof of the plague, 1641.

From the 6. of October, to the 13 of the ſame, —— 1109, whereof of the plague, —— 962. In the out pariſhes, —— 203, whereof of the plague, —— 184. In Bridewell 9. peſthouſe, 4.
Buried in all this weeke, 1312, whereof of the plague, 1146.

From the 13 of October, to the 20 of the ſame, —— 647, whereof of the plague. —— 540. In the out pariſhes, —— 119, whereof of the plague, —— 109. In Bridewell 6. peſthouſe
Buried in all the weeke, 766, whereof of the plague, 645.

Buried in all, within London and the liberties, ſince the ſicknes begin, 35167. whereof of the plague, 29402.

The number that hath died in the Citie of Weſtminſter, and the places following, ſince the ſicknes began in them.

Buried in Weſtminſter, 824. Whereof of the plague, 794.
Buried in the Sauoy, 198 Whereof of the plague, 179.
Buried in Stepney pariſh, 1962. Whereof of the plague 1901.
Buried at Newington-butts, 614. Whereof of the plague, 604.
Buried in Iſlington, 108. Whereof of the plague, 100.
Buried in Lambeth. 389. Whereof of the plague, 365.
Buried in Hackney, 192. Whereof of the plague, 190.
Buried in Redcliffe, 100. Whereof of the plague, 90.

¶ *The whole number buried within the 8. ſeuerall places laſt before-named, ſince the ſicknes began in them, is 4534. Whereof the number of the plague, is 3998.*

¶ And the full number that hath beene buried in all, both within London and the liberties, and the eight other ſeuerall places laſt before mentioned, is 40040. Whereof the number of the plague is, 32257.

¶ *The ſeuerall viſitation by the Plague in the City of Norwich.*

¶ In the yeere of our Lord, 1349. from the firſt of Ianuary to the laſt of Iune, there died of the plague within the Citie of *Norwich*, 57104. perſons, beſides Eccleſiaſticall Mendicants and Dominicks.

¶ From the firſt of Iune 1579. to the firſt of the ſame moneth, 1580. there died of the peſtilence in the City of Norwich. 4918. perſons.

¶ And from the 8 of April 1603. (which was the time that this laſt viſitation beganne in the City of *Norwich*) there hane died to the 29. of Iuly, of all diſeaſes, (as well Strangers as others) 387. And from the 29 of Iuly, to the 14 of October following, the number is ſet downe weekely.

From the 29 of Iuly, to the 6. of Auguſt, the whole number is 67. the number of Strangers, is 32, the number of the plague, is 55.
From the 6 of Auguſt to the 12. in all 73. Strangers 16. plague 60
From the 12 of Auguſt to the 19. in all 96. Strangers 31. plague 87.
From the 19 of Auguſt to the 26. in all 96. Strangers 31. plague 87
From the 26. to the 2 of Septem. in all 132. Stran. 53. plague 119.
From the 2 of Septemb. to the 9, in all 140. Strang. 38. plague 120.
From the 9 of Septemb. to the 16, in all, 218. Strang. 80. plague 204
From the 16 of Septemb. to the 23, in all 166, Strang. 70 plague 158
From the 23 of Septemb. to the 30. in all 169, Strang. 75. plague 161
From the 30 of Sept. to the 7 of Octob. in all, 182, Stran. 80 pla. 168
From the 7 of October to the 14, in all, 104. Strangers 62. plague 95.
The whole number, is 1832. Whereof of the plague, 1759.

At London printed by I. R. for Iohn Trundle, and are to be ſold at his ſhop in Barbican, neere Long lane end.

Figure 12.1 *A true bill* (1603). The Bodleian Libraries, University of Oxford, Firth. b.15. Image attribution CC-BY-NC 4.0

1593 ...'. Very similar lists of events can be found in other medical treatises, for instance in William Bullein's *A Comfortable Regiment* from 1562 (Jenner 2012: 262). After this overview, before finally presenting the actual mortality statistics for the present year of 1603, *A true bill* contains a prayer-like component embedded in the text: 'God of his mercy, as he did then, hold his heauy hand from vs, and giue vs true repentance, the onely meane to win his grace toward vs.' This underlines the special nature of the disease, depending wholly on the mercy of God.

The Red-Crosse: OR, Englands Lord haue mercy vpon vs (Anon. 1625, see Figure 12.2) was written by an anonymous author and published by John Trundle, who had published a number of Thomas Dekker's pamphlets and works of a sensational nature (Jenner 2012: 255). Printed during the year of the most fatal outbreak in seventeenth-century England, the 'Red-Crosse' of the title referred to the practice of marking the doors of infected houses by painting a red cross so that people would know to stay away. While this pioneering text is 'the earliest surviving example of a particular kind of inexpensive single-sheet textualization of the plague, almost all of which have "Lord Have Mercy Upon Us", or some variant thereof in the title', much of the content is, in fact, taken directly from *A true bill* (Jenner 2012: 255, 262), including the discussion about the causes and the historical overview of the disease. The new components include a remedy, 'A preseruation by way of defence, to be vsed in common Assemblies, and in open Aire', recommending the use of 'a piece of strong Tobacco in your hand to smell too; or the Root called Angelica, to bite on now and then, as occasion requireth'. It is not a recipe proper, as imperative verb forms are not used, but a recipe paraphrase, which was common in medical treatises of the time (Taavitsainen 2001). The lack of an effective cure for the plague meant that preventive medicine, such as the remedy in *The Red-Crosse*, was promoted (see Pahta & Ratia 2010: 98). At the end of the text, at the bottom of the right-hand column, is included '*A necessary Prayer for the present time*' (emphasis original).

This edition of *The Red-Crosse*, located at the British Library and found in EEBO, has an existing earlier copy from the same year at the Guildhall Library (see Jenner 2012: 256). The earlier edition has a more spacious layout, and a remarkable increase in the total number of plague victims can be seen when the two copies are compared: from 1,478 to 6,771. This underlines the ephemeral nature of these broadsheets: new editions were printed every Thursday in order to give up-to-date information to people yearning for it (see Slauter 2011: 4).

The first part of the title of *The Red-Crosse* is quite short and memorable. The bill highlights only the beginning of the long title, which

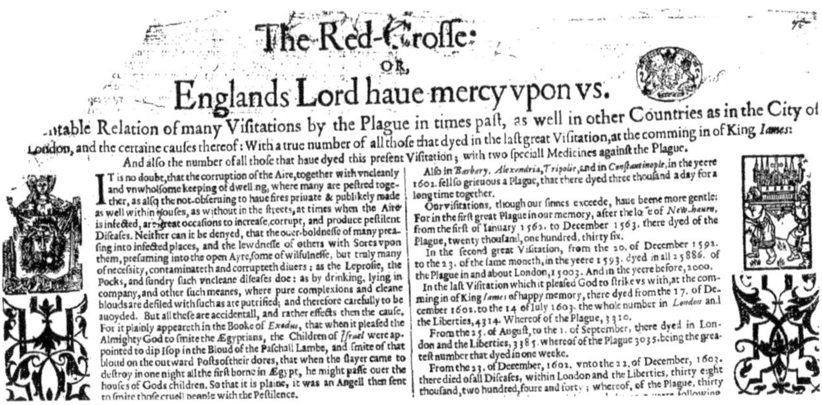

The Red-Crosse:
OR,
Englands Lord haue mercy vpon vs.

…ntable Relation of many Visitations by the Plague in times past, as well in other Countries as in the City of London, and the certaine causes thereof: With a true number of all those that dyed in the last great Visitation, at the comming in of King *Iames*: And also the number of all those that haue dyed this present Visitation; with two speciall Medicines against the Plague.

IT is no doubt, that the corruption of the Aire, together with vncleanly and vnwholsome keeping of dwelling, where many are pestred together, as also the not-obseruing to haue fires priuate & publikely made as well within houses, as without in the streets, at times when the Aire is infected, are great occasions to increase, corrupt, and produce pestilent Diseases. Neither can it be denyed, that the ouer-boldnesse of many pressing into infected places, and the lewdnesse of others with Sores vpon them, presuming into the open Ayre, some of wilfulnesse, but truly many of necessity, contaminateth and corrupteth diuers: as the Leprosie, the Pocks, and sundry such vncleane diseases doe: as by drinking, lying in company, and other such meanes, where pure complexions and cleane bloudsare defiled with such as are putrified; and therefore carefully to be auoyded. But all these are accidentall, and rather effects then the cause. For it plainly appeareth in the Booke of *Exodus*, that when it pleased the Almighty God to smite the Ægyptians, the Children of *Israel* were appointed to dip Isop in the Bloud of the Paschall Lambe, and smite of that bloud on the outward Posts of their dores, that when the slayer came to destroy in one night all the first borne in Ægypt, he might passe ouer the houses of Gods children. So that it is plaine, it was an Angell then sent to smite those cruell people with the Pestilence.

Also in *Barbary, Alexandria, Tripolie*, and in *Constantinople*, in the yeere 1602. fell so grieuous a Plague, that there dyed three thousand a day for a long time together.

Our visitations, though our sinnes exceede, haue beene more gentle: For in the first great Plague in our memory, after the lo[illegible]e of *New-hauen*, from the first of Ianuary 1562. to December 1563. there dyed of the Plague, twenty thousand, one hundred, thirty six.

In the second great Visitation, from the 20. of December 1592. to the 23. of the same moneth, in the yeere 1593. dyed in all 25886. of the Plague in and about London, 15003. And in the yeere before, 2000.

In the last Visitation which it pleased God to strike vs with, at the comming in of King *Iames* of happy memory, there dyed from the 17. of December 1602. to the 14 of Iuly 1603. the whole number in *London* and the Liberties, 4314. Whereof of the Plague, 3310.

From the 25. of August, to the 1. of September, there dyed in London and the Liberties, 3385. whereof of the Plague 3035. being the greatest number that dyed in one weeke.

From the 23. of December, 1602. vnto the 22. of December, 1603. there died of all Diseases, within London and the Liberties, thirty eight thousand, two hundred, foure and forty; whereof, of the Plague, thirty [illegible]

Figure 12.2 The upper part of *The Red-Crosse* (1625). © British Library Board, General Reference Collection C.20.f.5.(69)

demonstrates a verbal emphasis instead of a visual one (see Figure 12.2). With regard to decoration, the margins in *The Red-Crosse* are more elaborate and wider in comparison to *A true bill* (1603) and they also display small illustrations at the top with religious imagery, moving even further away from the simple layout of official bills.

During the next major outbreak of the plague epidemic in 1636, *The Red-Crosse* was reprinted by H. Gosson with very few changes (Anon. 1636a).[5] The long title is shorter, as it does not contain the reference to 'the last great Visitation, at the comming in of King *Iames*' of the 1625 edition. The 'two speciall Medicines' – that is using tobacco or angelica root as preventives and a prayer – are not mentioned in the title, although they can be found in the text. What is new in the 1636 edition is the relatively large empty space on the page after the weekly statistics for the reader to fill in later. The barely visible handwritten inscriptions of added dates and numbers show that the bill was indeed used for this function.

A comparative bill *LORD haue mercy vpon vs* (Anon. 1636b, see Table 12.1) is the only one in the material with a genuinely short and 'catchy' title, which was a novelty of the seventeenth century (Shevlin 1999: 55). The decorative style of the broadsheet is further enhanced by the use of blackletter in the headings and the title. The title is highlighted by a frame embellished with skulls. On both sides of the frame religious

[5] For instance, the reference to the outbreaks 'in *Barbary, Alexandria, Tripolie*, and in *Constantinople*, in the yeere 1602' is missing.

advice is given, including 'Watch & pray, for you know not when the Lord will come.' About half of the text consists of recipes indicated by the verb *take*, representing the text type of instruction. These recipes are divided into two kinds: 'Preservative from Infection', printed on the left side of the broadsheet (see Example 3), and 'Preservative when infected', on the right.

(3) By Drinke.
TAke worme-wood, and herbe of grace, and steepe them all night in a pint of beere, with a lemmon sliced, and drink them in the morning fasting. (Anon. 1636b: LORD haue mercy vpon vs)

The recipes are followed by a longer, instructive passage under the heading 'A special meanes to preserve health' with religious content. The rest of the text is reserved for the well-known poem 'LIke to the Damaske Rose you see' (five stanzas), here titled 'The Brevity of mans Life, as well by reason of this, as all other Diseases'. The poem deals with the transient nature of human existence but in a generic way, with no actual reference to disease. There is also a shorter poem, 'Of mans resurrection'. The numerical data on the plague victims is pushed to the margins and printed in a smaller font than the rest of the text. Plenty of room has been left for the reader to add more numbers accordingly. The text is practice oriented, containing both religious and medical advice.

A similar emphasis on religion and medicine is maintained in *LONDONS LORD HAVE MERCY VPON VS*, represented by three editions in the material (H. C. 1637, Anon. 1665a, Anon. 1665b). The 1637 edition has an illustration of plague-stricken London with a skeleton and carts pulling corpses right under the long title at the centre of the text. This same illustration was present in the later 1665 edition of the text and, with minor alterations, in texts 6 and 8 (Anon. 1665c, Anon. 1666), at the same location on the page. The mortality statistics are presented in the margins. In the later editions from 1665, more space was needed to cover the new outbreaks of the plague, so the lower middle part of the page also displays this information. The 1637 edition begins with a short recipe manifested by the use of imperative verbs: *take*, *cut*, *put*, and *drinke*, which is followed by a long verse and an equally long prayer. The prayer is not the same as in *The Red Crosse*, but a contemporary one referring, for instance, to the drought that affected the south of England from 1634 to 1637: '. . . thou hast proved his Prophets to be false Prophets, by sending downe these sweet and comfortable showers of raine upon the earth, . . .'. In a similar manner, the poem in *LONDONS LORD HAVE MERCY VPON VS* also refers to recent events:

(4) When sixe yeares since, a little Plague God sent,
He shoke his rod to move us to repent:
Not long before that time, a dearth of corne,
Was sent to us to see if we would turne:
And the last Summer none deny it can,
The beasts did suffer for the sinne of man:
Grasse was so short and small, that it was told,
Hey for foure pound a load was daily sold. (H. C. 1637: LONDONS LORD HAVE MERCY VPON VS)

The reference to 'a little Plague' is to the epidemic of 1630. The summer drought of 1636 is also mentioned. The two editions of this same text from 1665 look strikingly different from each other, the first having no decorations. The long verse, partly shown in (4), has been edited in both to better reflect the year of 1665: 'sixe yeares since, a little Plague' has been changed to 'Seventeen years' and 'the last Summer' with reference to the drought has been replaced with a more general 'And after that'. Close to the end of the poem, the 1637 edition says: 'And now againe he doth with us begin, T' increase the Plague, as we increase in sinne'. In the 1665 editions, this is reformulated as follows: 'The Plague among us is not yet removed, Because that sin of us is still beloved.' Instead of a prayer, the 1665 editions contain recipes and some recipe paraphrases. When these texts under scrutiny are analysed together, the remedies given in them are, almost without exception, new, adding to the topical nature of the bills.

The decorated later edition of *LONDONS LORD HAVE MERCY UPON US* (Anon. 1665b) included a novel section that helped the reader to better understand the current development of the epidemic for the past week: 'Increased in the Burials', 'Parishes clear of the Plague', and 'Parishes Infected' (Figure 12.3).

The phrases 'Increased/Decreased in the Burials this Week' mark the beginnings of statistical analysis; this new feature was also present in two other broadsheets published the same year, *The Mourning-Cross* and *Londons Loud Cryes to the Lord by Prayer*. Slauter (2011: 2) claims that based on contemporary letters and diaries, this feature was of utmost importance to readers because interpreting the data in the bills could be difficult.

Buried this week of all Difeafes, 1787. Of the Plague, 1414. Increafed in the Burials, 399.
Parifhes clear of the Plague, 20. Parifhes Infected, 110.

Figure 12.3 A section containing statistical analysis in *LONDONS LORD HAVE MERCY UPON US* (Anon. 1665b). © British Library Board, General Reference Collection 74/C.20.f.4.(123)

As a genre, bills of mortality are very flexible as certain elements could be added or omitted depending on what was emphasised or how much space there was to use. For example, the 1665 edition of *LONDONS LORD HAVE MERCY UPON US* (Anon. 1665b) presents weekly statistics for 1665 instead of a prayer, which was present in the earlier 1637 edition, taking up the exact same spot of the text. The bills often had small print and tight margins, and the 1637 copy of *LONDONS LORD HAVE MERCY VPON VS* does not display the years entirely chronologically, as 1592 is presented after 1625 and before 1630. In comparison, in the 1665 editions chronological order is retained.

Of all the texts examined here, *The Four Great Years of the Plague* (Anon. 1665d) is the only one with a spacious layout. It has decorations solely at the top and bottom margins: an angel and two crossed bones. Only the major outbreaks of 1593, 1603, 1625, and 1636 are listed, with added numbers from '*Stepney, Redriff, Islington, Newington, Lambath, Hackney, Covent Garden*, St. *Margrets Westminster*.' (emphasis original) The long title highlights the statistical function of the broadsheet: 'Compared by the Weekly Bills of Mortality Printed every Thursday in the said years, by which its Increase and Decrease is plainly discerned in all those Years.'

With the great visitation of 1665, *The Red-Crosse* was reprinted under a new name, *The Mourning-Cross* (Anon. 1665e; see Figure 12.4). The long title is more descriptive of the contents than that of its predecessor, *The Red-Crosse* (Anon. 1625, 1636a). For example, causes and history of the disease components are included in 'Containing The certain causes of Pestilential Diseases' and 'an Accompt of several modern Plagues or Visitations in times past'. The use of italics in the title draws attention to both place and time and underlines the ephemeral nature of the text: '*England*'s Lord have Mercy upon Us', 'in the City of *London*', '*August* 29. 1665'. This practice of highlighting relevant textual items becomes more common in the second half of the century (see also Figure 12.5). The prayer advertised in the long title is the same prayer included in *The Red-Crosse*, but the earlier editions do not mention it in the title. Although the text was printed under a new name, the main difference lies in the layout. Instead of two columns decorated at the margins, the text is divided horizontally into three different sections. The first section and the whole text are dominated visually by an image of a cross (see Figure 12.4).

Content-wise, the first section of *The Mourning-Cross* is identical to *The Red-Crosse* (1625 and 1636 editions), but the paragraph on London 'to have had as great blessings as ever had Jerusalem' has not been included, making the tone of the text more negative. Another paragraph missing is the one on the change of Princes, which information was no longer

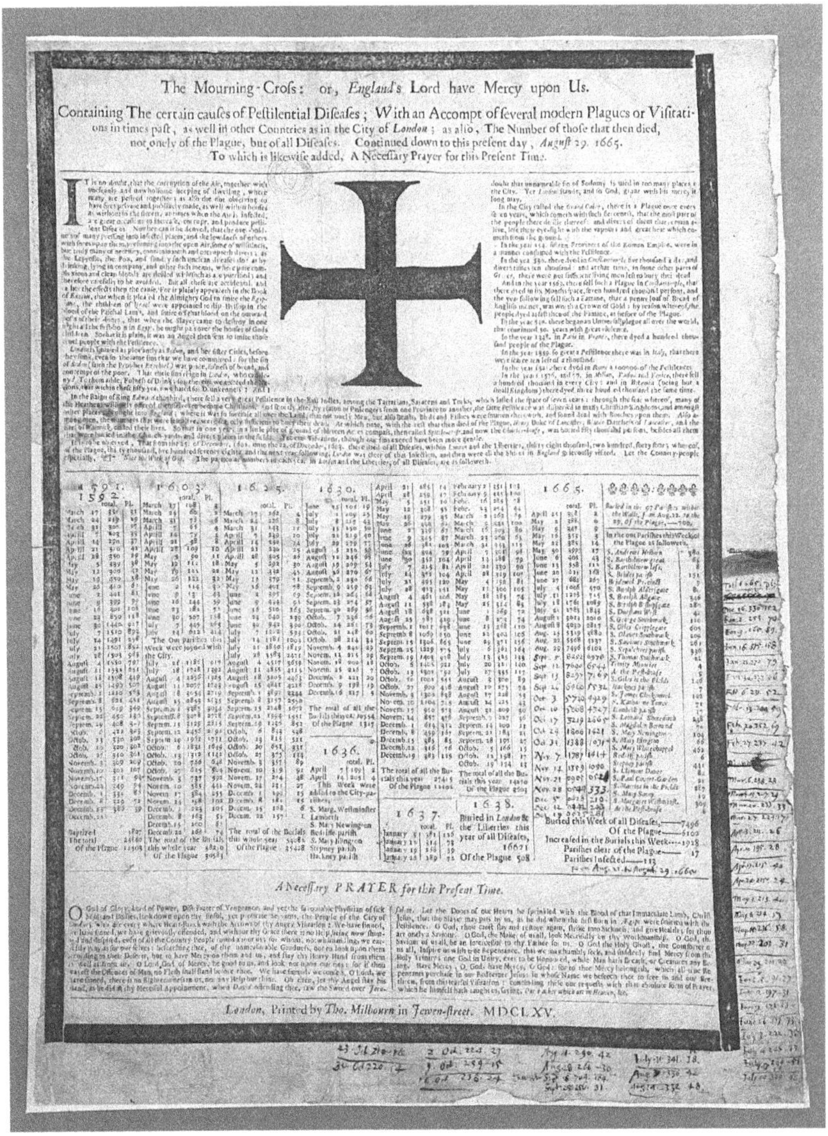

The Mourning-Crofs: or, *England's* Lord have Mercy upon Us.

Containing The certain caufes of Peftilential Difeafes; With an Accompt of feveral modern Plagues or Vifitations in times paft, as well in other Countries as in the City of *London*; as alfo, The Number of thofe that then died, not onely of the Plague, but of all Difeafes. Continued down to this prefent day, *Auguft* 29. 1665.
To which is likewife added, A Neceffary Prayer for this Prefent Time.

A Neceffary PRAYER for this Prefent Time.

London, Printed by *Tho. Milbourn* in *Jewen-ftreet*. MDCLXV.

Figure 12.4 *The Mourning-Cross* (1665). Guildhall Library, City of London

deemed important in 1665. A paragraph referring to King William and to the year of 1066 was also excluded. At the end of this first section, new content about the total number of the diseased from 1602 to 1603 was added with the phrase 'Note the Work of God' following it. The phrase

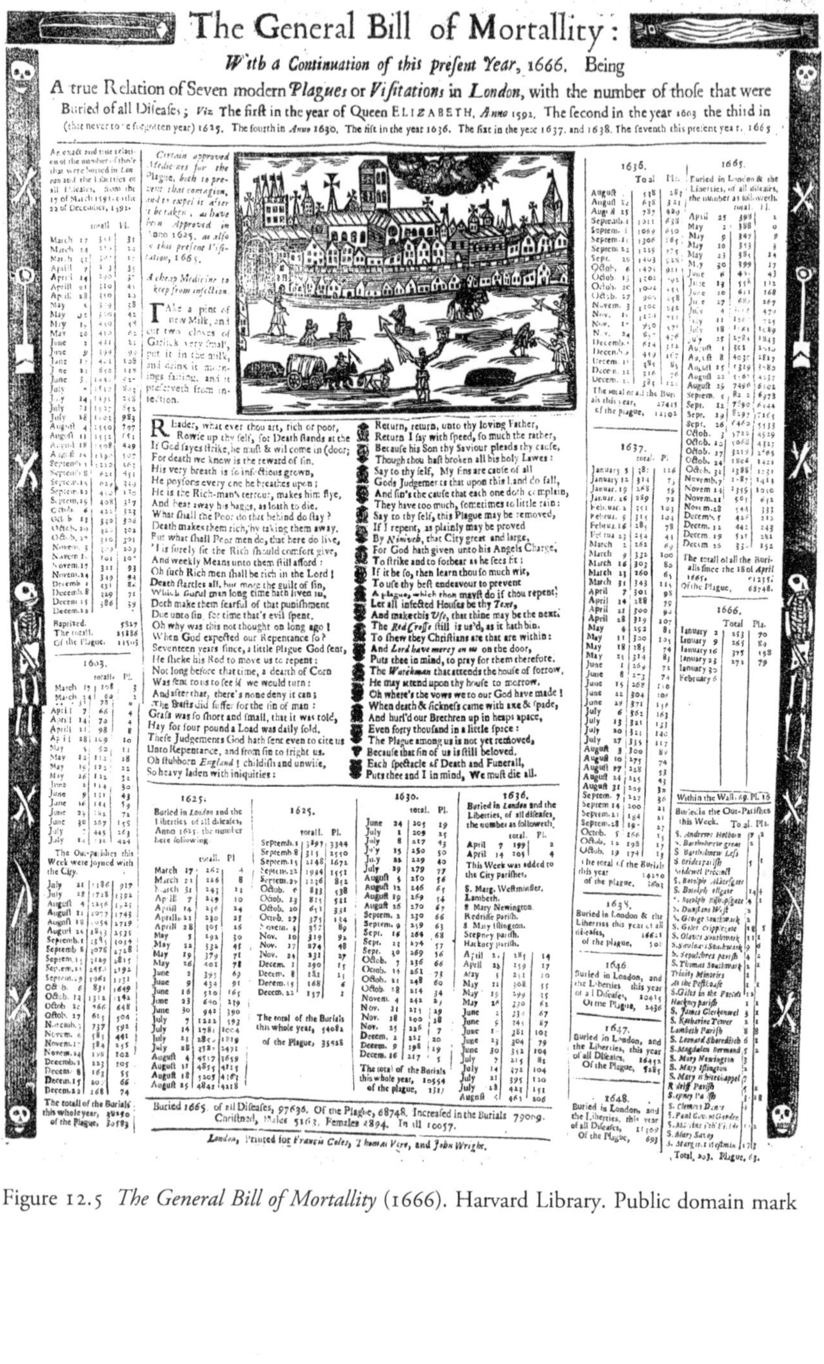

Figure 12.5 *The General Bill of Mortallity* (1666). Harvard Library. Public domain mark

was also present in the earlier editions of *The Red-Crosse* (1625 and 1636), but embedded in the surrounding text, whereas in *The Mourning-Cross* (1665) it is highlighted with italics and a manicule preceding it right above the second horizontal line (see Figure 12.4).

The Mourning-Cross also differs from its predecessor by its functions: it is a comparative bill containing mortality statistics from several years. The middle section of the bill is dedicated to these numbers. The years of visitations are in a bigger font so that they stand out in the text; this is a common feature in comparative bills.[6] Although the years can be easily spotted in the text, the actual numbers need to be scrutinised with care due to the size of the print. Weekly statistics are provided for the years 1591, 1603, 1625, 1630, 1636, 1637, and 1665. The data for 1638 includes only totals, as the number for diseased of the plague was a low 508 for that year. The statistics for 1665 are given until 29 August, and handwritten notes have been added to a blank space specifically designed for this purpose: weekly numbers from 5 September to 19 December.[7] After the weekly statistics for the year 1665 and the total numbers for 'the 97 Parishes within the Walls', the list continues with 35 out-parishes, including the Pest-house, which is not present in earlier bills. This copy of *The Mourning-Crosse* was put to use, as even outside the textual frame handwritten inscriptions have been added to include later numbers to the 1665 data, probably from January to December 1666. The prayer at the bottom of the page is the same one included in the previous versions, but the layout makes it stand out much more.

Londons Loud Cryes to the Lord by Prayer (Anon. 1665c) is dominated by a long prayer with references to the Bible in the margins. Otherwise the broadsheet looks very similar to the illustrated editions of *LONDONS LORD HAVE MERCY VPON VS* (Anon. 1637, 1665b), with the illustration of London and elaborately decorated margins. The year 1592 has been later inscribed by hand under 1591. Curiously, the number for 'baptized' has been included under the first two years, 1591 and 1603, but not for the later outbreaks.

The last text of the dataset, *The General Bill of Mortallity* (Anon. 1666, see Figure 12.5), has identical decorations in the margins to *LONDON'S*

6 An exception to this rule is *Londons Loud Cryes to the Lord by Prayer* (Anon. 1665c). The layout of this text is very tight and some of the years are not emphasised: the oldest outbreak of 1592 included in the comparative data and other minor epidemics containing only annual data (see Table 12.1).

7 This feature can also be found in *LONDON'S Lord have mercy upon us* (Anon. 1665a), where, in addition to leaving a considerable amount of empty space at the right-hand margin, dates for the coming eight weeks have been provided covering the rest of the year 1665.

Lord have mercy upon us (Anon. 1665a), with skeletons, shovels, and crossed bones. The illustration of London is also the same. The probable reason for the similarities in the layout is that both bills were printed for Francis Coles, Thomas Vere, and John Wright. The recipe titled '*A cheap Medicine to keep from infection*' is also identical (emphasis original). However, it is the only recipe on the page because this later bill also covered the outbreak of 1666, or at least the first weeks of January with empty spaces for the reader to fill in the rest, which meant that less space could be reserved for recipes.[8] Visually, this last text is a typical specimen of the London bill of mortality, with features of *memento mori* and the illustration of London. A combination of different elements from statistical data to a recipe and a verse shows how the genre has developed from the first, visually plain specimen (Figure 12.1) to elaborate broadsheets containing multiple functions (Figure 12.5).

12.4 Conclusions

One of the main findings of this study is how London bills of mortality broadsheets adapted to the recurring plague epidemics in the course of the seventeenth century. The bills had a crucial role in providing indispensable information for the citizens of London and the surrounding areas. A closer examination of the texts revealed that the early exemplars of the genre borrowed much of their content from earlier texts, especially medical treatises, in the discussions of the origin of the disease and the description of historical plague epidemics. Later a new layer of information was added to the genre when the plague years of the late sixteenth century and the seventeenth century up to 1666 were statistically compared to each other. In time, medical advice and prophylactics gained prominence in the bills. The presence of religious guidance in the form of prayers and religion- or death-related imagery became even more pronounced. As the analysis illustrated, even poems were in part rewritten to better reflect the ongoing situation. It could be said that, for the most part, the later texts discarded non-essential information in order to include the maximum amount of topical information on the page: statistics for different years of the epidemic, recipes, and religious advice, to name the most important items. Later the numerical data became more detailed by including the increase

[8] For some reason, text 8 (Anon. 1666) includes the numbers for 'Christned', divided by sex, for the year 1665 and the total number for 'Baptized' for the year 1592, although this information is generally not given in the bills analysed for this study.

or decrease in the numbers as well as listing 'infected' or 'clear' parishes. The comparative bills were also sometimes updated by adding new parishes to the statistics. By 1665, it seems that the focus had shifted somewhat and the bills started to cover increasingly more areas than just the London parishes.

The overall appearance of the bills becomes quite uniform. Many of these broadsheets are decorative and display in the upper middle part an illustration of plague-stricken London, and also have elaborate margins with *memento mori*; the first examples of the use of these visuals appear in 1637 in the analysed material. A shared component in all of these texts is the inclusion of total numbers at the end of the section dedicated to each month or year. This feature is not highlighted in the early texts, but later, from 1665 onwards, the total numbers are emphasised with italics, for example. In general, later texts visually highlight important information, that is certain keywords such as dates, locations, and the number of burials. One of the novel features is leaving empty spaces on the page to allow for the reader to fill in by hand new information about plague casualties. What the readers were first and foremost interested in were the statistics of the plague epidemic, but the recipes and religious advice clearly had a function too. To further investigate these functions, a thorough analysis of a larger dataset of plague broadsheets would, however, be needed. The various components act almost as independent items that can be moved around to create a broadsheet for the public eagerly waiting for new information. The bills of mortality, written by anonymous authors, could be continuously updated and created in collaboration to render them something topical and of interest to their readers.

REFERENCES

Anon. 1582. *The number of all those that hath dyed in the Citie of London & the liberties of the same [. . .]*. London: J. Charlewood.

Anon. 1603a. [TEXT 1, by 'Henry Chettle']. *A true bill of the whole number that hath died in the cittie of London, the citty of Westminster, the citty of Norwich, and diuers other places*, [. . .]. London: Printed by I.R. for Iohn Trundle.

Anon. 1603b. [TEXT 1]. *A true bill of the vvhole number that hath died in the cittie of London, the citty of VVestminster, the citty of Norwich, and diuers other places, [. . .]*. London: Printed by I. R[oberts] for Iohn Trundle.

Anon. 1625. [TEXT 2]. *The Red-Crosse: or, Englands Lord haue mercy vpon vs [. . .]*. London: Printed for Iohn Trundle.

Anon. 1636a. [TEXT 2]. *The red-crosse, or, englands lord have mercie upon us [. . .]*. London: Printed for H. Gosson.

Anon. 1636b. [TEXT 3]. *Lord haue mercy vpon vs. A speciall remedy for the plague.* London: Printed [by R. Young and M. Flesher] for M. S[parke] Junior.

Anon. 1665a. [TEXT 4]. *LONDON'S Lord have mercy upon us. [. . .].* Printed at London.

Anon. 1665b. [TEXT 4]. *LONDONS LORD HAVE MERCY UPON US. [. . .].* London: Printed for Francis Coles, Thomas Vere, and John Wright.

Anon. 1665c. [TEXT 6]. *Londons loud cryes to the Lord by prayer: [. . .].* London: Printed for T. Mabb, for R. Burton, and R. Gilberson.

Anon. 1665d. [TEXT 7]. *The Four great years of the plague, viz. 1593, 1603, 1625, and 1636 [. . .].* London: Printed for Peter Cole [. . .].

Anon. 1665e. [TEXT 5]. *The mourning-cross: or, England's Lord have mercy upon us [. . .].* London: Printed by Tho. Milbourn in Jewen-street.

Anon. 1666. [TEXT 8]. *The general bill of mortallity: with a continuation of this present year 1666. [. . .].* London: Printed for Francis Coles, Thomas Vere and John Wright.

Balmford, James. 1603. *Short dialogve concerning the plagves infection. Published to preserue bloud, through the blessing of God.* London: [R. Rield] for Richard Boyle.

Biber, Douglas. 1988. *Variation across speech and writing.* Cambridge: Cambridge University Press.

Buck, Peter. 1977. Seventeenth-century political arithmetic: Civil strife and vital statistics. *Isis* 68(1): 67–84. www.jstor.org/stable/230374 (accessed 28 October 2020).

Claridge, Claudia. 2013. From page to screen: The relevance of encoded visual features in the *Lampeter Corpus*. In Anneli Meurman-Solin & Jukka Tyrkkö (eds.), *Principles and practices for the digital editing of diachronic data.* Helsinki: Varieng. https://varieng.helsinki.fi/series/volumes/14 (accessed 17 May 2022).

Dekker, Thomas. 1625. *A Rod for Run-awayes.* London: [By G. Purslowe] for Iohn Trundle.

Fissell, Mary E. 2007. The marketplace of print. In Mark S. R. Jenner & Patrick Wallis (eds.), *Medicine and the market in England and its colonies, c. 1450–c. 1850*, 108–32. Basingstoke; New York: Palgrave Macmillan.

Greenberg, Stephen J. 1997. The 'Dreadful Visitation': Public health and public awareness in seventeenth-century London. *Bulletin of the Medical Library Association* 85(4): 391–401.

Greenberg, Stephen. 2004. Plague, the printing press, and public health in seventeenth-century London. *Huntington Library Quarterly* 67(4): 508–27.

H. C. 1637. [TEXT 4, by Crouch, Humphrey]. *LONDONS LORD HAVE MERCY VPON VS [. . .].* London: Printed for Richard Harper.

Jenner, Mark S. R. 2012. Plague on a page: *Lord Have Mercy Upon Us* in early modern London. *Seventeenth Century* 27(3): 255–86.

McConchie, R. W. 2013. Some reflections on early modern printed title-pages. In Anneli Meurman-Solin & Jukka Tyrkkö (eds.), *Principles and practices for the digital editing of diachronic data*. Helsinki: Varieng. https://varieng.helsinki.fi/series/volumes/14 (accessed 17 May 2022).

Munkhoff, Richelle. 1999. Searchers of the dead: Authority, marginality, and the interpretation of plague in England, 1574–1665. *Gender & History* 11(1): 1–29.

Pahta, Päivi, & Maura Ratia. 2010. Treatises on specific topics. In Irma Taavitsainen & Päivi Pahta (eds.), *Early Modern English Medical Texts: Corpus description and studies*, 73–100. Amsterdam: Benjamins.

Paltridge, Brian. 1996. Genre, text type, and the language learning classroom. *ELT Journal* 50(3): 237–43.

Porter, Stephen. 2009. *The Great Plague*. Stroud: Amberley.

Ratia, Maura. 2013. Investigating genre through title-pages: Plague treatises of the Stuart period in focus. In Anneli Meurman-Solin & Jukka Tyrkkö (eds.), *Principles and practices for the digital editing of diachronic data*. Helsinki: Varieng. https://varieng.helsinki.fi/series/volumes/14 (accessed 17 May 2022).

Ratia, Maura, & Carla Suhr. 2017. Visual and verbal communication in title-pages of early modern medical texts. In Matti Peikola, Aleksi Mäkilähde, Hanna Salmi, Mari-Liisa Varila, & Janne Skaffari (eds.), *Verbal and visual communication in Early English texts (Utrecht Studies in Medieval Literacy)*, 67–93. Turnhout: Brepols.

Shevlin, Eleanor F. 1999. 'To reconcile book and title, and make 'em kin to one another': The evolution of the title's contractual functions. *Book History* 2 (1): 42–77.

Slauter, Will. 2011. WRITE UP YOUR DEAD: The bills of mortality and the London plague of 1665. *Media History* 17(1): 1–15.

Stage, Kelly J. 2011. Plague space and played space in urban drama, 1604. In Rebecca Totaro & Ernest B. Gilman, *Representing the plague in early modern England*, vol. 14, 54–75. London: Routledge.

Suhr, Carla. 2011. *Publishing for the masses: Early modern English witchcraft pamphlets*. Mémoires de la Société Néophilologique de Helsinki 83. Helsinki: Société Néophilologique.

Sullivan, Erin. 2011. Physical and spiritual illness: Narrative appropriations of the bills of mortality. In Rebecca Totaro & Ernest B. Gilman, *Representing the plague in early modern England*, vol. 14, 76–94. London: Routledge.

Swales, John M. 1990. *Genre analysis: English in academic and research settings*. Cambridge: Cambridge University Press.

Taavitsainen, Irma. 2001. Middle English recipes: Genre characteristics, text type features and underlying traditions of writing. *Journal of Historical Pragmatics* 2(1): 85–113.

Taavitsainen, Irma. 2004. Transferring classical discourse conventions into the vernacular. In Irma Taavitsainen & Päivi Pahta (eds.), *Medical and scientific writing in early modern English*, 37–72. Cambridge: Cambridge University Press.

Thomas, Keith. 1973. *Religion and the decline of magic*. Studies in Popular Beliefs in Sixteenth- and Seventeenth-Century England. Harmondsworth: Penguin.

Watt, Tessa. 1991. *Cheap print and popular piety 1550–1640*. Cambridge: Cambridge University Press.

Wear, Andrew. 2000. *Knowledge and practice in English medicine, 1550–1680*. Cambridge: Cambridge University Press.

Werlich, Egon. 1976. *A text grammar of English*. Heidelberg: Quelle & Meyer.

CHAPTER 13

Advertising Proprietary Medicines in Pamphlets

Carla Suhr

A new player emerged in the English medical marketplace in the second half of the seventeenth century: proprietary medicines. Pamphlets advertising various pills, elixirs, salts, and powders comprised as much as around a fifth of all new medical titles printed in the period 1650–1690 (Fissell 2007: 116–17). These 'early modern infomercials', as the historian Mary E. Fissell characterizes them (2007: 120), informed the public of the 'singular virtues' 'never found out before' of particular medicines, described the 'wonderful cures' performed by them, and indicated the appropriate dosages for use. Sometimes they also engaged in heated disputes about the effectiveness of the cures or the true 'ownership' of the medicines.

Pamphlet advertisements of proprietary medicines are fascinating examples of specialized texts that straddle two (or more) functions: while promoting the products is the primary aim (even if it is not voiced as such), these texts also appropriate established (learned) medical knowledge and discourse conventions and impart them to the general public. As such, pamphlet advertisements can be considered a new hybrid genre incorporating both old and new structural elements and linguistic features. The old components were modeled on or repurposed from existing genres of medical writing, while new ones were invented for new overtly promotional requirements. So far these texts have been considered mostly by medical historians (e.g. Porter 1989; Styles 2000; Fissell 2007; Wallis 2008; Mackintosh 2018), but they have garnered little attention from historical linguists (although see Mullini 2010; Ratia & Suhr 2011). In this chapter, I will conduct a move analysis (Swales 2004) of thirty-two pamphlet advertisements from the period 1660–1700 in order to identify the structural elements of this new hybrid genre. Furthermore, I will look for the origins of the identified elements in earlier, established medical genres by referring to earlier research on the structural elements characteristic of recipes and treatises. The comparison will also show which elements are completely new. This case study of one hybrid genre will thus demonstrate the innovativeness of late seventeenth-century medical professionals, who developed a new medical genre from existing ones to make best use of the possibilities afforded to them by the changes in the contemporary medical marketplace.

13.1 Genre Analysis and Advertisements for Proprietary Medicines

According to the already iconic definition by Swales (1990: 58), a genre is made up of communicative events with a shared rationale, which is recognized by expert members of a discourse community. The rationale – that is, the communicative purpose of a genre – 'shapes the schematic structure of the discourse and influences and constrains choice of content and style' (Swales 1990: 58). For Bhatia (1993: 21), the communicative purpose of a genre is reflected in the 'interpretive cognitive structuring of the genre' representing the 'accumulated and conventionalized social knowledge available to a particular discourse or professional community'. Both definitions emphasize the role of recognized conventional structures and stylistic decisions for achieving the communicative purpose of a genre. Genres also reflect the beliefs and values of the discourse or professional communities and even societies at large (Tardy & Swales 2014: 166), which is why genre analysis has established its place as a part of discourse analysis. Rhetorical moves in Middle English and Early Modern English medical genres have been analyzed in several studies (see e.g. Mäkinen 2006; Taavitsainen 2001, 2011).

Both Swales and Bhatia recognize that genres are not static but are shaped by their users; this is also reflected in the fact that genres can become mixed with or embedded in other genres (Bhatia 2005). According to Bhatia (2005: 220), modern advertising genres are especially prone to 'colonize' or invade 'the territorial integrity' of professional and academic informative genres. He suggests that the reason for this lies in the fact that the most popular strategy found in promotional genres is to describe a product in a positive manner, thereby combining the advertising purpose with an informative purpose; a shared informative purpose makes it easier for the genres to be mixed into genres that have been labeled as *infomercials*, *infotainment*, or *advertorials* (Bhatia 2005: 221). As Fissell's (2007: 120) characterization of early modern pamphlet advertisements of proprietary medicines as 'infomercials' demonstrates, the 'colonizing' of informative texts by promotional purposes was taking place already in the seventeenth century. This study will shed some light on how this 'colonizing' of informative texts takes place in a new genre.

The method chosen for analyzing this new genre of proprietary medical advertisements is *move analysis* (Swales 2004; Tardy & Swales 2014), which seeks to identify stretches of text that serve a particular rhetorical function. The Swalesian concept of moves has a clear parallel with the concept of macrostructures, which has also been used as the methodological framework in genre analytical studies (see e.g. Borde 2015). Move analysis has been used to analyze a variety of modern genres, including academic and professional genres (see e.g. Maswana, Kanamaru, & Tajino 2015 on research articles, Lorés-Sanz 2016 on abstracts), but also hard-sell print advertisements (Bhatia 2005) and legal news reports (Ge 2016). Recently, move analysis has also been employed in the analysis of modern mixed genres such as online science news (Zhang 2018) and advertorials (Zhou 2012). Historical genres investigated with this method include late modern English death notices (Borde 2015) and patent specifications (Groom & Grieve 2019). Caren auf dem Keller (2004) analyzes the structure of medical advertisements in eighteenth-century newspapers.[1] Identifying the moves of these pamphlet advertisements of medicines and comparing them to structures found in earlier informative genres of medical writing will reveal how an overtly advertising purpose 'infiltrates' traditional informative genres such as recipes and treatises on specialized topics to the extent that a new hybrid genre is formed.

Proprietary medicines were a new element in the very fluid early modern medical marketplace, which was populated by patients with different financial means and medical practitioners with varying levels of formal medical learning. Furthermore, medical texts were increasingly available for both learned and lay audiences. The wealthy and middle-class patients were just as likely to rely on physicians, apothecaries, midwives, or untrained medical entrepreneurs (often called quacks by the professional physicians), such as Humphrey Nendick (d. 1707) or Anthony Daffy (d. 1680) (see Figures 3–6 and 14 in the Image Gallery). The universal medicines prepared by both university-trained and self-taught medical practitioners took the form of pills, powders, and elixirs, and as these were sold in a variety of outlets, the patients never met the medical professional whose name was on the package. These proprietary medicines were too expensive for the poorer sort, even though they were

[1] It should be noted that of the three historical studies mentioned here, only Groom and Grieve (2019) mention move analysis as their method. Borde (2015) and auf dem Keller (2004) both refer to structural elements as the objects of their analyses. However, despite the different terminology, the methodologies are in essence the same.

often advertised as affordable, so they must be considered semi-luxury or even luxury products (Haycock & Wallis 2005: 2). The manufacturers or 'owners' of the medicines named in the pamphlets most likely wrote the pamphlet texts themselves; only eight of the thirty-two pamphlet advertisements investigated in the present study are anonymous. Proprietary medicines were promoted in handbills posted on walls and in pamphlets distributed in the street, but also by shouting in the street and word of mouth. Figure 14 in the Image Gallery shows the title page of Anthony Daffy's pamphlet advertisement for his *Elixir Salutis* (1675). Advertisements of services and products such as medicines gradually found their way into newspapers by the late seventeenth century (Brownlees 2011: 166).[2] In the eighteenth century, advertisements for proprietary medicines were a staple in newspapers (Mackintosh 2018: 232). An analysis of almost 3,000 advertisements in the Zurich English Newspaper Corpus (ZEN) of eighteenth-century newspapers found that 13 per cent of them advertised medical products, many of which were branded by including a proper name in their label (auf dem Keller 2004: 61, 63–4).

Medical historians, who were the first scholars to pay attention to ephemeral texts such as handbills and pamphlets that advertised the services and products of quacks, note that the language of these texts is characterized by hyperbole (see e.g. Porter 1989). Linguistic studies have taken note of the frequent use of affective features and even speech-like informal structures, as well as the use of first- and second-person pronouns and text-internal and text-external deixis as strategies to amplify the authority of the author (Mullini 2010; Ratia & Suhr 2011). In eighteenth-century medical advertisements in newspapers, the tradition of hyperbole was still present, seen in the frequent use of adjectives like *great*, *excellent*, *infallible*, *perfect*, and *famous* (auf dem Keller 2004: 90–1). Despite this, by the late eighteenth century the preferred style for advertising proprietary medicines in newspapers avoided hyperbole and preferred bland, factual writing that aligned the advertisers with orthodox therapies and regular practitioners (Mackintosh 2018: 234). Testimonials and case reports were used only sparingly (auf dem Keller 2004: 105), but reassurances of the consistent and correct composition of the medicines

[2] However, medical advertisements do not appear to be very common: Brownlees (2011: 169) analyzed a sample of twenty-six numbers of the *London Gazette* from 1681 and found only one medical advertisement. Book advertisements were by far the most frequently advertised product with twenty-two advertisements.

continued, with the name on the packaging given as proof of quality (Mackintosh 2018: 234). The repetition of advertisements in newspapers made proprietary medicines one of the first examples of branding (Styles 2000; Mackintosh 2018: 234). It should be noted, though, that branding can be considered to have begun already with pamphlets, which were often reprinted and revised regularly.

13.2 Materials and Methods

The primary material of this study consists of thirty-two texts advertising various proprietary medicines, published in England between 1660 and 1700 and available in the *Early English Books Online* (EEBO) database (http://eebo.chadwyck.com). These texts share the same communicative purposes of promoting a particular medicine and informing the readers of, for example, the properties of the medicine and where it could be obtained. The authors, when named, were also the manufacturers of the medicines or the owners of the secret recipes for the medicines. The texts were identified from bibliographies of previous scholarship and by using relevant keywords as database search terms. When possible, only first editions of the texts were considered. There are two instances of the same product advertised twice in separate pamphlets, but in these cases the texts are not identical. For example, in 1668 Constantine Rhodocanaces published a pamphlet of twenty-seven pages describing his *alexicacus* or spirit of salt; three years later his advertisement for the same product was only one sheet long. Despite some repetition, the texts are so different that both are included in this study.

The length of the advertisements ranges from one sheet to thirty pages (c. 500–10,000 words), though most commonly the pamphlets are eight or sixteen pages long. Publications that consist of only one sheet or page are arguably not really pamphlets, but rather broadsheets or handbills, although I have included them in this analysis as they are structured in the same way as pamphlets and shared the same promotional function. There are eight such texts in the material. Separate title pages (found in twelve texts) were not included in the analysis, but prefatory material indicated with a label addressing the reader (in eight texts) was included.

As discussed by Groom and Grieve (2019: 208–9), traditional move analysis is inherently qualitative, as close reading is necessary to identify sections of texts serving particular rhetorical functions. This was the case with this study as well. Text-structuring cues such as section headings or titles were useful in differentiating between moves, and other layout features such as changes in type size or font or empty space, initial capitals, as well as pointing devices such as manicules and asterisks (cf. auf dem Keller 2004: 97–9), were also used as visual signals of borders between structural elements.

In move analysis, individual *moves* can range from single clauses up to a paragraph and have various realizations (*steps*) (Swales 2004: 228–9). However, in the material for this study, *moves* usually take up at least one paragraph and often span several paragraphs, though in the shorter texts some moves can be very short. A move such as *testimonial* can consist of several testimonies of successful treatments, but in such cases it was only counted as one instance of the move. However, if another move, such as *directions for use*, occurs between two testimonials, the testimonials were considered to be two separate moves. Thus, moves can occur more than once in a text, but never consecutively. Noting the order of moves gives information about their preferred locations in the texts and also of patterns of co-occurrences, though a full-fledged quantitative analysis of the frequencies and co-occurrence patterns of moves falls outside the scope of this study.

The rhetorical functions of moves can be realized in multiple different ways within the move, and this is why, for each move, I also took note of the most common realizations (*steps*). For example, *sales information* can include information about packaging, pricing, and locations of vendors. It should be noted, though, that the primary focus of the study was on identifying the moves of the texts rather than the complete repertoire of strategies for realizing them.

Once the moves and their typical steps had been identified, I looked for potential sources and models for them in other early modern medical texts, many of which had roots in medieval traditions. I compared the moves of pamphlet advertisements to descriptions of the elements of vernacular recipes (Stannard 1982) and descriptions of the discourse forms of medical texts of the sixteenth and seventeenth centuries outlined in the descriptions of the categories of the *Early Modern English Medical Texts* corpus (EMEMT; see Taavitsainen & Pahta 2010), which contains a representative sample of medical texts from this period. Apart from Jerry Stannard's recipe elements (Stannard 1982), there has been no comprehensive study of the moves of early modern English medical genres; the corpus category descriptions of discourse forms are the closest available approximation to such an overview, supplemented by Wear's (2000) monograph on early modern English medicine. The most immediate models of pamphlet advertisements seem to be in specialized texts describing particular methods or therapeutic substances (see Pahta & Ratia 2010); indeed, that is the category in which examples of pamphlet advertisements are placed in the corpus, but there are also parallels to medical textbooks that had their origins in medieval *practica* or *compendia* (Wear 2000: 117). I also compared my findings to auf dem Keller's (2004) analysis of the structure of medical advertisements in eighteenth-century newspapers.

13.3 Results and Analysis

In this section I will describe the moves identified in the material and make some observations about possible precursors found in earlier medical texts. Through close reading I identified seven moves in advertisements for proprietary medicines: *endorsement*, *symptoms*, *virtues*, *directions for use*, *testimonials*, *addressing critics and competitors*, and *sales information*.

As shown in Table 13.1, only three of the moves, *virtues*, *directions for use*, and *sales information*, are found in almost all of the pamphlets, so they can be considered more or less compulsory elements. The order of the moves varies, though some tendencies could be identified. The moves are discussed in the order in which they tend to appear in the pamphlets.

13.3.1 Endorsement

Endorsement is a versatile move that tends to be the first element in pamphlet advertisements. It is found in twenty-four of the thirty-two texts, and in eighteen cases it is the first move. This move serves to raise interest in the promoted product and to set it apart from other, competing medicines. The move also establishes the credentials of both the product and its manufacturer. Typical steps or strategies for realizing this move include references to noble clients, the approval of eminent physicians, a classical secret medicine only recently discovered, the extensive travel or

Table 13.1 *Occurrences of the seven moves (total number of texts = 32)*

Move	Number of texts in which the move occurs
Endorsement	24
Symptoms	8
Virtues	30
Directions for use	26
Testimonials	16
Addressing critics and competitors	15
Sales information	31

experience of the manufacturer, considerations of the public good rather than personal gain, and general usefulness of the medicine for the public at large. William Sermon demonstrates many of these strategies in the advertisement for his pill:

(1) Friendly reader,
Having through the wonderful Goodness and Mercy of the Almighty God, by long experience in searching the great Volume of Nature, by a diligent inspection, observing the property of each Distemper, with the nature and occult quality of Metals, Minerals, and Vegetables; some years past arrived to the sublime preparation of this most excellent Medicine, whose transcendent Virtues (of late) have been known to many persons of great worth. A Medicament so exceeding rare as admits no Rival for the performance of the foresaid Cures, &c. the want of which every year causeth great numbers of Men, Women, and Children to descend untimely to their Graves. (William Sermon, *An Advertisement Concerning Those Most Famous Cathartique and Diuretique Pills*, 1671: 1)

In the opening paragraph to the pamphlet, Sermon points out his own long experience and diligence in medical matters, refers rather vaguely to 'many persons of great worth' who were aware of his pill, and claims that his medicine is not only 'most excellent' but also 'exceeding rare' and better than all others in curing illnesses and ailments and thereby saving innumerable lives. The hyperbole evidenced by premodifiers such as *wonderful*, *great*, *sublime*, *transcendent*, and *exceeding* is very characteristic of endorsements.

Similar strategies for endorsing a new medicine or medical procedure can be seen already in the sixteenth century in medical treatises focusing on promoting specific cures or methods as viable medical procedures for other medical professionals. In medieval recipes there is no *endorsement* move. The parallels between the communicative functions of the earlier treatises and pamphlets advertising finished products to potential customers are clear, and therefore it is easy to understand how the *endorsement* move became a conventionalized move in pamphlet advertisements within the first decades of the new genre. Thomas Witherden was clearly aware of some of the conventional strategies for realizing this move, but he played on the readers' expectations by refusing to engage in these strategies:

(2) Though I have not impudence to brag of great Travels, long Journeys, many Voyages, and what Wonders I have done beyond Sea; nor am ambitious to shew large Parchments, Broad-Seals, &c.

not sinistrously covetous of popular Applause; yet modesty will justly allow me so much confidence, to tell the World, that I have (for these many years) been my own Physician and Patient [. . .]. (Thomas Witherden, *Elixir Salutis*, 1679: 1)

Witherden claims that his competitors' references to travel and markers of approval are 'impudence' and 'ambition', instead emphasizing the fact that he has tested his cures himself. Witherden, too, makes heavy use of descriptive premodification, but seems to be doing it in an ironic fashion to show his awareness of the hyperbolic overuse of this feature by other authors.

13.3.2 Symptoms

As suggested by the label, this move describes how particular illnesses or conditions can be identified by the symptoms exhibited by the patient. However, as many of the medicines claimed to be universal panaceas, it could be considered superfluous – and indeed, the move is not very common. It is only found in eight texts. According to Wear (2000: 113–15), medieval and early modern remedy books did not contain information about symptoms because they assumed that lay people were able to self-diagnose. Authors of pamphlet advertisements who drew on remedy books as the models for their texts probably made the same assumption and therefore did not consider *symptoms* a necessary move.

The length of the *symptoms* move varies depending on how many diseases or conditions the authors choose to describe. The sparsest realizations consist of a simple phrase indicating the ailment to be treated: 'For any pain in the *Stomach*, and bad *Digestion*, or *Reluctancy* [. . .]' (Salvatore Winter, *Directions for the Use of My Elixir*, 1664: f. A2). A common strategy was to save space by giving only a few examples of conditions and the symptoms associated with them. Headings were often used to distinguish between different sets of symptoms:

(3) The Symptomes of the Fits of the Mother
IT arises with a trembling on the left side, with cold windy Vapours, and after the cold fit is over, (the which, sometimes lasteth an hour two or three) then an hot fit ariseth, one after another, that the party is all in a Water with it [. . .]. (Lionel Lockyer, *An Advertisement Concerning those most Excellent PillsCalled Pillulae Radijs Solis Extractae*, 1664: 3)

Lockyer's description combines medical terminology such as 'cold windy Vapours' and 'hot' and 'cold fit', which draw on humoral theory, with concrete and easily understood description of where the fits start and how long they can last.

Symptoms is a move that can also be found in textbooks on the practice of medicine and in specialized texts on specific medicines, which take pains to explain the symptoms of the conditions that can be cured by the medicine or procedure described in the texts. Connecting the signs of a condition with medical theory was considered an aspect of learned discourse such as textbooks on the practice of medicine, which made this information available also to literate lay people (Wear 2000: 116–17). In specialized texts on specific medicines, discussing symptoms and linking them to medical theory gave the authors authority, as they implied a higher level of learning.

In Stannard's (1982) classification of medieval vernacular recipe elements, there is no element similar to *symptoms*; the closest one is *purpose*, which states what ailment the recipe is intended for by naming either the ailment or a symptom, but it does not entail a full discussion of the symptoms, and actually aligns most closely with just the headings found in a *symptoms* element. Wear (2000: 106) notes that what modern medicine considers a symptom of a disease was often viewed as a disease in early modern medicine, and the labeling practice apparent in headings found in the *symptoms* element bears this out. Headings, especially when accompanied by other layout features such as changes in typeface or empty space, made it easy for potential customers to see at a glance whether purchasing the pamphlet would be worth their while.

13.3.3 Virtues

Symptoms were usually followed by *virtues*, which is a move found in all but two of the pamphlet advertisements. This move explains how the medicine works to cure various conditions or what its effect is on different organs. As with *symptoms*, the condition is often indicated in a heading. Charles Peter shows that he is aware that descriptions of symptoms were frequently expected, but he moves directly to the virtues of his tincture after briefly explaining his decision to skip the *symptoms* element:

(4) STONE in the Kidneys, Ureters, Bladder, and Neck of the Bladder I need not name the Symptoms; every unhappy Mortal, who has felt this Distemper, knows to their cost how great the Torment. Yet, God be praised, this *Cordial Tincture* can clear the Body from Stones, brings away great Quantities of Gravel, hinders the coagulating of

Gravel and slimy Humours, (which generate Stones) hinders all retention of Humours in the Kidneys, Ureters, Bladder, and prevents Stoppages in the Neck of the Bladder. (Charles Peter, *The Cordial Tincture*, 1686: 6)

Virtues shares many features with *symptoms*, though the purposes of these two moves are clearly different. As in *symptoms*, authors distribute learned medical information to lay readers in the *virtues* element. In (4), Peter refers to not only specific medical conditions and organs, but also to particular processes causing these conditions. Unlike Lockyer in (3), Peter does not use any layman's terms in his explanation, but relies heavily on medical jargon and terminology. Interestingly, both Lockyer and Peter make use of humoral theory, which shows that this classical theory was still pervasive in the late seventeenth century, despite the emerging scientific thought style that emphasized experimentation over ancient authorities (see Taavitsainen & Schneider 2019).

Virtues have clear precursors in medieval recipes and early modern medical textbooks and specialized treatises. The recipe element *rationale* provides evidence that proves the efficacy of the recipe by explaining how the ingredients work in the cure, and sometimes even refers to humoral theory. The same applies to textbooks and specialized treatises as well. Perhaps having such clear models explains why *virtues* are practically an obligatory move in pamphlet advertisements of medicines.

13.3.4 Directions for Use

Another move that is found in almost all pamphlet advertisements is the *directions for use* (twenty-six texts), which gives information about how the medicine should be administered to patients of different gender, age, or general condition, and for different ailments. This move is an integral part already of medieval vernacular recipes: Stannard (1982: 60–5) lists the element he calls *application and administration* as one of the four required elements of recipes, and similar elements are also found in later medical genres that included recipes or described specific medical procedures. Example (5) demonstrates that the instructions for using proprietary medicines often nonetheless left some room for individual interpretation:

(5) Now in the *Griping* of the *Guts*, according to the strength of the Patient, may be taken four or five spoonfuls, less or more, as cause requires, and it must be repeated again in five or six hours, and the

same again the third time, if need require, and you not doubt of a cure. (Anon., *Elixir Magnum Vitae*, 1670–1680: 5–6)

The exact dosage is here to be decided by the person administering the cure, as is the question of whether a third dose is needed. This particular pamphlet seems to assume that the reader and potential customer is a medical practitioner rather than a patient looking to self-medicate. In example (6), the reader is clearly assumed to be the patient, but the author is still comfortable placing the responsibility for choosing the suitable dosage on the customer:

(6) You may use of them at your pleasure, whether late or early, or at any hour of the day, before meat, or after meat, or in the time of feeding; but being taken in time of Supper, they defend the head (as we have said) from those vapours and fumes that ascend to it in the night [. . .] The Dose is, Seven, Nine or Eleven [pills], and that three or four times a month, as necessity or the temper of the Body shall require. (Patrick Anderson, *Grana Angelica*, 1681: 1)

Anderson leaves it up to the patient to decide not only the dosage but also the time of taking the medicine. They also determine themselves whether it is necessary to repeat the cure. He may have intended to give the impression that his medicine is easy to use, as it does not require the patient to follow a strict schedule or rationing scheme. The vagueness of the instructions had the added benefit that the patient could be blamed for not taking the correct dosage if the medicine did not work as expected.

As with *virtues*, the *directions for use* move has clear precursors in medical recipes, the *application and administration* element. Earlier treatises on specific medicines also often contained comparable information. The linguistic features of the recipe model were also adopted: modal verbs such as *may* and *must* are common in this element, as are imperatives (see Chapter 15 in this volume). This placed the author in a position of authority, which could be further enhanced by the use of distancing strategies such as the passive voice (as in Example (4)) and the pronoun *we* when referring to the author (as in Example (5)).

13.3.5 Testimonials

Testimonials is a move that could take many forms in pamphlet advertisements. It is found in sixteen of the texts, and in nine texts the move is used more than once. In many cases *testimonials* are short summaries or anecdotes of success stories, as in this passage:

(7) *Worms.* The Porter at *Dorchester House* about three years ago being at the point of death, took one dose of this Medicine and voided a worm of twenty one foot long, and hath been well ever since. (Smart, *Smart's Aurum Purgans*, 1665: 3)

Smart included a number of similar testimonials that exhibited how his medicine had cured a variety of ailments, aiming for credibility without actually giving so much information that a specific person could be identified. Smart relies heavily on testimonials in his advertisement, as they make up almost half of his text. Other authors included fewer testimonials but embellished them with details and sometimes even a narrative structure. Still others reproduced letters from grateful customers in their texts as proof of the value of their medicine.

Testimonials can sometimes be found at the beginning of texts or directly following an initial *endorsement*, but more often they co-occur with *symptoms*, *virtues*, and *directions for use*. In longer texts, it is often the *testimonials* that take up most space rather than explanations of how the medicine effects its cure. This is clearly a move that was considered to have strong selling power that would convince readers to buy the product.

Though this element had no clear predecessors in medieval recipes, apart from brief references to classical authorities finding a recipe useful in the *incidental data* element, specialized medical treatises of the sixteenth and seventeenth centuries made increasing use of case studies as evidence of the efficacy and value of the procedures and medicines they described (see Taavitsainen 2011). These case studies, which are evidence of the new scientific thought style that valued empiricism over classical authorities, are clear models of the testimonials found in pamphlet advertisements and modern promotional genres. The *testimonial* move was evidently considered a conventional move in advertisements, as omitting it usually required a comment. Charles Peter, in (8), claims that he has turned down several offers for testimonials because his medicine does not need any, while Nathaniel Lomax uses a lack of space as his explanation in (9):

(8) And not a few have offer'd to certifie the wonderful effects wrought on them by it [the cordial tincture]; but 'tis below me to accept of so mean a thing; my own authority being sufficient to give *Credit* to this, or any other *Medicine*. (Charles Peter, *The Cordial Tincture*, 1686: 3–4)

(9) And, as to inserting names, and Letters of Cures as many do, I have not room [. . .] though I can prove plentifully [. . .]. (Nathaniel Lomax, *Delaun Reviv'd*, 1680: 10)

Both authors take pains to indicate that they have access to testimonials even though they are not included in their advertisement. Some authors who leave out this move go so far as to suggest that testimonials can be provided upon request.

Symptoms, *virtues*, *directions for use*, and *testimonials* often occur multiple times in medical pamphlet advertisements, when authors wish to describe the efficacy of their medicine for a number of different diseases with theory and examples and to tailor the recommended dosage to suit the ailments. As mentioned before, *symptoms* is not a very common move, but when present, it tends to precede the other three elements. The order of *virtues*, *directions for use*, and *testimonials* is more varied even within the same text, perhaps to add some variety to a text that might otherwise turn into a repetitive list. These four (or three, if we discount the rather rare *symptoms*) moves seem to form the core elements of the informative function of pamphlet advertisements, as they co-occur in different permutations when illnesses and their cures are described.

13.3.6 Addressing Critics and Competitors

The marketplace of proprietary medicines was an arena with fierce competition. This is reflected in the move labeled *addressing critics and competitors*, which is found in about half of the texts (fifteen of thirty-two). In this move, authors defended themselves against criticism or attempted to debunk or discredit their competitors by exposing them as quacks and counterfeiters. This element could be placed as the first move or following an *endorsement* in pamphlet advertisements, in which case the authors often use evocative language with exclamations and rhetorical questions in defense of their medicine or their own qualifications. When placed as the next to last move, a less common placement, the focus was more often on warning against the counterfeit medicines of competitors.

Authors had to be careful not to give away the 'secrets' of their medicine when they described its virtues, but that also left them open to claims of incompetence or fake medicines, especially when there was a similar medicine already on the market. For example, Anthony Daffy, Thomas Hinde, Thomas Witherden, and Daniel Woodward all produced and sold an Elixir Salutis. Everyone claimed ownership of the 'true' medicine and denounced the others as dangerous counterfeit medicines. Critics and competitors were not always named but referred to more vaguely, as in the following example:

(10) But some scandalously report, that these Pills are dangerous in the working, being too strong for any person but one of extraordinary strength of Nature. Secondly, That I have no skill in the Art of Physick; and that I have no other Medicine but this particular Receipt or Composition. But let all know, these are meer scandals, raised upon me by persons of an envious spirit; and especially by some of the same Faculty; who are afraid that this Medicine may in great measure eclipse that mercenary repute which they have gotten by fraud and several Artifices. (William Sermon, *An Advertisement Concerning those most Famous Cathartique and Diuretique Pills*, 1671: 21–2)

Sermon does not name his opponents, but he specifies complaints made against him: that his pills are dangerously strong, and that he is not a trained physician and therefore can only produce one medicine rather than a range of them. His critics are attacking his credentials and his product as faulty out of envy and fear that they will lose their customers to him, Sermon writes, and then goes on to discredit their practice as mercenary and fraudulent.

The fierce argumentation evident in the *addressing critics and competitors* move bears a resemblance to the controversies of the sixteenth and seventeenth centuries on topics related to politics, religion, and science. At first controversies took place in treatises, but they spilled into pamphlets as well, which allowed for faster reactions to volleys. In these controversies, authors picked apart their opponents' arguments and defended themselves against the specific criticism made against them, often referring to specific sections of texts published by their opponents (see Ratia & Suhr 2011). First-person pronouns are used to stress the authority of the writers, and readers are included in the argument by addressing them with second-person pronouns. The same strategies are employed on a smaller scale in pamphlet advertisements, too, as well as in other specialized treatises on particular medical procedures or substances.

13.3.7 Sales Information

The final move found in pamphlet advertisements is a completely new move not seen in earlier medical writing, yet it is found in all but one of the texts. *Sales information* was an absolutely necessary component of pamphlet advertisements, for it gave customers the practical information they needed to find and purchase the medicine. Usually this was the final element of a text, but in some texts where the element is very brief, it is placed near the beginning; in pamphlets advertising several medicines, the price of the medicine is mentioned in connection with each product. The information included in this move concerns the price of the product and the exact locations of its vendors; the latter information was often formatted as a list. In some cases the medicine could only be obtained from the author himself, but the most popular ones were sold in dozens of establishments, in London and other major cities. Furthermore, authors often offered to send the medicine outside London upon request. Comparing successive editions of pamphlets shows that the lists of vendors were regularly updated. Frequently authors also include descriptions of the containers or their seals – occasionally even a picture of the seal – so that customers could be sure that they bought the true medicine rather than a counterfeit version of it.

Not surprisingly, the *sales information* move was adopted into newspaper advertisements of medicines in the late seventeenth century. Auf dem Keller (2004: 101–2) calls this element the *standing details*. Her analysis of eighteenth-century news advertisements shows that also in medical news advertisements, information about where to purchase a medical product was a compulsory element.

13.4 Discussion

The analysis of the moves of the new genre of pamphlet advertisements of proprietary medicines has shown that the authors of these texts drew on a variety of traditions of medical texts as models for writing. Two moves, *virtues* and *directions for use*, are found already in medieval medical genres of recipes, remedy books, and *practica* books or compendia describing the proper practice of medicine. The *symptoms* move is found in medieval *practica* books as well, and in an abbreviated form in the *purpose* element of recipes. These three moves are also found in new genres that appear in the early modern period, specialized medical treatises describing particular procedures or therapeutic substances.

Many of the procedures or substances outlined in specialized medical treatises were also claimed to be secrets originating from classical antiquity, which is one of the strategies found in the *endorsement* move of pamphlet advertisements. Another two moves, *testimonials* and *addressing critics and competitors*, have also been found to be characteristic of contemporary specialized treatises, which therefore can be confirmed as the most immediate models for pamphlet advertisements. The fact that six of the seven moves found in pamphlet advertisements were present in several other contemporary medical genres is evidence of, on the one hand, the fuzziness of the borders between genres, but, on the other hand, also of the dynamic nature of genres: they change and mix according to the communicative needs of the discourse community that uses and produces them. Furthermore, medical writers were sufficiently familiar with all of these genres to be able to exploit them in the formation of a new hybrid genre.

However, pamphlet advertisements have one further move, *sales information*, that is not found in any other earlier or contemporary medical genre. This is the move that is most clearly related to the advertising function of the texts, as it provides the information on pricing and purchasing locations. This move is the only one found later in eighteenth-century newspaper advertisements of medicines (auf dem Keller 2004), though a more detailed analysis of auf dem Keller's rather vague *body text* category could reveal other similarities. A comparison of the seven moves identified for pamphlet advertisements and the nine rhetorical moves identified for modern hard-sell print advertisements (Bhatia 2005) reveals some similarities: both types of texts include a move for establishing the credentials of the advertised product or advertiser (the *endorsement* element in pamphlets), a move for detailing the product (the *virtues* and *sales information* moves in pamphlets), and a *testimonials* move.

Move analysis of a variety of genres has shown that moves should be considered a repertoire of options from which writers select only some to use in their texts, though there may be some obligatory elements. For example, Groom and Grieve (2019) identified seventeen rhetorical moves for late modern patent specifications, but found that only six of these moves are present in almost all of them. In pamphlet advertisements of proprietary medicines, only the *virtues*, *directions for use*, and *sales information* moves can be considered obligatory, though it seems that the *endorsement* and *testimonial* elements were also recognized as conventional moves, as some authors felt compelled to comment on their decision to omit them. The order of moves is usually also fluid, though *endorsements*, when found, tend to be the first move in an advertisement, and *sales information* typically comes at the end of the text. *Symptoms* tend to precede *virtues*, as they are logically connected, but *directions for use* and *testimonials* also co-occur with these moves in different combinations.

Previous studies of the linguistic features of pamphlet advertisements have remarked on their hyperbole, which serves as an affective feature, as well as the strong authorial presence and the frequent addresses to the reader. This study did not focus specifically on the linguistic features of the moves, but it did find that some linguistic features are prevalent in particular elements. First- and second-person pronouns and addresses to the reader appear in most moves. However, the interpersonality found in these texts is not dialogic in nature, for its function is to establish the author as the expert and source of knowledge. The imperatives and modals of possibility and necessity found especially in the *virtues* and *directions for use* further demonstrate the instructive nature of the pamphlets. The promotional function, on the other hand, is evident in the hyperbole in the descriptions found especially in the *endorsements*. Narratives can be found in *testimonials* that are made up of lengthy case studies. A more detailed analysis of linguistic features could identify further linguistic strategies for realizing the purposes of the individual moves.

13.5 Conclusion

This study has analyzed the moves found in seventeenth-century pamphlet advertisements of proprietary medicines and compared them to similar elements found in earlier and other contemporary medical genres. The analysis shows that pamphlet advertisements of proprietary medicines are a prime example of a hybrid genre that makes use of old, well-established conventions and novel contemporary developments in other medical genres. At the same time, a completely new move is added to satisfy the overtly promotional aspect of the texts, which is related to the changes that were taking place in the medical marketplace in the early modern period with the introduction of the first branded medicines.

Proprietary medicines became an enduring element of the medical marketplace, and texts advertising these products moved from pamphlets to other publication formats, specifically to newspapers, while pamphlet advertisements declined and disappeared. An obvious start for future studies is in the newspaper advertisements of medicines, which start to proliferate in the second half of the seventeenth century and become a common feature in the eighteenth. Comparing the moves found in pamphlet advertisements and the much shorter newspaper advertisements will reveal the enduring elements of medical advertisements first conceived by the opportunistic and innovative pamphlet writers.

REFERENCES

Bhatia, Vijay K. 1993. *Analyzing genre: Language use in professional settings.* London; New York: Longman.

Bhatia, Vijay K. 2005. Generic patterns in promotional discourse. In Helena Halmari & Tuija Virtanen (eds.), *Persuasion across genres: A linguistic approach*, 213–25. Amsterdam; Philadephia: Benjamins.

Borde, Sarah. 2015. Late Modern English death notices: Transformations of a traditional text type. In Birte Bös & Lucia Kornexl (eds.), *Changing genre conventions in historical English news discourse*, 103–33. Amsterdam; Philadephia: Benjamins.

Brownlees, Nicholas. 2011. *The language of periodical news in seventeenth-century England.* Newcastle upon Tyne: Cambridge Scholars Publishing.

Fissell, Mary E. 2007. The marketplace of print. In Mark S. R. Jenner & Patrick Wallis (eds.), *Medicine and the market in England and its colonies, c. 1450–c. 1850*, 108–32. Basingstoke; New York: Palgrave Macmillan.

Ge, Yunfeng. 2016. Sensationalism in media discourse: A genre-based analysis of Chinese legal news reports. *Discourse & Communication* 10(1): 22–39.

Groom, Nicholas, & Jack Grieve. 2019. The evolution of a legal genre: Rhetorical moves in British patent specifications, 1711 to 1860. In Teresa Fanego & Paula Rodríguez-Puente (eds.), *Corpus-based research on variation in English legal discourse*, 201–34. Amsterdam; Philadelphia: Benjamins.

Haycock, David Boyd, & Patrick Wallis. 2005. Quackery and commerce in seventeenth-century London: The proprietary medicine business of Anthony Daffy. *Medical History*, Supplement No. 25.

auf dem Keller, Caren. 2004. *Textual structures in eighteenth-century newspaper advertising: A corpus-based study of medical advertisements and book advertisements.* Aachen: Shaker Verlag.

Loréz-Sanz, Rosa. 2016. ELF in the making? Simplicity and hybridity in abstract writing. *Journal of English as a Lingua Franca* 5(1): 53–81.

Mackintosh, Alan. 2018. *The patent medicines industry in Georgian England: Constructing the market by the potency of print.* London: Palgrave Macmillan.

Mäkinen, Martti. 2006. Between herbals et alia: Intertextuality in medieval English herbals. PhD dissertation, University of Helsinki.

Maswana, Sayako, Toshiyuki Kanamaru, & Akira Tajino 2015. Move analysis of research articles across five engineering fields: What they share and what they do not. *Ampersand* 2: 1–11.

Mullini, Roberta. 2010. 'Gull'd by the enchanting tongues of *quack* and *zany*': The rhetoric of nostrum marketing in speech and print in early modern London. In Nicholas Brownlees, Gabriella Del Lungo, & John Denton (eds.), *The language of public and private communication in a historical perspective*, 359–76. Newcastle upon Tyne: Cambridge Scholars Publishing.

Pahta, Päivi, & Maura Ratia. 2010. Treatises of specific topics. In Irma Taavitsainen & Päivi Pahta (eds.), *Early Modern English Medical Texts: Corpus description and studies*, 73–99. Amsterdam; Philadelphia: Benjamins.

Porter, Roy. 1989. *Health for sale: Quackery in England, 1660–1850*. Manchester: Manchester University Press.

Ratia, Maura, & Carla Suhr. 2011. Medical pamphlets: Controversy and advertising. In Irma Taavitsainen & Päivi Pahta (eds.), *Medical writing in Early Modern English*, 180–203. Cambridge: Cambridge University Press.

Stannard, Jerry. 1982. Rezeptlitteratur as Fachlitteratur. In William Eamon (ed.), *Studies on Medieval Fachlitteratur*, 59–73. Brussels: Omirel.

Styles, John. 2000. Product innovation in early modern London. *Past & Present* 168: 124–69.

Swales, John. 1990. *Genre analysis: English in academic and research settings*. Cambridge: Cambridge University Press.

Swales, John. 2004. *Research genres: Explorations and applications*. Cambridge: Cambridge University Press.

Taavitsainen, Irma. 2001. Changing conventions of writing: The dynamics of genres, text types, and text traditions. *European Journal of English Studies* 5(2): 139–50.

Taavitsainen, Irma. 2011. Medical case reports and scientific thought-styles. In Francisco Alonso-Almeida (ed.), Special Issue: Diachronic English for specific purposes. *Revista de Lenguas para Fines Específicos* 17: 75–98.

Taavitsainen, Irma, & Päivi Pahta (eds.), *Early Modern English Medical Texts: Corpus description and studies*. Amsterdam; Philadelphia: Benjamins.

Taavitsainen, Irma, & Gerold Schneider. 2019. Scholastic argumentation in early English medical writing and its afterlife: New corpus evidence. In Carla Suhr, Terttu Nevalainen, & Irma Taavitsainen (eds.), *From data to evidence in English language research*, 191–221. Leiden: Brill.

Tardy, Christine M., & John M. Swales. 2014. Genre analysis. In Klaus P. Schneider & Anne Barren (eds.), *Pragmatics of discourse*, 165–87. Berlin: De Gruyter.

Wallis, Patrick. 2008. Consumption, retailing, and medicine in early-modern London. *Economic History Review* 61(1): 26–53.

Wear, Andrew. 2000. *Knowledge and practice in English medicine, 1550–1680*. Cambridge: Cambridge University Press.

Zhang, Yiqiong. 2018. Retailing science: Genre hybridization in online science news. *Text & Talk* 38(2): 243–65.

Zhou, Sijing. 2012. 'Advertorials': A genre-based analysis of an emerging hybridized genre. *Discourse & Communication* 6(3): 323–46.

CHAPTER 14

Persuasion in Hungarian Medical Recipes

Ágnes Kuna

> There is wondrous power for curing that in the skull of a dead man.
> (MBM-203)

Recipes constitute one of the most ancient genres of the medical text tradition, which has served as an important medium for sharing knowledge about healing since the very beginning of medication. Moreover, it also preserves and transmits sociocultural practices of healing as well as several other practical activities characteristic of particular ages and nations, thus functioning as a kind of 'cultural footprint' or 'mirror' (De la Cruz-Cabanillas 2020: 57–8). This continuity also underlies the social relevance of the genre (Heinemann 2000: 520).

In the sixteenth and seventeenth centuries, recipes were an especially prominent genre in medication and in the compilation and documentation of knowledge related to household activities (Leong 2018). This is testified to by recipe collections, remedy books preserved either in a handwritten form or in print, and also by knowledge and experiences shared in letters. Beyond sharing knowledge, such texts also foreground the function of persuasion by affirming the efficacy of a recommended therapy and by aiming for the creation of a positive attitude in the reader (McVaugh 1997: 216), which is linguistically well documented (e.g. Jones 1998; Taavitsainen 2001; Alonso-Almeida & Cabrera-Abreu 2002; Mäkinen 2011).

The goal of this chapter is to identify major patterns of persuasion in sixteenth- and seventeenth-century Hungarian recipes. It begins by offering an overview of the main features of sixteenth- and seventeenth-century healing and the related medical text tradition, highlighting the role of

This research was supported by the János Bolyai Research Scholarship of the Hungarian Academy of Sciences and by the ÚNKP-21-5-ELTE-223 New National Excellence Program of the Ministry for Innovation and Technology from the source of the National Research, Development and Innovation Fund, and also by the Hungarian Scientific Research Fund (Nr. K129040).

medical recipes as a genre in this context. This is followed by a demonstration of the material, methodology, and research questions of the investigation. The results section presents the most characteristic categories and linguistic constructions of persuasion in the material under study. Finally, the chapter ends with a short summary and concluding remarks.

14.1 The Sociocultural Background of the Hungarian Medical Discourse Domain in the Sixteenth and Seventeenth Centuries

The roots of Hungarian healing practices can be traced back to shamanism. However, apart from this early period, they have formed an integral part of the history of European medication, whose main features and stages are highlighted here in their relation to the corresponding medical text tradition.

Medication in Hungary in the sixteenth and seventeenth centuries was characterized by a high degree of heterogeneity. While the traditions of ancient Greco-Roman and Arabic medicine continued, folk healing also played a remarkable role, usually drawing on personal experiences, beliefs, and superstitions. In addition, the influence of organized religion ought not to be overlooked (Hoppál 1990: 699–701). Healing belonged to the spheres of both science and everyday practice, with the latter engaging a broad spectrum of society through a highly varied group of healers (see Figure 14.1). Apart from a small number of physicians, pharmacists, and barbers, most of the healing was carried out by specialists working among the people. Inevitably, this had an impact on the vernacular medical text tradition, in which scientific works accounted for a minority compared to popular recipe collections, remedy books, and herbarium books (Voigts 1982; Taavitsainen & Pahta 2004: 160).

The sixteenth and seventeenth centuries mark the first stage of Hungarian medical writing, providing the earliest surviving documents of considerable length. From the preceding periods, only fragmentary texts survive. As Szlatky observes:

> Manuscripts and printed books together characterize the first period of Hungarian medical literature, and any differences resulting from printed as opposed to manuscript forms are easily offset by similarities deriving from shared themes, modes of presentation and the medium of Hungarian. (Szlatky 1983: 384)

Scientific treatises did not appear in Hungarian in the sixteenth and seventeenth centuries. Thus, surgical practices were primarily shared in

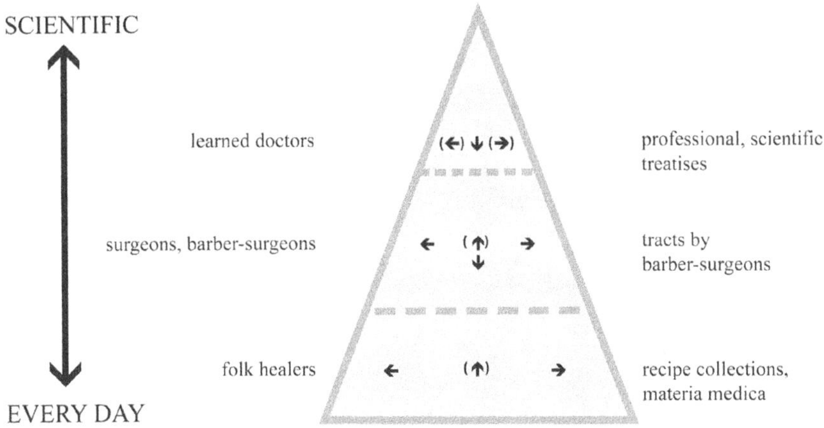

Figure 14.1 Correlations between the layered structures of medication and medical communication (sixteenth and seventeenth centuries)

recipe collections and other remedy books. From references made by contemporary authors, it is safe to infer that Hungarian-language medical literature must have included considerably more vernacular texts than those that are available to posterity (Szlatky 1980: 134).

Most of the surviving medical writings from this period are manuscripts (see Figure 14.2). The manuscripts were typically produced by compilation, translation, and copying, and have little in the way of a unifying principle. The professional standard of these compilations varies greatly, depending on the quality of the authors' sources and that of the translation. The key feature of these collections is that they served practical purposes. The texts are typically everyday recipe collections, remedy books, and herbarium books indicative of the scientific level of the era. In all of these texts, the genre of recipes plays a prominent role.

14.1.1 Recipe: Context for Persuasion

For millennia, recipes have been a central genre for sharing knowledge about healing and other practical everyday information. This holds true for the sixteenth and seventeenth centuries as well, with recipes permeating all levels of the medical text tradition (Taavitsainen 2001; Carroll 2004; Alonso-Almeida 2013). At this time, recipes played a key role in doctors' works, surgical documents, and everyday recipe collections alike.

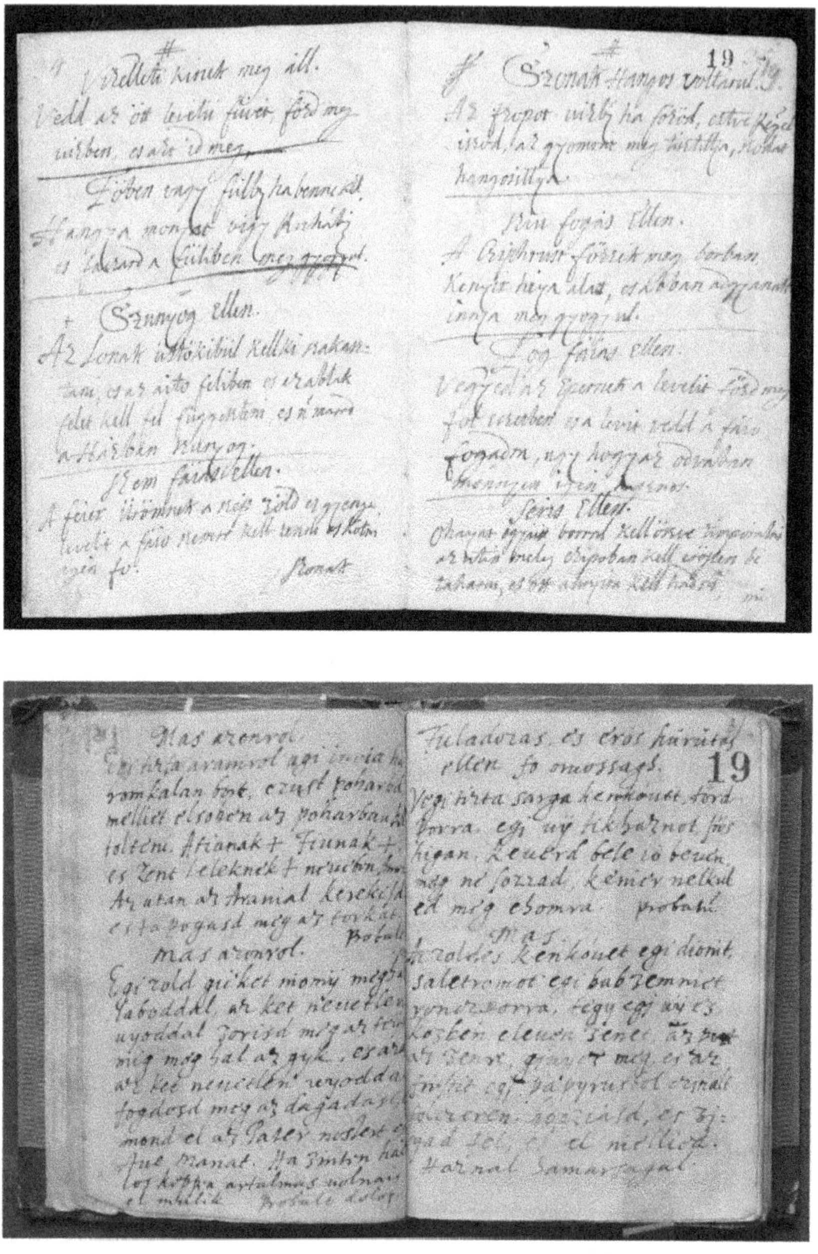

Figure 14.2 Illustrations of the manuscripts KP and HP

In the era under study, a recipe can be considered as a basic-level genre with several subtypes organized thematically (Hunt 1990: 16–17) or according to typical speech situations (e.g. therapeutic, herbal recipes, bloodletting, veterinary knowledge, dietary suggestions and beauty care, cookery recipes). They served as a key medium for sharing everyday knowledge ('household science') at the time (Leong 2018: 4) and had a much broader sphere of use than they do now. The basic or general theme of the genre is USEFUL KNOWLEDGE.[1] Thus, the notion of positive evaluation and a concomitant persuasive intention are already evident in a recipe's theme. USEFUL KNOWLEDGE is typically elaborated in relation to recommended actions ('this is how to do it'; Carroll 2004: 188). More specifically, recipes are instructions (Görlach 1992: 745; Taavitsainen 2001: 86) for the preparation of a substance, whether it is medicine, food, or some other everyday item (soap, wool, etc.).

Recipes include different types of typical information, though none of it is obligatory (Stannard 1982: 60–5). While subject to variation, the arrangement of this information follows a clear communicative principle or textual strategy, namely that of chronological sequencing (Taavitsainen 2001: 98). Prototypically, information occurring in sixteenth- and seventeenth-century recipes can be packaged into three functional units (Kuna 2016a: 205): (i) *heading* (what it is for: introducing an illness and its cure at a conceptual level); (ii) *section for instructions* (how much of what, and how: ingredients, measurements, instructions, methods, and tools); and (iii) *persuasion* (with an emphasis on efficacy and usefulness):

(1) *Ver hasrul* [heading].
Szedgied az cyprust, rutath, tongöri szölöt, eggiot fözd meg feier borban es igia meg. [section for instructions]
Probatum est. [persuasion] (TOK-176; emphasis added)
('Dysentery. Take cypress, rue and red currant, cook them together in white wine and let the patient drink it. This has been tried.')

The third functional unit, persuasion, is the focus of this chapter. In the analysis, however, I examine not only text-final persuasive units but rather the texts in their entirety, exploring persuasive communication. In the

[1] Conceptual categories/domains are marked by small caps, in line with the conventions of cognitive linguistics. A conceptual domain or frame is a coherent body of knowledge organized around a central concept (Croft & Cruse 2004: 17).

section below, I outline its linguistic and conceptual manifestations as well as its strategic character.

14.1.2 Persuasion in Recipes

The functional unit serving the purposes of persuasion by highlighting the recipe's efficacy has been broadly analysed in the literature, going by a variety of terms such as *efficacy statement*, *efficacy phrase*, *tag phrase*, and *stock phrase* (see e.g. Jones 1998; Alonso-Almeida & Cabrera-Abreu 2002; Mäkinen 2011). Efficacy phrases evaluate the medical value of a recipe and create a positive attitude toward it. As the earlier analyses have revealed, efficacy phrases have a variety of forms and roles. These expressions often signal the influence of a Latin source, which is characteristic of the genre; moreover, they also provide clues for textual organization. Prototypically, efficacy phrases appear toward the end of medical recipes (Cameron 1993: 40; Jones 1998: 201). However, other positions are also possible (Hunt 1990: 22–4; Taavitsainen 2001: 104–6; Alonso-Almeida & Cabrera-Abreu 2002: 140; Mäkinen 2011: 161–2).

Taking stock of previous studies on efficacy phrases but also departing from them in certain ways, the present analysis focuses on the linguistic and conceptual elaborations of persuasion, as well as the relationship between persuasion and evaluation in sixteenth- and seventeenth-century Hungarian medical recipes. Patterns of persuasive intent (and not the persuasive effect; Jucker 1997: 122–3) are considered in light of the contemporary sociocultural background of the texts.

In the analysis, persuasion is interpreted as a linguistic-conceptual strategic action aimed at changing the addressee's attitudes or behaviour, or at reinforcing her existing beliefs and conceptions with respect to a given phenomenon (Jucker 1997: 122; Virtanen & Halmari 2005: 5). In relation to attitudes, evaluation is a key aspect of persuasion, as indicated by the fact that one of the main ways of expressing persuasion is by using evaluating assertive speech acts (Ortak 2004: 149). Evaluation has both direct and indirect forms of instantiation, depending on whether the speaker expresses value attribution with an explicit linguistic symbol (e.g. *good*, *wonderful*) or opts for indirect construal by relying on background information (e.g. the authenticity of a person). Though linked to persuasion and its polarizing style of suggestive communication (cf. Ortak 2004: 155), value attribution may of course also receive expression by other speech acts, too. In the case of recipes, these include promises and prognostications related to the result of therapy (Alonso-Almeida & Cabrera-Abreu 2002: 145–51).

14.2 Research Data and Method

Owing to the lack of an electronic corpus of Hungarian medical language, the material of the present empirical research on persuasion in recipes consists of the transcripts of five handwritten recipe collections for everyday use,[2] as well as the earliest surviving handwritten remedy book in Hungarian, *Ars medica* (ca. 1577). The latter has been made available in a software-based form as well (Szabó & Bíró 2000), which serves as a basis for the analysis of this remedy book. Although the selected works (see Table 14.1 and sources) cannot showcase the medical discourse domain of the era in its entirety, they still supply representative material for the study of major patterns of expressing a persuasive intent. This representativity comes from the fact that they comprise a high number of recipes (approximately 15,000–18,000) and display characteristic features of recipes of that time. The overwhelming majority (more than 95 percent) of the texts are related to healing; however, household know-how (about hunting and bee-keeping) also occurs in some of them, especially in the recipe collections.

The analysis of persuasion adopts a pragmatic perspective (Pelclová & Lu 2018) and primarily follows qualitative principles. The latter is in part justified by the fact that no electronic corpus of Hungarian medical recipes is available at present; therefore, methods for a corpus-based pragmatic study of persuasion cannot be applied (e.g. Mäkinen 2011). Additionally, the choice of qualitative methods also results from the goals of the analysis. Specifically, the exploration of genre-specific conceptual patterns invites qualitative analytical methods. The coding and mapping of patterns do, however, facilitate quantitative analyses and contribute to the goal of allowing persuasion to be searched for and studied also in a quantitative manner.

Over the course of analysis, I adopted a multistep procedure. Conceptual categories (codes)[3] associated with persuasion were established

[2] Work on compiling the sixteenth- and seventeenth-century subcorpus of the *Corpus of Medical Hungarian* is in progress (Kuna 2016b). Several manuscripts have received literal and normalized transcriptions, but they are not yet publicly available. This is the reason why the present analyses are based on Hoffmann's (1989) literal transcriptions of the recipe collections. References to examples correspond to the numbering conventions of the source. The recipe collections are not variations of a single manuscript, as only a few of the recipes are shared by all of the collections.

[3] The terms *conceptual category* and *code* are used interchangeably here. Although in linguistics *code* has several meanings, in the present chapter it is adopted in accordance with the terminology of qualitative software-based analysis.

Table 14.1 *Data about the manuscripts under study*

Title of the manuscript[a]	Number of recipes	Word count	Abbreviation[b]
Ars medica	Not known	192,913 words	AM
Testi orvosságok könyve	399	12,693 words	TOK
Kis patika	156	4,875 words	KP
Házi patika	262	8,210 words	HP
Medicusi és borbélyi mesterség	1,426	43,131 words	MBM
Mindenféle orvosságoknak rendszedése	232	13,862 words	MOR
TOTAL	6,877 (+AM)	275,684 words	

[a]For English translations of the titles, see sources.
[b]For specifying the source of each example, I use these abbreviations along with the recipe number or the numerical structure of the manuscript itself.

at multiple levels. First, I used a sample consisting of around 5,000 recipes to study acts of persuasion as functionally distinct textual units within recipes (Kuna 2016a: 214–16). In this earlier work, which was oriented toward text typology, it was already highlighted that persuasion formed part of an overall text-producing strategy. For the analysis of this strategy, a preliminary system of categories was subsequently set up, aimed at describing typical conceptual categories of persuasion in recipes. This procedure involved taking stock of and categorizing linguistic constructions associated with a persuasive intent and positive communication, in a way that was informed by related analyses in the disciplines of rhetoric and psychology, as well as studies of early and modern-era medical communication.

After setting up a system of categories, its validity was tested by eight Master of Arts (MA) students of psychology taking a course on suggestive communication in a medical context. Two students identified their own coding categories for words or phrases they regarded as having persuasive or suggestive force. They also provided descriptions for the coding categories. The codes described by the two students overlapped considerably with my own coding criteria. After the conflation and re-editing of the two lists of coding categories, six other students encoded the same 100 recipes (4,285 words) with the help of precise code descriptions. With the exception of one coder, intercoder agreement was in the range of 60–90 percent. In 2018, an MA student of linguistics again performed the coding process. With regard to the marking of passages in the texts and the main conceptual categories, her work resulted in intercoder agreement exceeding 80 percent with my own analysis. It should be noted that in this system a persuasive phrase can receive multiple codes. Beyond coding the conceptual-linguistic categories of persuasive expressions, I also marked the position of each persuasive phrase within a recipe, with the aim of determining the positional distribution of such phrases (see Section 14.3.2). The coding procedure is illustrated in the following example:

(2) *Ha az örménygyükeret megsütüd, megtöröd, vajban megfőzöd, az ótvart megkened véle,* ***meggyógyul vele szépen.*** (MBM-120; emphasis added)
('When you fry horse-heal, crush it, cook it in butter, and spread it on impetigo, **it heals nicely with this.**')

In (2), a total of three codes are associated with the quotation *meggyógyul vele szépen* ('it heals nicely with this'). With regard to distribution, it is text-final; in terms of content, it profiles GOOD, NICE, as well as HEALING (see Section 14.3.3). The entire analysis followed the same principle. In the five recipe collections, 2,912 phrases (quotations) were classified as pertaining to persuasion, and a total of 4,170 code designations were made.

After the codes were updated to their final versions, the subsequent qualitative analysis was performed with the software ATLAS.ti 7.2, which is able to visualize the co-occurrence or overlap of code categories, and also lists coded linguistic representations. This way, it was possible to retrieve typical linguistic constructions expressing a persuasive intent, which can be later integrated into the automatic query of expressions with a persuasive function in an electronic corpus.

This idea was put to the test in the analysis of *Ars medica*. The codes set up and validated by employing multiple coders as well as the software-based analysis served as a basis for the study of *Ars medica*, which I performed on the electronic edition of the remedy book (Szabó & Bíró 2000). This part of the present study incorporated the use of the proprietary search engine of ATLAS.ti to retrieve the linguistic representations of the conceptual categories, as supplied by ATLAS.ti. This change of method was made necessary by the fact that *Ars medica* is hardly amenable to qualitative analysis by ATLAS.ti, as the software is ill-suited for the study of such lengthy documents. The setting up of codes and the linguistic representations emerging from the analysis of recipe collections made it possible to search for tokens in this extensive work, and thus to collect linguistic representations related to the conceptual-linguistic category of persuasion.

I used a lemmatized search to retrieve token clusters. For example, in the case of USEFULNESS (*hasznosság*), I searched for more than twenty word-forms related to the category (e.g. *haszn**, *hat**). The same procedure was adopted for all the other categories as well; that is, I examined possible linguistic representations identified by earlier analyses and searched for (as well as manually filtered) them individually. This was partly made necessary by the fact that not all of the tokens were related to persuasion; moreover, it sometimes happened that the search engine displayed two searched-for tokens in the same window, at the same time. Therefore, frequency could only be calculated on the basis of manual checking of tokens. When it comes to personal names, geographical names, and similar categories, my work was aided by the word list of *Ars medica.* Ultimately, I identified and analysed a total of 3,884 phrases related to persuasion in the remedy book.

By using the material and methods described above, I sought to answer the following questions: With what frequency do persuasive phrases occur in recipes? In which position or in which part of the recipes do they occur? How can they be described in terms of conceptual-linguistic categories? What co-occurrences do these categories display? What role is played by the concept of VALUE, including both its positive and its negative poles, in the expression of persuasive intent? Do acts of persuasion have a prototype in Hungarian medical recipes of the sixteenth and seventeenth centuries? In what follows, I discuss the results of my analysis in terms of their relevance for these issues.

14.3 Trends of Persuasion in Sixteenth- and Seventeenth-Century Hungarian Recipes: Results

14.3.1 Frequency of Persuasive Phrases

Based on the analysis, a total of 6,796 persuasive phrases were identified in the six manuscripts. Their distribution is presented in Figure 14.3.

In the case of the five recipe collections analysed by ATLAS.ti, I conducted a further survey to find out the 'density' with which persuasive phrases occurred in particular manuscripts, in order to facilitate comparisons. The frequency of persuasive phrases in recipe collections was compared in terms of three numerical indices. F1 concerns the average number of phrases per recipe, measured by dividing the number of persuasive quotations in the manuscript by the number of recipes. The second index, F2, specifies the average number of persuasion-related code designations

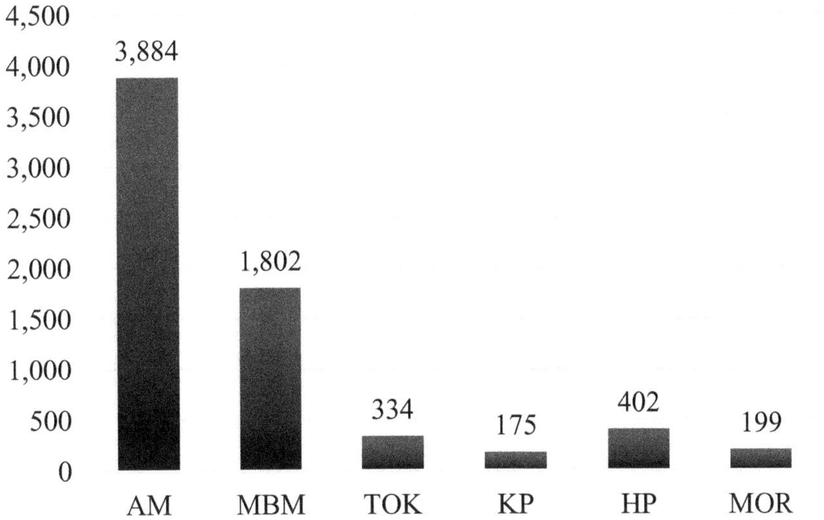

Figure 14.3 The numerical distribution of persuasive phrases in the recipe collections

per recipe, measured by dividing the number of persuasion-related code designations in the manuscript by the number of recipes. Finally, the third index, F3, highlights the frequency of occurrence of persuasive phrases with respect to the number of word tokens (the number of persuasive quotations divided by the number of word tokens in the manuscript, multiplied by 100 for the sake of ease of exposition). The values of the three figures in particular manuscripts are presented in Figure 14.4.

As we can see, in MBM, KP, and HP, on average there is more than one persuasive quotation per recipe. Of course, this does not mean that every recipe would have a persuasive part (some of them have none, while others include several). In the recipe collections TOK and MOR, by contrast, F1 falls below 1; that is, on average there is fewer than one persuasive phrase in the recipes. F2, for its part, concerns the question of how often the conceptual categories co-occur, typically enhancing each other's effect. This index is the highest in MBM and HP, around 2. This means that on average two categories are combined in particular quotations in every recipe. F2 is at its lowest in TOK and MOR, with values around 1. This means that generally just one code designation is associated with each quotation. Looking at F3, we can see that persuasive phrases have the highest share with respect to the number of word tokens in HP (4.8), MBM (4.1), and KP (3.5). By contrast, the F3 values of TOK (2.4) and

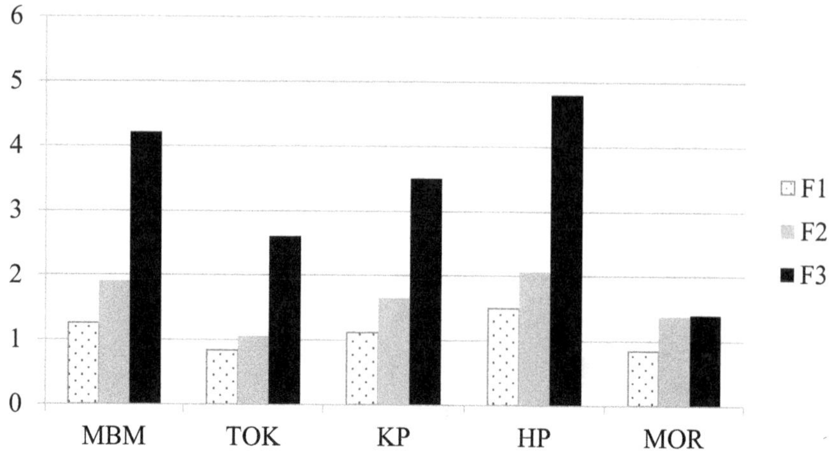

Figure 14.4 Values of F1, F2, and F3 in the recipe collections

MOR (1.4) are much lower. Based on the three figures, the elaboration of persuasive acts is more intense in MBM, KP, and HP than in TOK and MOR.

14.3.2 The Positional Distribution of Persuasive Phrases in the Texts

I examined the distribution of linguistic representations of persuasion in the five recipe collections analysed by ATLAS.ti. The results are shown in Figure 14.5.

As can be seen, the text-final position is the most dominant, making up 43 percent, or 50 percent when the penultimate position[4] is also included. In close correlation with the directing of attention, persuasive communication puts a premium on information in first and last positions (Miller & Campbell 1959); essentially, this can be interpreted as a positioning operation. When the first position (also prominent in terms of positioning) is also taken into account (15 percent), then the three positions have a share of 65 percent in total. The relatively high proportion of persuasive phrases in text-medial position can be primarily ascribed to the frequency

[4] The penultimate position was marked in cases where a persuasive part in text-final position was immediately preceded by another persuasive part and separated from other passages by an interpunctuation mark in the manuscript, cf. Example 4. Such efficacy phrases are closely connected to text-final persuasion, which is why the latter position can be said to have a share of 50 percent.

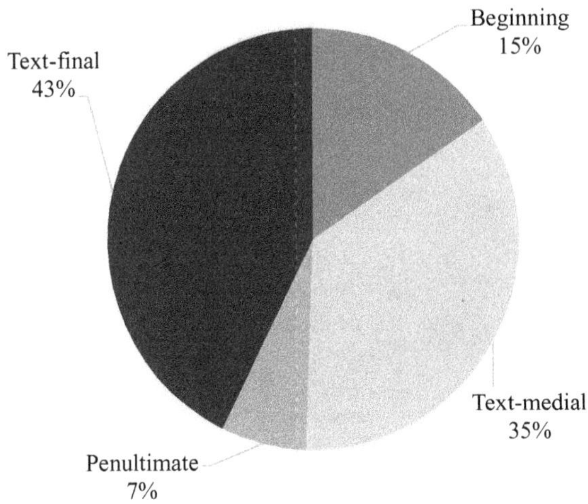

Figure 14.5 The distribution of persuasive phrases in recipes included in recipe collections

and general scope with which the concept of GOOD is linguistically elaborated (see Section 14.3.3). To summarize, positioning is a key factor for persuasion in the recipes, with special prominence attached to text-final and text-initial positions.

14.3.3 Conceptual Categories of Persuasion and Their Co-occurrences in Medical Recipes

Over the course of qualitative analysis, I explored the conceptual construal of persuasion in recipes along the lines of ten main classes and twenty-five subcategories. For their detailed presentation in terms of semantic features, including several illustrative examples, see Kuna (2018). In the present chapter the categories are only discussed in a summary fashion, and presented in Table 14.2,[5] with solely the frequency and co-occurrence of categories (as revealed by software-based investigations) receiving in-depth analysis.

Based on the software-supported analysis, the ten main codes related to persuasion have the frequencies in the remedy book and in the five recipe collections shown in Figure 14.6.

[5] The numbers do not indicate chronological order; rather, they only aid the process of coding and illustration. A slight difference with respect to Kuna (2018) is that after a software-based analysis of the entire material, categories 9 and 10 came to be included.

Table 14.2 *Conceptual categories of persuasion*

1. GENERAL POSITIVE VALUE	
1.1. GOOD, NICE, BEAUTIFUL	(3) *Főszédelgésről* ***igen jó, jó*** (MBM-33) ('For dizziness, it is **very good, good**')
1.2. USEFUL	(4) *Ez is próbált dolog,* ***hasznos való*** (MBM-9) ('This is also a tested thing, **useful**')
1.3.WONDER, WONDERFUL	(5) ***csuda*** *hasznát érzi* (MBM-845) ('feels its **miraculous** benefit')
1.4.CLEVER, WISE	(6) *kövessed amaz* ***bölcznek*** *mondását* (HP-195) ('follow the advice **of that wise man**')
1.5.IMPORTANT, FAMOUS	(7) *Ezek oly* ***fö dolgok,*** *az mellieknek massa nem talaltatik.* (KP-156) ('These are **important things** which have no parallels')
1.6.FORTUNE/LUCK	(8) ***Szerenczéd liszen puskádhoz.*** *Probatum est.* (HP-202) ('**You will have luck with your gun**. It has been tried.')
1.7.OTHER (EFFORTLESSNESS)	(9) ***minden erőltetés nélkül*** *kitisztítja az rosz nedvességet* (MBM-508) ('it cleans the bad humidity **without strain**')
2. INTENSITY	(10) E*s ottan meg indittia, ha még* ***uas auagi aczel erejü giomor uolnais*** (KP-73) ('And then it sets it in motion, even when **the stomach has the power of iron or steel**')
3. TESTEDNESS	(11) ***Probalth dologh*** *egjnehanzor sok ieles ferfiakon* (TOK-311) ('**This thing has been tried** a couple of times on several outstanding men')
4. CERTAINTY	
4.1. CERTAIN, TRUE [+]/[–]	(12) ***bizony*** *orvosság* (AM I.97b) ('it is an ***unfailing*** cure'
4.2. DOUBT	(13) *de lehet* ***ketsegh*** *az olyan beteghez* (AM I.157a) ('but **doubt** may affect a patient like that')
5. TIME FACTOR	
5.1. SPEEDINESS	(14) *haznal* ***hamarsagal*** (KP-29) ('it brings benefits **soon**')
5.2. BELATEDNESS	(15) ***soha*** *megh nem gyogyulhat* (AM I.105a) ('s/he can **never** recover')
6. RESULT OF THERAPY	
6.1. HEALING	
6.1.1. HEALING, RECOVERY	(16) *köszvénybül* ***meg gyogyét*** (HP-91) ('**it cures you** of gout')
6.1.2. PASSING OF THE DISEASE	(17) *csudalatossan* ***ki vonysa a' genieseget, es megh tiztettia*** (MOR-21) ('miraculously **it removes pus, and cleans it**')

Table 14.2 (*cont.*)

6.1.3. POSITIVE CHANGE	(18) elmenek **tiztulast es uidulast *zerez*** (KP-23) (**'it cleans and cheers up** the mind')
6.1.4. OTHER	(19) *melegen a tyúkoknak adod,* ***sokat tojnak tőle.*** (MBM-138) ('if you give it to the hens while it is warm, **they will lay lots of eggs from it**')
6.2. FATAL OUTCOME	(20) *hamar megh hal az ember* (AM I.137a) ('the man **will die** soon')
7. AUTHENTICITY/CREDIBILITY	
7.1. THE RECIPE'S AUTHOR	(21) ***Magam*** *probal**tam*** *dolog* (KP-5) ('A thing **I** have tested **myself**')
7.2. THIRD PERSON	
7.2.1. SPECIFIC FAMOUS PERSON	(22) ***Reverius híres doktor*** *írja* (MBM-706) ('**the famous doctor Reverius** writes this')
7.2.2. GENERAL, NON-SPECIFIC PERSON	(23) ***Minden doktorok dicsírik*** *ezt a füvet* (MBM-1248) ('**All doctors praise** this herb')
7.2.3. REFERENCE TO GOD	(24) *ketsegnelkul* ***Isten akarattiabol*** *megh allattia az fenet* (TOK-227) ('without doubt, **God willing,** it will stop the problem')
8. EMOTIONAL INVOLVEMENT	
8.1. POSITIVE EMOTIONAL EFFECT	(25) ***Barátom, nem tréfa ez. Ezt observáld bár meg. Köszvényes barátom, próbáld meg, nem hagysz hazugságban, ebben is, hidd el bár*** (MBM-840) ('My friend, this is no joke. Observe this. My gouty friend, try it, you won't find me lying about this either; believe me')
8.2. NEGATIVE EMOTIONAL EFFECT	(26) *Agy velenek penigh* ***semmi ugy nem art,*** *minth az emztetlensegh* (AM I.2a) ('**Nothing is as bad** for the brain as indigestion')
9. ARGUMENTATION, JUSTIFICATION	(27) *eczuetest ne igiek,* ***mert*** *hamar megh eozül miatta* (TOK-354) ('should not drink anything with vinegar **because** his hair will grow grey because of it')
10. OTHER (e.g. geographical place, prayer, incantation)	(28) *es jol lösz:* ***X9XX5XOCX3X*** (HP-208) ('and will be good: ***X9XX5XOCX3X***')[6]

[6] Charms and prayers may form a part of persuasive, suggestive communication. However, they occur very rarely in the recipes under study (see category 10 in Figure 14.6).

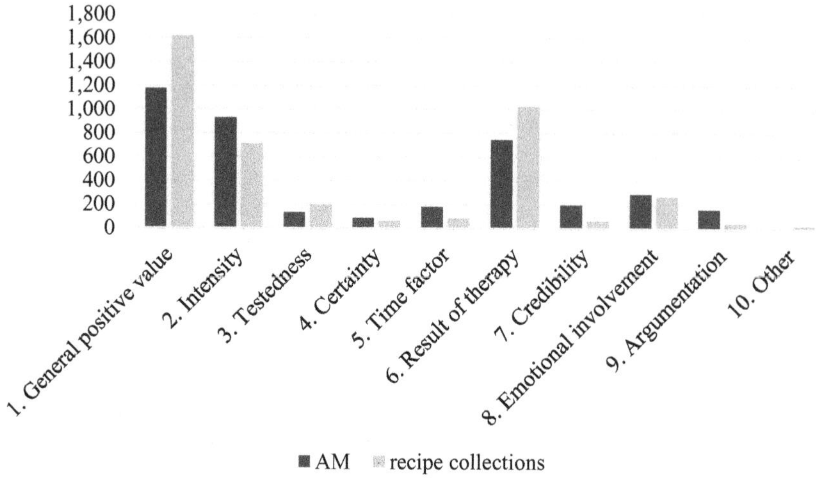

Figure 14.6 The frequency of categories related to persuasion in *Ars medica* and in the recipe collections

As Figure 14.6 shows, 1. GENERAL POSITIVE VALUE is the most frequent category in *Ars medica* and in the recipe collections. Also prominent are the elaborations of 2. INTENSITY and the 6. RESULT OF THERAPY. In the recipe collections, 1. GENERAL POSITIVE VALUE and 6. RESULT OF THERAPY are expressed more frequently, whereas in the remedy book, the linguistic representations of 7. AUTHENTICITY/CREDIBILITY are more common. This may be explained by genre-specific features, by the sources used by authors (and the schemas they follow), and the scholastic style alike (Taavitsainen & Pahta 1998: 167–74). Generally speaking, though, it can be concluded that the proportions of patterns of persuasion are remarkably similar between the recipe collections and the remedy book. This is most probably linked to the fact that each text was written for non-professional people, and they are based on a similar text tradition, following similar patterns. Unfortunately, scientific treatises in Hungarian are not available from the era under study, hence they cannot serve as a standard of comparison (cf. Mäkinen 2011: 171–5).

The examples in Table 14.2 and 14.3 both show that a given persuasive phrase may well be associated with many categories and receive multiple codes. For example, in (29), which is the heading of a recipe, the concepts of 1.5 IMPORTANCE/FAMOUS, 2. INTENSITY, and 3. TESTEDNESS are combined:

(29) *Akarmi fele forma közueny ellen fö probált oruossag.* (KP-18)
('It is a major tested medicine against any kind of gout.')

The ATLAS.ti software makes it possible to study co-occurrences across main and subcategories in the five recipe collections under study, and I analysed the clustering of all of the categories. Here, however, I only present co-occurrences in terms of the ten main categories (see Table 14.3), with colour coding to indicate the frequencies of the co-occurrences.

Looking at relationships across main categories, we can see that they typically do not co-occur with themselves. Exceptions in this regard concern 1. GENERAL POSITIVE VALUE and 6. RESULT OF THERAPY. The multiple elaborations (58 times in both cases) presumably have an accentuating function. To a lesser extent, the categories of 7. AUTHENTICITY/CREDIBILITY and 8. EMOTIONAL INVOLVEMENT also

Table 14.3 *The clustering of the main categories in the recipe collections*

	1.	2.	3.	4.	5.	6.	7.	8.	9.	10.
1.	58									
2.	546	0								
3.	18	21	0							
4.	10	10	2	0						
5.	22	41	0	0	0					
6.	199	209	3	25	65	58				
7.	33	24	13	2	0	8	8			
8.	59	64	1	11	2	68	7	2		
9.	14	12	0	0	0	9	3	29	0	
10.	7	8	3	0	0	0	11	0	0	0

1 – 20
21 – 50
51– 100
100 – 200
200 –

1. GENERAL POSITIVE VALUE
2. INTENSITY
3. TESTEDNESS
4. CERTAINTY
5. TIME FACTOR
6. RESULT OF THERAPY
7. AUTHENTICITY/CREDIBILITY
8. EMOTIONAL INVOLVEMENT
9. ARGUMENTATION
10. OTHER

co-occur with themselves. As shown by Table 14.3, 1. GENERAL POSITIVE VALUE and 6. RESULT OF THERAPY are often combined (in 199 instances), and these two categories are also the most likely to be elaborated in conjunction with 2. INTENSITY (in 546 and 209 instances, respectively). Further, it can be established that 8. EMOTIONAL INVOLVEMENT is often combined with 1. GENERAL POSITIVE VALUE (59 instances), with 2. INTENSITY (64 times), and with 6. RESULT OF THERAPY (68 instances). Moreover, a close relationship between 5. TIME FACTOR and 6. RESULT OF THERAPY can also be discerned (65 co-occurrences).

The analysis shows that the concept of 2. INTENSITY is almost always combined with some other category, and even particular subcategories. Most frequently 2. INTENSITY co-occurs with 1. GENERAL POSITIVE VALUE (546 instances) and especially its subcategories 1.1 GOOD/NICE/BEAUTIFUL (403 instances), 1.2 USEFUL (87 times), and 1.5 IMPORTANT/FAMOUS (33 instances). 2. INTENSITY also often co-occurs with 6. RESULT OF THERAPY (209 instances), more specifically its subcategory of 6.1.3 POSITIVE CHANGE (205 instances). Furthermore, 2. INTENSITY co-occurs with the subcategory 5.1 SPEEDINESS (41 instances) of 5. TIME FACTOR, and with the subcategory 8.1 POSITIVE EMOTIONAL EFFECT (40 instances) of 8. EMOTIONAL INVOLVEMENT (64 instances). Clustering as a tendency may be put down to the fact that the linguistic elaboration of 2. INTENSITY can be linked to various constructions in recipes (e.g. enhancement, expression of degree, hyperbole, lengthiness, ALL–NOTHING, and the extremes of other scales). In addition, it also highlights the fact that persuasion and its conceptual-linguistic construal are fundamentally related to more intense elaboration, which is iconically manifested in the expressions involved.

14.3.4 Persuasion and Value

The results of analysis also point to the fact that the operation of polarization (value attribution) is central for the function of persuasion in recipes. This finding is in line with research on persuasion in the modern and historical era (Ortak 2004; Östman 2005; Mäkinen 2011), and also with the definition of persuasion that refers to a change of attitude, typically also involving/activating explicit or implicit value attribution.

Based on the manuscripts under study, elaboration of the positive pole is much more dominant than that of the negative pole in recipes of the era. This can be seen in data on both frequency of occurrence and co-occurrences. In the recipe collections, a positive outcome is highlighted 1,034 times, but a negative one only 17 times; in *Ars medica*, these figures are 649 and 93, respectively. Furthermore, it can be observed that the concept of 6.1 HEALING receives extensive metaphorical construal (Kuna 2014), whereas a negative outcome is generally expressed literally. The positive pole's predominance is also suggested by the fact that our present-day interpretive horizon opens up the complex category of 1. GENERAL POSITIVE VALUE, which proves to be the most frequently attested category in both the recipe collections and *Ars medica* (see Figure 14.6). By contrast, GENERAL NEGATIVE VALUE does not appear as a separate code; instead, it is subsumed by 6.2 FATAL OUTCOME and 8.2 NEGATIVE EMOTIONAL EFFECT, at a much lower frequency rate. In sixteenth- and seventeenth-century recipes, persuasion is typically associated with positive value attribution, in harmony with a positive attitude, the intention of creating trust, and the goal of the genre. On top of this, polarization also plays a role in the recipe's theme (USEFUL KNOWLEDGE) and in the elaboration of 6. RESULT OF THERAPY, the timing of therapy (5. TIME FACTOR), and 8. EMOTIONAL INVOLVEMENT. Here again, the positive pole is primarily foregrounded. Less directly, the concept of VALUE is also bound up with references to concrete persons or God, as the persons involved and God evoked a positive attitude in the era under study. Thus, polarity is also implied by the category of 7. AUTHENTICITY/CREDIBILITY.

14.3.5 The Prototype for Persuasion in Recipes

Based on the analysis, it is possible to outline the prototype for persuasion in Hungarian recipes, which basically conforms to what we know from the literature about efficacy phrases in other languages (see Section 14.1.2). This prototype has the following properties: it is positioned at the end of recipes; it is intimately related to the script evoked by recipes and by the concept of healing; relatedly, it has a considerably general scope (not being restricted to particular illnesses); it may stand by itself or in conjunction with other persuasive patterns; and it typically foregrounds a positive value. Accordingly, the prototype for persuasion in recipes is most directly linked to the codes 1.2 USEFULNESS, 3. TESTEDNESS, and 6.1.1 HEALING/RECOVERY. Finally, the analysis suggests that the prototype is not directly linked to the most frequent category, which is represented by the subcategory 1.1 GOOD, evoking a positive attitude in the most general way.

14.4 Conclusion

This chapter's aim was to explore categories related to persuasion in sixteenth- and seventeenth-century medical recipes on the basis of Hungarian texts. I analysed five recipe collections with the qualitative software ATLAS.ti and one remedy book by using the proprietary search engine of its electronic edition. The process of categorization prioritized semantic rather than formal criteria. At the same time, as a result of software-based analysis, it became possible to list linguistic representations instantiating particular categories, which may be put to use in corpus-based searches in the future.

The research has revealed the fact that persuasion constitutes a characteristic strategy of text production underlying Hungarian medical recipes in the era. Persuasive parts in the Hungarian texts under study are remarkably similar to medical recipes produced in other languages in the same era, which follows from the way in which these texts were created and how knowledge was transmitted at the time. The analysis has also shown that evaluative language is fundamental for the persuasive function of recipes. In the Hungarian sample, the positive pole clearly dominates, in close relation to the goal of the genre; that is, the sharing of knowledge.

One limitation of the present study is that, in the absence of a corpus of medical Hungarian, it was not possible to analyse the recipe collections and the remedy book with precisely the same methodology. Thus, with regard to *Ars medica*, no results have been produced concerning the distribution of persuasive phrases, the co-occurrence of categories, and the frequency of persuasive phrases with respect to the number of word tokens. A further limitation is that the study offers no insight into what features and historical developments characterize persuasion-related categories in various discourse domains. The reason is that no learned treatises written in Hungarian are available from the era under study; these did not begin to appear until the eighteenth century.

Despite these limitations, the analysis has the advantage of extending the interpretation of persuasion as strategic action to historical texts, studying it from the perspective of the speaker's persuasive intent, taking the genre of recipes as a point of departure. For this purpose, qualitative software-based analysis was performed, which allows one not only to present particular categories but also to find out about their frequency rates and co-occurrence tendencies. In addition, the analysis also opens up possibilities for comparison with studies focusing on other languages, with the prospect of reaching a better understanding of medical recipes in pan-European and cross-cultural dimensions.

SOURCES

AM = Váradi Lencsés, György: *Ars Medica*, c. 1577. In Szabó & Bíró (2000).

HP = *Házi patika* [Home pharmacy]; Oct.Hung.485; c. 1663. In Hoffmann (1989): 227–46.

KP = Váradi Vásárhelyi, István: *Kis patika* [Little pharmacy]; Duod.Hung 66. 1628. In Hoffmann (1989): 211–25.

MBM = Becskereki Váradi Szabó, György: *Medicusi és borbélyi mesterség* [Medical and barber profession]; Nr. 5295. 1668–1703. In Hoffmann (1989): 341–434.

MOR = *Mindenféle orvosságoknak rendszedésse* [Classification of medicaments]; Oct.Hung.87; second part of seventeenth century. In Hoffmann (1989): 459–72.

TOK = Szentgyörgyi, János: *Testi orvosságok könyve* [Book of medicine for the body]; Oct.Hung.500; c. 1619. In Hoffmann (1989): 173–201.

REFERENCES

Alonso-Almeida, Francisco. 2013. Genre conventions in English recipes, 1600–1800. In Michelle Di Meo & Sara Pennell (eds.), *Reading and writing recipe books 1550–1800*, 68–92. Manchester: Manchester University Press.

Alonso-Almeida, Francisco, & Mercedes Cabrera-Abreu. 2002. The formulation of promise in medieval English medical recipes: A relevance-theoretic approach. *Neophilologus* 86: 137–54.

Cameron, Malcom Laurence. 1993. *Anglo-Saxon medicine*. Cambridge: Cambridge University Press.

Carroll, Ruth. 2004. Middle English recipes: Vernacularisation of a text-type. In Irma Taavitsainen & Päivi Pahta (eds.), *Medical and scientific writing in late medieval English*, 174–95. Cambridge: Cambridge University Press.

Croft, William, & Alan D. Cruse. 2004. *Cognitive linguistics*. Cambridge: Cambridge University Press.

De la Cruz-Cabanillas, Isabel. 2020. Early modern English recipe as a mirror of the time period. *Studia Neofilologiczne* 16: 47–60.

Görlach, Manfred. 1992. Text-types and language history: The cookery recipe. In Matti Rissanen, Ossi Ihalainen, Terttu Nevalainen, & Irma Taavitsainen (eds.), *History of Englishes. New methods and interpretations in historical linguistics*, 736–61. Berlin: Mouton De Gruyter.

Heinemann, Wolfgang. 2000. Textsorte – Textmuster – Texttyp. In Klaus Brinker, Gerd Antos, Wolfgang Heinemann, & Sven Frederik Sager (eds.), *Text- und Gesprächslinguistik. Ein internationales Handbuch zeitgenössischer Forschung*, vol. 16(1), 507–23. Berlin: Walter de Gruyter.

Hoffmann, Gizella (ed.). 1989. *Medicusi és borbélyi mesterség. Régi magyar ember- és állatorvosló könyvek. Radvánszky Béla gyűjtéséből* [Old Hungarian books on the healing of people and animals. From the collection of Béla Radvánszky]. Szeged: JATE/MTA.

Hoppál, Mihály. 1990. Népi gyógyítás [Ethnomedicine]. In Mihály Hoppál (ed.), *Magyar Néprajz* vol. 7, 693–724. Budapest: Akadémia Kiadó.

Hunt, Tony. 1990. *Popular medicine in thirteenth-century England: Introduction and texts*. Cambridge: D. S. Brewer.

Jones, Claire. 1998. Formula and formulation: 'Efficacy phrases' in medieval English medical manuscripts. *Neuphilologische Mitteilungen* 99: 199–209.

Jucker, Andreas H. 1997. Persuasion by inference. Analysis of a party political broadcast. In Jan Blommaert & Chris Bulcean (eds.), Political linguistics. Special issue of *Belgian Journal of Linguistics* 2: 121–37.

Kuna, Ágnes. 2014. Illness-conceptions in the persuasive sections of Hungarian medical recipes from the 16th and 17th centuries. In Martin Hilpert & Susanne Flach (eds.), *Yearbook of the German Cognitive Linguistics Association*, vol. 2, 51–68. Berlin: Mouton De Gruyter.

Kuna, Ágnes. 2016a. Genre in a functional cognitive framework: Medical recipe as a genre in 16th and 17th century Hungarian. In Ninke Stukker, Wilbert Spooren, & Gerard Steen (eds.), *Genre in language, discourse and cognition*, 193–224. Berlin: Mouton De Gruyter.

Kuna, Ágnes. 2016b. A Magyar Orvosi Nyelv Korpusza [Corpus of Hungarian Medical Texts]. *Magyar Orvosi Nyelv* 16(1): 26–30.

Kuna, Ágnes. 2018. Patterns of persuasion in Hungarian medical discourse domain from the 16th and 17th centuries. In Jana Pelclová & Wei-lun Lu (eds.), *Persuasion in public discourse: Cognitive and functional perspectives*, 21–42. Amsterdam; Philadelphia: Benjamins.

Leong, Elaine. 2018. *Recipes and everyday knowledge: Medicine, science, and the household in early modern England.* Chicago; London: Chicago University Press.

Mäkinen, Martti. 2011. Efficacy phrases in Early Modern English medical recipes. In Irma Taavitsainen & Päivi Pahta (eds.), *Medical writing in Early Modern English*, 158–79. Cambridge: Cambridge University Press.

McVaugh, Michael Rogers. 1997. Bedside manners in the Middle Ages. *Bulletin of the History of Medicine* 71(2): 201–23.

Miller, Norman, & Donald T. Campbell. 1959. Recency and primacy in persuasion as a function of the timing of speeches and measurements. *Journal of Abnormal and Social Psychology* 59(1): 1–9.

Ortak, Nuri. 2004. *Persuasion. Zur textlinguistischen Beschreibung eines dialogischen Strategiemusters*. Tübingen: Max Niemeyer Verlag.

Östman, Jan-Ola. 2005. Persuasion as implicit anchoring. The case of collocations. In Helena Halmari & Tuija Virtanen (eds.), *Persuasion across genres: A linguistic approach*, 183–212. Amsterdam; Philadelphia: Benjamins.

Pelclová, Jana, & Wei-lun Lu (eds.). 2018. *Persuasion in public discourse: Cognitive and functional perspectives*. Amsterdam; Philadelphia: Benjamins.

Stannard, Jerry. 1982. Rezeptliteratur als Fachliteratur. In William Eamon (ed.), *Studies on Medieval Fachliteratur*, 59–73. Scripta 6. Brussels: Omirel.

Szabó, T. Attila, & Zsolt Bíró. 2000. *Ars Medica Electronica: Váradi Lencsés György (1530–1593)*. CD-Rom. BioTár Electronic, Gramma 3.1. & 3.2.

Szlatky, Mária. 1980. Magyar nyelvű, kéziratos orvosló könyvek a 17. századból [Hungarian medical manuscripts from the 17th century]. *Magyar Könyvszemle* 96(2): 131–48.

Szlatky, Mária (ed.). 1983. *Minden doktorságot csak ebből késértek Szemelvények orvosi kézikönyvekből* [Excerpts from medical reference books]. Budapest: Magvető Kiadó.

Taavitsainen, Irma. 2001. Middle English recipes: Genre characteristics, text type features and underlying traditions of writing. *Journal of Historical Pragmatics* 2(1): 85–113.

Taavitsainen, Irma, & Päivi Pahta. 1998. Vernacularisation of medical writing in English: A corpus-based study of scholasticism. *Early Science and Medicine* 3 (2): 157–85.

Taavitsainen, Irma, & Päivi Pahta. 2004. Vernacularisation of scientific and medical writing in its sociohistorical context. In Irma Taavitsainen & Päivi Pahta (eds.), *Medical and scientific writing in late medieval English*, 1–19. Cambridge: Cambridge University Press.

Virtanen, Tuija, & Helena Halmari. 2005. Persuasion across genres: Emerging perspectives. In Helena Halmari & Tuija Virtanen (eds.), *Persuasion across genres: A linguistic approach*, 3–24. Amsterdam; Philadelphia: Benjamins.

Voigts, Linda. 1982. Editing Middle English medical texts: Needs and issues. In Trevor Levere (ed.), *Editing texts in the history of science and medicine*, 39–68. New York: Garland.

CHAPTER 15

Persuasion in Early Modern English Medical Recipes

Martti Mäkinen

(1) But Galen is flat against this preposterous custome of drinking thus fasting; averring, that to drink strong drink fasting, is very hurtfull for the nerves and nervous parts, and withall, hasteneth and procureth to the body many dangerous diseases, as Epilepsie, Apoplexie, and many others. It is therefore farre better for thy health to eat a little before thou drinke. (Hart, Klinike, Or the Diet of the Diseased, 1633: 113)[1]

Persuasive passages appealing to reason like in (1) characterise Early Modern English medical texts, especially in the more theoretical subgenres of the medical register, like treatises on specific topics and textbooks.[2] Persuasion – that is, linguistic behaviour that aims at changing or strengthening the audience's thinking or behaviour (Virtanen & Halmari 2005: 3) – is a common textual feature that is prominently present in the more practically oriented medical genres. Even recipes, which are often studied as specimens of instructive texts, attest to persuasion, for instance in the form of efficacy phrases (Jones 1998; Mäkinen 2011).

The study of persuasion in texts focuses on the means and strategies to alter the audience's attitude and on bringing about a change in the minds of text recipients. Students of historical texts are in the unfortunate position that the effect of persuasion on the audience, the perlocutionary effect, is usually beyond the researcher's reach (Jucker 1997). Nevertheless, the ways in which authors attempt to persuade the audience can be studied with some certainty also in texts without access to the audience's reactions or responses (Virtanen & Halmari 2005: 7).

There are no texts with a persuasive function only, nor are there texts that would not be persuasive. Thus, persuasion in itself is often implicit,

[1] All texts cited in the examples are from the *Early Modern English Medical Texts* corpus (EMEMT; Taivitsainen et al. 2010).

[2] This chapter adopts the categories of EMEMT (Taavitsainen et al. 2010).

and it can never be associated exclusively with linguistic phenomena (Östman 2005: 191). Persuasion is also affected by the situation, and the experience of persuasion is created jointly by the author and the audience, implying that it is not only a linguistic phenomenon (Virtanen & Halmari 2005: 4). The ubiquitousness of persuasion is also manifested in the fact that there are no genre labels that would identify persuasive texts. Even if persuasion is a communicative function, and communicative functions are often the means to identify text functions and genres (Swales 1990), persuasion is not a distinguishing feature between genres.

This chapter draws on investigations on emotive features in scientific writing (Taavitsainen 1994), discourse structure in early medical texts (Taavitsainen & Pahta 1997), metadiscursive practices in early English medicine (Taavitsainen 2000), text type features of Middle English recipes, including evidentials (Taavitsainen 2001a, 2001b), promises in Middle English recipes (Alonso-Almeida & Cabrera-Abreu 2002), transferring classical discourse conventions into the vernacular (Taavitsainen 2004), metadiscourse in Middle English recipes (Quintana-Toledo 2009), interpersonal reference, authorities, and classical terminology in medical recipes (Marttila 2011), and efficacy phrases (Mäkinen 2011), as well as a case study of persuasion in one medical preface (Mäkinen 2021). It complements the prior research on early modern medical recipes[3] by investigating persuasion in Early Modern English recipes in the genres outside recipe collections and *materia medica* literature.

An earlier study has investigated the use of efficacy phrases as a persuasive element in early modern recipe collections (Mäkinen 2011), but recipes also carry other persuasive elements. Using the *Early Modern English Medical Texts* (EMEMT) corpus (Taavitsainen et al. 2010), the present analysis looks into ways by which persuasion is interlaced with the informative and instructive contents of recipes, combining the Aristotelian concepts of *ethos*, *pathos*, and *logos* with a survey of modern metadiscourse practices (Hyland 2005, 2009, 2017). The approach has been applied earlier on a medieval medical preface (Mäkinen 2021), and the method provides a useful linguistic inventory in the form of metadiscourse items as expressed in the three elusive rhetorical strands, thus identifying quantifiable linguistic items that can be reanalysed with respect to the rhetorical concepts.

[3] The studies on persuasion that have informed the current chapter are Kuna (2014), which investigates the illness conceptions in Hungarian recipes, and Mäkinen (2011), which studies the types and distribution of efficacy phrases in English recipes (category 3) in EMEMT.

15.1 Background

15.1.1 Historical Setting of Medicine in England until 1700

Medieval medicine in classical and vernacular languages had been text centred: ancient authorities – Galen, Aristotle, Ibn Sina, Haly Abbas, and so on – were the canon of the science, and new texts were either translations, copies, or compilations of the Greek and Latin originals, at times disseminated also through Arabic authors' texts (Talbot 1967: 36, 44; Siraisi 1990). In England and in Europe, empiricism and first-person observation began to win ground around and especially after 1550, spelling a departure from the Galenic worldview and medicine, even if the ancient authorities were not forgotten immediately.

By the seventeenth century Galenism had been challenged and rejected by Paracelsian and Helmontian medicines that promoted chemical remedies, partly due to advances in chemistry (Wear 2000: 39, 353). However, the following extract from *Pharmacopaeia Londinensis* shows that the competing medical schools co-existed and were accepted by the medical audience for a time:

(2) We here present the World with a Translation of the London Dispensatory, lately Reformed by the Fellows now living, of the Colledge of Physicians: **being a Compendious Collection of the choicest Medicaments, whether Gallenical or Chymical yet known or in Request.** (Pharmacopaeia Londinensis, Preface, 1678; emphasis added)

The Galenic discipline still retained some support until the end of the seventeenth century and beginning of the eighteenth; that is, the paradigm shift in the natural sciences was taking place very slowly. Looking at medical practice itself, very little changed from a practitioner's, let alone from a patient's, point of view between 1500 and 1700 (Wear 1998 [1992]: 296).

15.1.2 Theoretical Background

The classical modes of persuasion – ethos, pathos, and logos – appeal to the audience through the character of the author (convincing the audience about the author's value as a source of knowledge), through the audience's emotions, and through logical reasoning, respectively. Persuasive discourse is aimed at (re)producing, reinforcing, and transmitting ideologies (Jucker 1997; Chaemsaithong 2011). The focus in persuasion is on the speaker/author and their attempts to prompt an action, an emotion, or a resolve in the audience (Kinneavy 1971: 21). Persuasion is thus a communicative purpose, which is, according to Swales (1990: 58), the basis for defining a genre. Nevertheless, persuasion is never the only purpose of any text, or in other words, persuasion is never overt in texts, albeit in some genres it can be more obvious than in others (Östman 2005: 200). The implicitness of persuasion leads to two conclusions: no linguistic feature is only persuasive, and any linguistic feature that can be identified as persuasive is always a member of another functional category as well. Therefore, persuasive linguistic features will always carry multiple functions. This conclusion concurs with the idea of multiple agendas of texts, persuasion being one of them.

As neither persuasion nor the Classical rhetorical concepts can be mapped to precise linguistic features, the linguistic study of persuasion presents a challenge. Therefore, help is sought in metadiscourse analysis. Metadiscourse comprises all the linguistic means used by an author to comment on a text, guide the readers to navigate through the text, and create a relationship with them. Metadiscourse consists of 'comments about the evolving text rather than about the subject matter. [. . .] These comments have two main functions: textual and interpersonal' (Taavitsainen 2000: 193). Hyland (1998, 2005, 2009, 2017) has identified metadiscourse inventories of linguistic features that either facilitate the audience's process of reading, or create a relationship between the author and the audience, explicitly or implicitly (Quintana-Toledo 2009: 21). These inventories have inspired the research aims of this study.

This chapter remaps metadiscourse items onto rhetorical concepts as a means to triangulate the linguistic data, as this may give us new insights into the concept of persuasion. Remapping metadiscourse items provides a normalised method to observe persuasion in texts, irrespective of the texts analysed. It is acknowledged that the study of persuasion in modern genres has ventured beyond Classical rhetorics lately (e.g. the rhetorical move analysis of research articles; see Nwogu 1997; Swales 2004), or even attempted departing from it and its terminology (New Rhetoric, see Perelman 1979; Ritivoi 2008). Nevertheless, the current approach provides a new way to look at existing analyses within Classical rhetorics, creating more 'resolution' by adding the metadiscourse apparatus.

15.2 Method

Ethos is concerned with the credibility of authors as the source of knowledge and how they appear to the audience. In the case of medieval medicine, the author's credibility was in the use of the ancient sources, in a manner that was deemed correct. *Logos*, on the other hand, is the appeal through the audience's sense of reason. Nevertheless, in the case of early scientific writing, a lot rested on the repetition of the ancient authors' ideas and words; that is, *logos* in the literal sense of the word. Thus, there is a reason to argue that *logos* functions on two different levels of persuasion, the appeals through reason, but also through the character of the author, who appears as the steadfast preserver of the ancient learning. Which one applies in each case depends on the disciplinary underpinnings of the text at hand: is it Galenic or Paracelsian/Helmontian?

Even if we cannot map the rhetorical facets to precise linguistic phenomena, we can analyse linguistic phenomena and reanalyse them with respect to the Aristotelian concepts. Metadiscourse items capture the majority of the passages that contain persuasive elements in recipes, and the kind of persuasion that takes place outside metadiscourse is mainly connected to the professionalism of authors and their meticulousness in the repetition of the expected recipe structure. The position of metadiscourse items seems to be culturally or contextually conditioned: for example, Kuna (2014: 56) notes that the persuasive sections in early modern Hungarian recipes are often situated towards the end of recipes. In the current material, metadiscourse items are found both at the beginning, with or after the purpose of the text, and at the end of recipes, but especially attitude markers and boosters may occur also within the recipe, in the preparation and administration of the medicine.

The metadiscourse classes annotated in the text and examined are (see Hyland 2005: 50–4):

- Attitude markers
- Boosters or emphatics
- Transition markers
- Endophoric markers
- Engagement markers
- Evidentials
- Code glosses
- Hedges
- Modal verbs
- Efficacy phrases (not included in Hyland's metadiscourse inventory)

These classes are not tied to specific linguistic features. According to Hyland (2005: 37), the text-producing communities' practices and contexts must be the starting points in the analysis of metadiscourse, therefore also in this study the analysis begins with a qualitative element, which then identifies the relevant linguistic phenomena.

The one item studied beyond Hyland's metadiscourse classes, efficacy phrases, vouches for the beneficial outcome of the therapy (Jones 1998; Mäkinen 2011). This item may overlap with the metadiscourse classes studied, and this is duly noted in the analysis.

In the reanalysis of the metadiscourse class, the relevant questions per each item are:

- Does the class reflect the rhetorical concepts?
- Does the class reflect more than one of the rhetorical concepts?

The reanalysed linguistic features provide a closed set of items, which makes it easier to replicate the study. Compared to qualitative rhetorical analyses, the current method thus improves the reproducibility of research and standardisation of the premises.

The analysis also provides a quantitative overview of the trends in medical recipes in different genres over the sixteenth and seventeenth centuries. The unit of analysis in the overview is a recipe, and the presence or absence of a metadiscourse class is treated as a binary variable. In other words, the number of different metadiscourse classes is normalised per recipe, answering the question: *What percentage of metadiscourse classes are attested in this recipe?* The percentages are then summed for all the recipes in a given genre and period and divided by the number of the recipes. The result – the mean of percentages – gives us an idea of the variety of metadiscourse classes used in a given period and genre. This is a necessary approach, as often metadiscourse items are multiword items, and therefore normalisation per word count is challenging and does not provide a reliable point of comparison. Also, recipes are of different length, and usually the more metadiscourse items a recipe attests to, the longer it is, which makes normalisation per word count even more challenging. Using the recipe as the unit of analysis provides us with an idea of what kind of variety is normal in a recipe in a given medical genre. As this study focuses on the attestation of metadiscourse items in recipes, it is not interested in the intensity of persuasion that they carry.

The data was collected from *Early Modern English Medical Texts* (1500–1700), a two-million-word multigenre corpus (Taavitsainen et al. 2010). The focus was on recipes in texts that are not identified as recipe collections as such; that is, excluding the corpus category 3.[4]

[4] Recipe collections and *materia medica* (category 3 in EMEMT) are a genre that is well studied, also partly with respect to the current research problem (e.g. Mäkinen 2011). The number of recipes they contain is also enormous compared to the number of recipes elsewhere, thus they will require a study of their own. Therefore, category 3 was excluded from the current study.

The recipes were collected manually from the texts in the categories of general treatises and textbooks (category 1), treatises on specific topics (category 2), regimens and health guides (category 4), surgical and anatomical treatises (category 5), and *Philosophical Transactions* (category 6).[5] The collected sample of recipes comprises 95,400 words in 48 texts.[6] The total number of recipes analysed is 963.

Extraction of recipes excluded any other instructive passages with therapeutic purposes. In other words, only items that (1) state the (medical) purpose, (2) list the ingredients, and (3) contain an instance of the imperative verb phrase *take* (or one of its synonyms) qualified as recipes in this study. These recipes were annotated for the metadiscourse items in focus by first generating a uniquified wordlist of all the recipes, and then tagging the potentially metadiscourse-relevant words by a find-and-replace command. After this, the resulting text files were proofread, any overlapping tags or errors were cleaned out, and missing tags were added.

15.3 Analysis

This section will present the observed metadiscourse categories and analyse them with respect to the Aristotelian categories (Section 15.3.1), and present a quantitative overview of the observations, commenting on the emerging trends in the data (Section 15.3.2).

[5] The EMEMT Appendix is not within the scope of this study.

[6] The texts that have provided recipe samples to this study are (the text identifications listed here are the short titles used in EMEMT: 292–343):

> 1525 *Handy warke of surgery*; 1525 *Seynge of uryns*; 1528 *Secrete of secretes*; 1539 *Myrrour or glasse of helth, plague*; 1540 *Byrth of mankynde*; 1546 *Boke of chyldren*; 1547 *Breuiary of helthe*; 1552 *Against sweatyng sicknesse*; 1562 *Bulleins bulwarke*; 1563 *Enchiridion of chirurgerie*; 1574 *Oleum magistrale*; 1575 *Treatise of chyrurgerie*; 1578 *Poore mans iewel*; 1584 *Vertue of nitre*; 1585 *Mithridatium*; 1596 *Booke of obseruations*; 1596 *Lves venerea*; 1596 *Key of philosophie*; 1602 *Cure of struma*; 1603 *Treatise of the plague*; 1604 *Complexions castle*; 1612 *Childbirth*; 1612 *Nvrsing of children*; 1612 *Whole art of chyrvrgerie*; 1616 *Preseruation of eyesight*; 1617 *Svrgions mate*; 1631 *Planetary ovres*; 1632 *Praxis medicinae*; 1636 *Certain necessary directions*; 1652 *Discourse of the secrets*; 1653 *De morbis puerorum*; 1662 *Sixth book of practical physic*; 1665 *Food and physic;* 1665 *Directions for the plague*; 1672 *Philosophical Transactions 7, 4098–5001*; 1676 *Of wounds*; 1682 *English remedy*; 1685 *Smallpox*; 1687 *Philosophical Transactions 16, 298* and *408–410*; 1691 *Plain and easie method*; 1693 *Marrow of chirurgery*; 1695 *Storehouse of physical practice;* 1695 *Compleat method of curing*; 1696 *Miscellania, tract 1*; 1697 *Continuation of the account of distempers*; 1697 *Art and nature*; 1698 *Physico-medical essay concerning alkaly and acid*; 1698 *Novum lumen chirurgicum.*

15.3.1 Inventory of Metadiscourse Items and Their Relevance in Persuasion

15.3.1.1 Attitude Markers

Attitude markers express the author's stance towards and evaluation of the propositional knowledge:

(3) In this disease we will **rather** vse pills then Electuaries (1632 Praxis medicinae)

(4) Or this, which I did learne of an old Parisian Priest, **who vaunteth himselfe to be very expert** in healing any kind of burning (1612 Whole art of chyrvrgerie)

Like evidentials (see below), attitude markers occur either at the beginning of a recipe, before the list of ingredients, or at the end, where a commentary on a recipe's desired effect may take place (as in efficacy phrases). Attitude markers are often accompanied by a booster that emphasises the stance expressed by the attitude marker (e.g. the word *very* in Example 4). Rhetorically, the majority of attitude markers defend the position adopted or praise the sources used and the medicines described. Therefore, they point towards logos by indicating the quality of the premises, or towards pathos by conveying to the readers that they are an audience to a high-quality exposition and exquisite remedies.

15.3.1.2 Boosters

Boosters or *emphatics* emphasise the certainty or force of a proposition, or evaluate the topic at hand:

(5) A **Never failing** Remedy for the Bite of a Mad Dog (1687 Philosophical Transactions 16, 408–10)

As previously mentioned, boosters occur frequently with attitude markers. As the author is the origin of any attitude expressions, boosters augment and enhance the audience's perception of the author; therefore the relevant mode of persuasion is ethos.

15.3.1.3 Transitions

Transition markers label stages in text, or sequence it, often in the order of a series of actions that would be typical of recipes. Common items in recipes are *then* (marking a new phase in the recipe procedure), *item*, *or*, and *and* in Examples 6–9; the first two invariably mark the beginning of a new recipe, and *and* often introduces the progress of the recipe preparation.

A less common item is *hereafter*, functioning as a frame marker for topic shift (10):

(6) & set them in freshe grese to putrifie, **then** frye them and strayne them (1546 Boke of chyldren)

(7) **Item** take of myrrhe/ castorium/ and storax/ of eche one dram-/ (1540 Byrth of mankynde)

(8) **or** take Myrrh, Galbanum, Ammoniac (1691 Plain and easie method)

(9) +R. Water Cresses, Sorrell, and Wormewood, of each one handfull, bruise them well, **and** broyle them in three quarts of Whey or new milke, **and** adde thereto a little suger and saffron, **and** let the sicke drinke thereof as often as hee will. (1617 Svrgions mate)

(10) but then it is good to fortifie each Dose, by some drops of the Essence or Tincture whereof we shall speak **hereafter**. (1682 English remedy)

Transitions are somewhat neutral as regards the rhetorical modes, yet they are not rhetorically unimportant. Itemisation and frame marking are a sign of an organised mind, clear argumentation, and care for the reception of the text and the quality of the end product. Therefore, all the three modes of persuasion are activated in and by transition markers.

15.3.1.4 Endophoric Markers

Endophoric references retrieve text and meanings from other *loci* in the current text; they may also refer to the whole work, beyond the current passage. *Anaphoric references* usually reactivate an earlier passage in the audience's mind, thus providing the reference with its meaning. In the current material, they often refer to the ingredients of the recipes, or to an instructive or theoretical passage earlier in the text:

(11) But if any of the great vaines be wou-ded, then **the cure aforesaid** is not sufficient. (1563 Enchiridion of chirurgerie)

(12) TAke tosted Nitre (which is **the seconde way of preparinge spoken of**) (1584 Vertue of nitre)

Cataphoric references usually introduce a new recipe:

(13) you shall doe in **thys maner**. Take Sanguinis draconis (1563 Enchiridion of chirurgerie)

Endophoric references are ubiquitous in the material, especially in the form of anaphoric references to the ingredients of the current recipe. For this reason they were eventually ignored in the quantitative treatment of the data; nevertheless, even though they are not discussed in this chapter, they are virtually everywhere.

15.3.1.5 Engagement Markers

Self-references signal the authorial presence in the text – the author is accessible to the reader and more intimately present:

(14) because **I** am of opinion that they might have been cured by the Method (1695 Compleat method of curing)

Self-references include all the cases of first-person singular pronouns, but also any noun phrases used to refer to the author. The uses of inclusive and authorial *we* are treated separately below.

Reader references address and engage the audience directly. Co-occurrence with self-references or inclusive *we* can be seen as an attempt to establish common ground or rapport with the audience:

(15) IF the wounde be great in the fleshe [. . .] **you** shall beginne **your** cure (1563 Enchiridion of chirurgerie)

Inclusive and authorial we are used, but not often. The inclusive use seems to occur in recipe procedures, as is exemplified here:

(16) Sometimes also, if the Disease run out to a length, **we** add Guaiacum (1676 Of wounds)

The authorial *we* provides an author reference, in the plural, even if the texts referred to in this study never have multiple authors. With reference to the information conveyed to the audience, the verb *speak* seems to be the preferred verb:

(17) hitherto **we** haue spoken of the Similer disease, now **we** will speake of organicall (1616 Preseruation of eiesight)

The last case of engagement markers is metadiscursive *imperatives* (i.e. imperatives other than the recipe-defining *take* or its synonyms), often in the preparative procedure or administration of the medicine. The most common of these by far is *let*:

(18) stop this Vessel close, and **let** it stand three Days and three Nights (1696 Miscellania, tract 1)

Engagement markers reanalysed with respect to Aristotelian rhetorical concepts point at ethos and pathos: they create a positive image of the author and the audience. The author appears as one with the authority to convey the valuable and often protected information about medical recipes to the audience (appeal through ethos), but often also as one who can count the audience among their peers. This aims at creating rapport with the intended readers, and it is therefore an appeal to the audience's emotions, that is, pathos.

15.3.1.6 Evidential Markers

Evidentials index, refer to, and assess sources of knowledge outside the current text, even if the last function is almost reduced to mere praise of the sources used. Evidentials identify the sources and relate the author's attitude towards the named sources:

(19) **Risius writeth in his great booke of Distillations** (1596 Key of philosophie)

The evidentials do not always refer as explicitly to the sources of information, and therefore they may require the shared knowledge of the medical practitioners and apothecaries to be understood (20):

(20) This remedy is set down by **Galen** (1603 Treatise of the plague)

(21) A soueraine and excellent Remedie taken out of **Alexis** (1603 Treatise of the plague)

Evidentials can usually be found at the end of a recipe, after information on the administration of the medicine, where also efficacy phrases often can be found. Another common location is the rubric of the recipe (21), which can extend over several lines like an introduction. Evidentials attest to the learnedness of the author and also support the claims made within the prevailing theoretical framework. The use of them, therefore, point towards ethos in the modes of persuasion, but also towards logos, both in the rhetorical and literal sense of the word (cf. the discussion in Section 15.2).

15.3.1.7 Code Glosses

Code glosses explain terms or passages in a language other than English. This is a telling sign of the author's consideration of the audience and their familiarity with medical terminology and foreign languages:

(22) into a certain kind of Vessels we call Lacteal **or milky Veins** (1698 Novum lumen chirurgicum)

Even if glosses often explain or even translate terms, they are also used for other purposes, like in Example 23. This is a passage in which one would expect a gloss, but which seems to be used to maintain the secrets of the trade, still ensuring that the intended audience receives the correct sense of the term (technically this is not a gloss, but it fits the function of the category):

(23) mixe them with pix Liquida (**it is not Tarre: you cosen, doe know the right pix LIquida**) (1584 Vertue of nitre)

At times code glosses resemble lists of alternatives for an effective ingredient. In Example 24, it would be impossible to know whether a gloss or an alternative is intended without the shared expert knowledge (it is a case of a gloss):

(24) poulder of Yreos roote, and Galanga roote, and **Lazer or Assa dulcis** (1584 Vertue of nitre)

In the light of these examples, code glosses are used to help the reader but also to indicate the superior position of the author, emphasising their authority and therefore pointing towards ethos. Nevertheless, some glosses or explanations of terms are not helpful in deciphering the referent of the term, or at least they require initiation in the tradition of the discipline. Therefore, they are inclusive for readers who are familiar with the terms and exclusive for others. Among the former the *loci* can invoke a sense of belonging among the intended audience; that is, they point towards pathos.

15.3.1.8 Hedges

Hedges dilute the author's commitment to the claim, or define requisite conditions that need to prevail in order to make the claim true. In recipes, hedges often condition the outcome of the therapy:

(25) This will Effect the Cure in a few Days, **provided** the Humours be not too Venemous, and the Parties keep themselves Temperate (1696 Miscellania, tract 1)

(26) **Some** find benefit by Shaving the Head, and by applying to the forepart of it a Plaister (1695 Storehouse of physical practice)

In the current recipes, hedges are relatively uncommon. They lessen authors' certainty, but they also safeguard their face. This is the case in Example 26: not all will find help in this remedy, but it is not unheard of.

This makes the author appear more reasonable and well informed in their claims, and therefore the main mode of persuasion in hedges is ethos.

15.3.1.9 Modals

Modal verbs are only one aspect of modality; the other manifestations of modality, like adjectives and adverbs expressing, for instance, necessity or possibility, have been categorised under attitude markers in this study. Modal verbs are used for several purposes, such as marking obligation:

(27) both the Letting of Blood and Purging **must** be reiterated (1695 Compleat method of curing)

(28) And to the wounded bone you **shall** vse Vnguentum aureum (1563 Enchiridion of chirurgerie)

They can signal possibility, permission, or even recommendation:

(29) They that are of a weak Constitution **may** take a Scruple or half a Dram of Salt of Vitriol [. . .] (1695 Storehouse of physical practice)

(30) TAke the purest Storax that you **can** get (1596 Key of philosophie)

Modal verbs are fairly frequent in efficacy phrases, where they signal the commitment of the treatment to a positive outcome or refer to the inevitability of the event of healing:

(31) and he **shall** be healed (1697 Art and nature)

Modality in early modern medical recipes is a complex issue and requires a study of its own. An overview of the modal auxiliary types in early modern medical texts (also in recipes partly coinciding with the current data) has been provided by Hiltunen and Tyrkkö (2011: 53–4), and modality specifically in medical recipes has also been commented on by Kopaczyk (2013: 282–3), and more recently by Alonso-Almeida and Álvarez-Gil (2020). Nevertheless, modality as such is not the scope of this chapter; rather, modal verbs are studied here due to their link to persuasion: authors use modal verbs to signal specific senses of verbs and to modify the audience's perception of them and also the propositional content of the text. The facets of persuasion at play are therefore ethos and logos.

15.3.1.10 Efficacy Phrases

Efficacy phrases may describe the outcome of a therapy; that is, they can describe the medicine's future effect, or make a promise of it, provided that the conditions set out in the recipe are fulfilled. Efficacy phrases can also be realised as a stock phrase, often in Latin, noting the end result or that the medicine is tried and tested. They occur both at the beginning, like in Example 32, and at the end of recipes in Examples 33–35:

(32) **An experiment often approued of Rasis** for the vomyte of chyldren. (1546 Boke of chyldren)

(33) yee shall mingle the powder of blacke Hellebore; put it in the eares, **and it cureth those infirmities.** (1631 Planetary ovres)

(34) Then boyle all together to a consistence. **Et fiat Cataplasma.** (1602 Cure of struma)

(35) and give two drachmes thereof to bee drunke in red wine, or Pome-Citerne water. **Probatum est.** (1631 Planetary ovres)

The different proof phrases may mean that the author of the text has actually tried and tested the recipe in practice (Mäkinen 2011: 170), but they may also be a reference to ancient and medieval medical authorities and the scholastic tradition (Jones 1998). Rhetorically, efficacy phrases indicate the soundness of the sources (ancient authorities) or the first-hand experience of the author, and therefore they are manifestations of logos and ethos.

15.3.2 Quantitative Observations on Metadiscourse Items in Recipes

The current section will move on from the relevance of metadiscourse items in the study of persuasion pointed out in Section 15.3.1 and elaborate the notion by quantified observations of the items.

Figure 15.1 provides an overview of the development of metadiscourse classes, including modal verbs, and efficacy phrases, in medical recipes outside recipe collections and *materia medica* literature in the sixteenth and seventeenth centuries. The figure includes all 963 recipes analysed. For Figure 15.1, the texts of each EMEMT category were merged for each century. Note that recipes are not present in all categories studied in the sixteenth and seventeenth centuries, and in particular that recipes cannot be found in all categories in equal quantities.[7]

Figure 15.1 illustrates the variety[8] of persuasion in medical recipes as expressed through metadiscourse items: the higher the percentage, the

[7] This is not a fault in the corpus: after all, it was not designed to be representative of recipes in all categories.

[8] Variety in Figure 15.1 is presented by the percentage: as indicated in Section 15.3, the percentage shows what portion of the available metadiscourse classes was in use in the recipes of a genre.

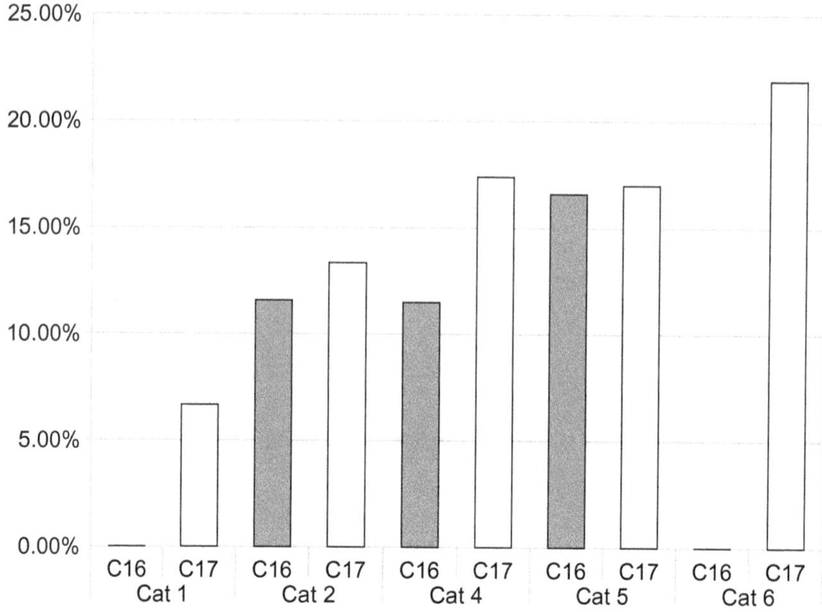

Figure 15.1 Variety of persuasion: percentage of available persuasion indicators / recipe
Legend: C16 = sixteenth century, C17 = seventeenth century
Cat1 = General treatises and textbooks; Cat2 = Treatises on specific topics; Cat4 = Regimens and health guides; Cat5 = Surgery and anatomy texts; Cat6 = *Philosophical Transactions*

more metadiscourse classes have been in used in the recipes of a genre. As was seen in Section 15.3.1, metadiscourse features, modal verbs, and efficacy phrases are relevant to persuasion and they can be reanalysed according to the three classical persuasive strands. Therefore, the presence of a metadiscourse item in a recipe is also a marker of persuasion, or, to paraphrase that, persuasion in medical recipes often takes place in elements that can be identified as metadiscourse items.

Figure 15.1 shows that categories 2 and 5 (Treatises on specific topics and Surgery and anatomy texts, respectively) maintain their level of using persuasive elements in comparison between the centuries. For categories 1 and 6 (General treatises and textbooks; *Philosophical Transactions*) we have no points of comparison in the sixteenth century, as the text samples in category 1 do not carry any recipes prior to 1600, and the category of *Philosophical Transactions* did not exist before the latter half of the seventeenth century. Category 4 (Regimens and health guides) is the only one that shows clear evolution in the variety of persuasion within recipes, with an increase from circa 12 per cent of available items to circa 17 per cent. The increased variety also implies an increase in the length of recipes. Unfortunately the development in category 4 would need to be corroborated with more data, as there are only two texts in the sixteenth century and one in the seventeenth century with recipes.

Secondly, differences between the categories can be observed regarding the frequency of metadiscourse classes. The scarcity of metadiscourse in category 1 is especially striking, as is the towering column of recipes in *Philosophical Transactions*. The latter must be left with just one comment: the category comprises a total of six recipes, and therefore would need more data to be reliable. However, the lack of persuasive elements in category 1 indicates that the recipes in the category merely contain the purpose, ingredients, and procedure (possibly also administration), but no exposition that would argue for the ingredients, the medicine, or the outcome of the therapy. In the current material, the number of metadiscourse classes directly correlates with the length of persuasive passages in recipes, and their absence entails the absence of overtly persuasive text. Nevertheless, one cannot conclude that the texts in category 1 would employ less persuasion than the other categories studied; rather, in the texts of category 1 the persuasive features related to recipes are manifested in the surrounding exposition in which the recipes are embedded.

Figures 15.2–15.5 illustrate the development of metadiscourse items in categories 1, 2, 4, and 5; *Philosophical Transactions* has been left out as a category, as the recipes are few, and there is no point of comparison in the sixteenth century. Category 1 is included, in order to provide a fuller view of the situation in the seventeenth century.

Figure 15.2 presents the development in the use of attitude, booster, and evidential markers in recipes from the sixteenth to seventeenth centuries. In all categories that provide information on both centuries (categories 2, 4, and 5), we can see boosters increasing when moving to the latter part of the period. However, both attitude markers and evidentials either increase or decrease, but never in the same direction in one category. In effect, one could say that there seems to be a negative correlation between the two markers: when attitude markers increase, evidentials decrease, and vice versa. Looking back at the reanalysis of metadiscourse items in Section 15.3.1, an increase in attitude markers would imply movement towards logos and pathos in persuasion, whereas an increase in evidentials would imply movement towards logos and ethos. If persuasion through the appeal to reason (logos) behaves in the same way in all categories, then an increase

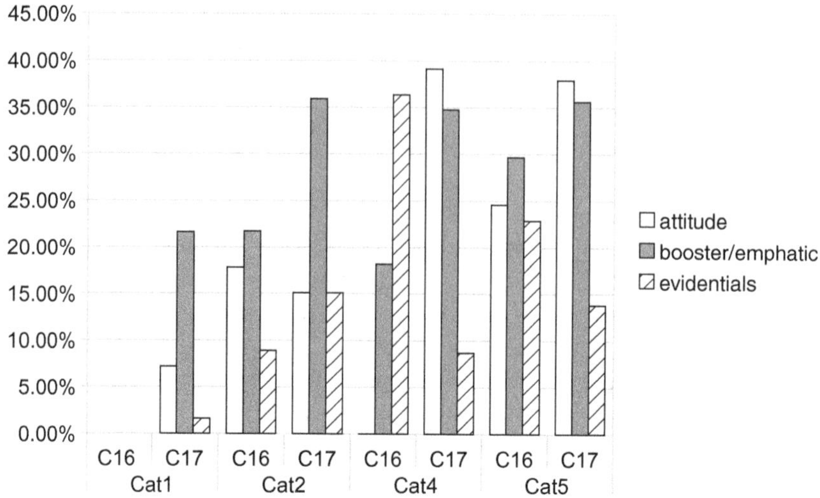

Figure 15.2 Percentage of recipes with attitude, booster, and evidential markers
Legend: C16 = sixteenth century, C17 = seventeenth century
Cat1 = General treatises and textbooks; Cat2 = Treatises on specific topics; Cat4 = Regimens and health guides; Cat5 = Surgery and anatomy texts

in evidentials points towards the appeal through the person of the author (ethos) as the preferred persuasive strategy (category 2), and, conversely, appeal to the audience's emotions (pathos) would be marked by increase in attitude markers (categories 4 and 5).

Figure 15.3 presents the development of engagement markers, code glosses, and hedges. Engagement markers seem to increase in categories 2, 4, and 5 towards the end of the period studied. Simultaneously, the use of code glosses is decreasing, and the use of hedges is minutely increasing. As argued in Section 15.3.1, even the minutest changes seem to imply a movement from ethos-focusing persuasion (code glosses) towards ethos and pathos-preferring persuasion (engagement markers and hedges); a shift from a world of discourse where there is no need for hedges to one that creates and uses them. One could also argue that later texts are intended more for colleagues and a professional audience than for an audience that would professionally stand on a lower tier of the hierarchy.

Figure 15.4 shows the development in the use of obligation-expressing modal verbs *must* and *shall*, and the modal verb *may*, expressing possibility, permission, recommendation, and (in this material rarely) hedging. *May* seems to be far more common in almost any period and category than *must*

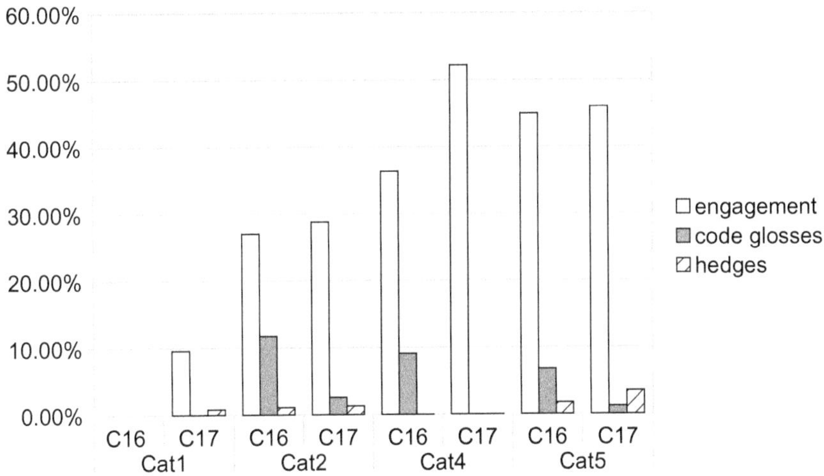

Figure 15.3 Percentage of recipes with engagement markers, code glosses, and hedges
Legend: C16 = sixteenth century, C17 = seventeenth century
Cat1 = General treatises and textbooks; Cat2 = Treatises on specific topics;
Cat4 = Regimens and health guides; Cat5 = Surgery and anatomy texts

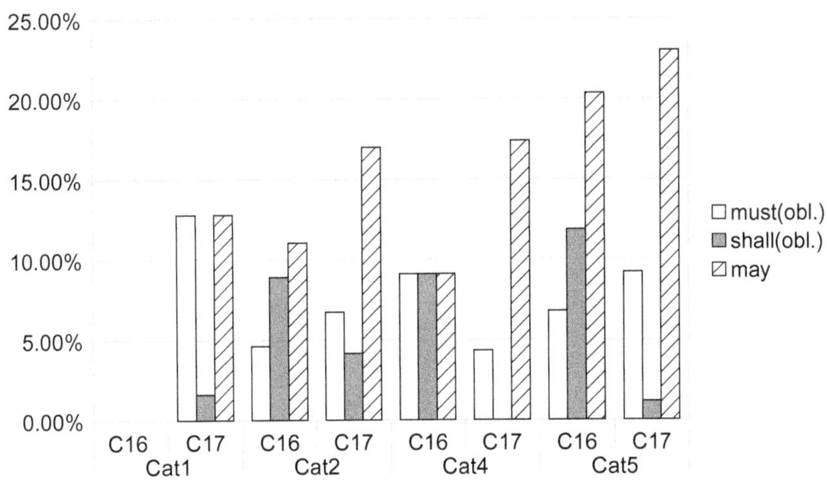

Figure 15.4 Percentage of recipes with modal verbs *must*, *shall* (obl.), and *may*
Legend: C16 = sixteenth century, C17 = seventeenth century
Cat1 = General treatises and textbooks; Cat2 = Treatises on specific topics;
Cat4 = Regimens and health guides; Cat5 = Surgery and anatomy texts

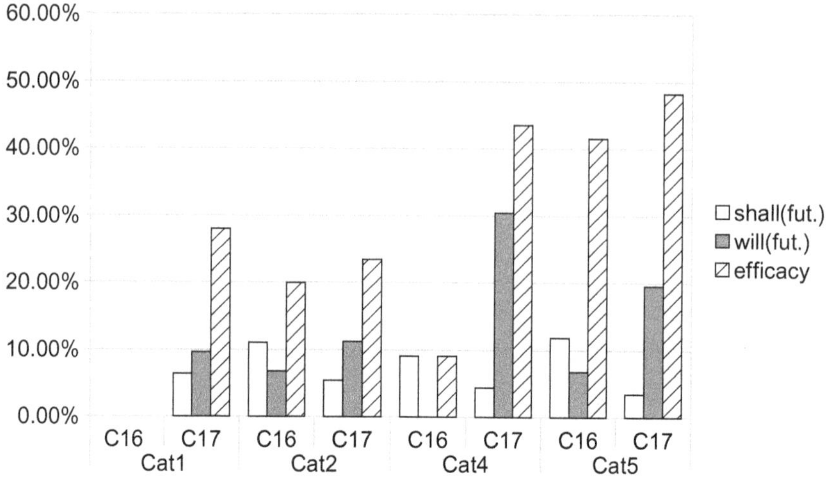

Figure 15.5 Percentage of recipes with modal verbs *shall* (fut.), *will* (fut.), and efficacy phrases

Legend: C16 = sixteenth century, C17 = seventeenth century
Cat1 = General treatises and textbooks; Cat2 = Treatises on specific topics; Cat4 = Regimens and health guides; Cat5 = Surgery and anatomy texts

and *shall*, and even if categories 2 and 5 show an increase in the use of *must* from the sixteenth to seventeenth centuries, the total of obligation-expressing modals decreases in all categories towards the end of the period studied. It seems fairly clear that the trend in modality is to move away from deontic modality and towards epistemic modality (this becomes also apparent in Figure 15.5). In terms of persuasion, there is a movement from a more authoritarian ethos towards an ethos that can weather failures and discussion, or at least can prepare for potentially face-threatening situations by creating a margin for errors through language.

Figure 15.5 gives the development of the modal verbs *shall* and *will* expressing futurity, and the use of efficacy phrases. The modals used to express the commitment of the medicine to its future effect are closely connected with efficacy phrases, thus the inclusion of the three features in Figure 15.5. The presence of efficacy phrases increases in all categories, and so does the total percentage of futurity-expressing modals, even if individual modals may decrease from the sixteenth to seventeenth centuries. In rhetorical terms, we can see the joint effort of appeal through *ethos* and *logos*: in efficacy phrases the author makes a promise about future events, and vouches for the soundness of the evidence.

15.4 Discussion

The analysis of metadiscourse features in recipes and their reanalysis in rhetorical terms have proved to be a usable method, even if a labour-intensive one. As metadiscourse items are not always single-word items, using normalised frequencies was deemed somewhat misleading. Also, the persuasive effect can never be calculated from individual words or even from singular metadiscourse items. Persuasion is always a coefficient of language use and the cultural context, and thus the current approach may render the persuasive elements in fragments that cannot provide the full picture. Nevertheless, the approach reveals something concrete about the elusive concept of persuasion, and at least it can aid in achieving a closer look at the mechanics of persuasion, if not the full view.

In this study, the presence of metadiscourse features per recipe was recorded, making a recipe the basic unit of analysis. Admittedly, that unit is not uniform across corpus texts: the more metadiscourse features a recipe carries, the longer and more varied it becomes. The length of recipes is a factor that was not accounted for in the design of the study. Nevertheless, it may bear relevance for similar studies in the future. In this study, the focus was on the number of metadiscourse classes per recipe, and that is directly related to the kind of persuasion a recipe employs. In recipes with more than one metadiscourse class, one could say that the metadiscourse items express the sum of the persuasive intent of the author. For example, attitude markers tend to co-occur with boosters; that is, the author's evaluative comment is often reinforced by a booster adjusting the force or the degree of the comment. Also, efficacy phrases tend to co-occur with modal verbs expressing future actions. The length of recipes is at play also in cases where mere skeletons of recipes (a list of ingredients and a verb indicating the desired manner of preparation) are embedded in the surrounding exposition, which often contains the persuasive features that we do not see in the recipe itself. This may be a genre-governed feature, but it could also be an authorial preference.

We see an increase too in the diversity of different metadiscourse classes used in the material. The potential reasons for this can be found in the evolving and emerging paradigms of medicine: in the sixteenth century, the developing science still leaned to some extent on Galenism, whereas Paracelsian ideology and chemical medicines were inventions of the seventeenth century. Nevertheless, we know that for a time in the latter century the two paradigms co-existed, and the trends observed in a text corpus may reflect exactly this.

In individual EMEMT categories, we can see a development away from one facet of classical rhetoric and movement towards the other facets, and these developments may vary from one category to another. The clearest indicators are the ones related to the use of modal verbs, which seem to imply a movement towards epistemic modality and away from deontic modality. All these changes seem to be moving the author's self-image towards a less authoritative tone of voice, at least when studying the metadiscourse items and modal verbs. We can also detect genre variation between the different categories of EMEMT, manifested in the ways persuasion is included in or excluded from the recipe text.

15.5 Conclusion

Persuasion is an elusive concept, and it seems that the present attempts to pinpoint persuasion to singular linguistic features can generate new knowledge on the phenomenon, but the prerequisite for that is a fairly cumbersome qualitative analysis. On the other hand, the current study has taught us something about the persuasiveness of metadiscourse items, and how they function as constituents of the persuasive coefficient of a text.

Looking at individual linguistic items creates a somewhat atomised view of persuasion, and in this case the persuasive effect of a whole text is always something else than the sum of its parts. Recipes in longer texts pose additional difficulties. Sometimes it means that recipes are completely drained of the persuasive features, as persuasion itself takes place elsewhere in the text. At other times, it is difficult to draw the line between the recipe and the exposition in which the recipe is embedded. Therefore it is, and should be, a different experience to study recipes in recipe collections than in other medical texts: embedded recipes are never the main item or focus of the text.

In the future, studies of metadiscourse and persuasion in medical recipes could provide comparisons between medical genres, and also between the medical register and other registers. The qualitative character of many an approach to persuasion is an issue that could be addressed. The current data set also offers further possibilities for studying, for instance, the authors' relationship with the audience, and the information accumulated in the study, considering persuasion from multiple angles, should lend itself also to visualisations of the phenomena.

REFERENCES

Alonso-Almeida, Francisco, & Francisco J. Álvarez-Gil. 2020. 'So that it may reach to the jugular': Modal verbs in Early Modern English recipes. *Studia Neofilologiczne* XVI, Special issue: Instructional writing across times and languages, 61–88.

Alonso-Almeida, Francisco, & Mercedes Cabrera-Abreu. 2002. The formulation of promise in medieval English medical recipes: A relevance-theoretic approach. *Neophilologus* 86: 137–54.

Chaemsaithong, Krisda. 2011. Discursive control and persuasion in early modern news discourse: The case of English witchcraft pamphlets and their prefaces (1579–1621). *English Text Construction* 4(2): 228–56.

Hiltunen, Turo, & Jukka Tyrkkö. 2011. Verbs of knowing: Discursive practices in early modern vernacular medicine. In Irma Taavitsainen & Päivi Pahta (eds.), *Medical writing in Early Modern English*, 44–73. Cambridge: Cambridge University Press.

Hyland, Ken. 1998. Persuasion and context: The pragmatics of academic metadiscourse. *Journal of Pragmatics* 30: 437–55.

Hyland, Ken. 2005. *Metadiscourse: Exploring interaction in writing*. London; New York: Continuum.

Hyland, Ken. 2009. *Academic discourse: English in a global context*. London: Continuum International.

Hyland, Ken. 2017. Metadiscourse: What is it and where is it going? *Journal of Pragmatics* 113: 16–29.

Jones, Claire. 1998. Formula and formulation: 'Efficacy phrases' in medieval English medical manuscripts. *Neuphilologische Mitteilungen* 99(2): 199–210.

Jucker, Andreas H. 1997. Persuasion by inference: Analysis of a party political broadcast. In Jan Blommaert & Chris Bulcaen (eds.), *Belgian Journal of Linguistics*. 11, Special edition: Political linguistics, 121–37.

Kinneavy, James L. 1971. A theory of discourse: The aims of discourse. Englewood Cliffs, NJ: Prentice-Hall.

Kopaczyk, Joanna. 2013. Formulaic discourse across Early Modern English medical genres. In Andreas Jucker, Daniela Landert, Annina Seiler, & Nicole Studer-Joho (eds.), *Meaning in the history of English. Words and texts in context*, 257–300. Studies in language companion series 148. Amsterdam: Benjamins.

Kuna, Ágnes. 2014. Illness-conceptions in the persuasive sections of Hungarian medical recipes from the 16th and 17th centuries. *Yearbook of the German Cognitive Linguistics Association* 2: 51–68.

Mäkinen, Martti. 2011. Efficacy phrases in Early Modern English medical recipes. In Irma Taavitsainen & Päivi Pahta (eds.), *Medical writing in Early Modern English*, 158–79. Cambridge: Cambridge University Press.

Mäkinen, Martti. 2021. Rhetorical re-analysis of metadiscourse items in Henry Daniel's Middle English prologue to *Liber uricrisiarum*. In Letizia Vezzosi (ed.), *Current Issues in Medieval England*, 171–94. Berlin: Peter Lang.

Marttila, Ville. 2011. New arguments for new audiences: A corpus-based analysis of interpersonal strategies in Early Modern English medical recipes. In Irma Taavitsainen & Päivi Pahta (eds.), *Medical writing in Early Modern English*, 135–57. Cambridge: Cambridge University Press.

Nwogu, K. N. 1997. The medical research paper: Structure and functions. *English for Specific Purposes* 16(2): 119–38.

Östman, Jan-Ola. 2005. Persuasion as implicit anchoring: The case of collocations. In Helena Halmari & Tuija Virtanen (eds.), *Persuasion across genres: A linguistic approach*, 185–212. Philadelphia: Benjamins.

Perelman, C. 1979. *The New Rhetoric and the humanities*. Dordrecht: Reidel.

Quintana-Toledo, Elena. 2009. Middle English medical recipes: A metadiscursive approach. *Studia Anglica Posnaniensia* 45(2): 21–38.

Ritivoi, A. D. 2008. Rhetorics: New Rhetorics. In W. Donsbach (ed.), *The international encyclopedia of communication*. https://doi.org/10.1002/9781405186407.wbiecr093.

Siraisi, Nancy. 1990. *Medieval and early Renaissance medicine: An introduction to knowledge and practice*. Chicago: University of Chicago Press.

Swales, J. M. 1990. *Genre analysis: English in academic and research settings*. Cambridge: Cambridge University Press.

Swales, J. M. 2004. *Research genres: Explorations and applications*. Cambridge: Cambridge University Press.

Taavitsainen, Irma. 1994. On the evolution of scientific writings between 1375 and 1675: repertoire of emotive features. In Francisco Fernández, Miguel Fuster Márquez, & Juan Jose Calvo (eds.), *Papers from the 7th International Conference of English Historical Linguistics, Valencia, Sept. 1992*, 329–42. Amsterdam; Philadelphia: Benjamins.

Taavitsainen, Irma. 2000. Metadiscursive practices and the evolution of early English medical writing 1375–1550. In John M. Kirk (ed.), *Corpora galore: Analyses and techniques in describing English*, 191–207. Amsterdam: Rodopi.

Taavitsainen, Irma. 2001a. Evidentiality and scientific though-styles: English medical writing in Late Middle English and Early Modern English. In Maurizio Gotti & Marina Dossena (eds.), *Modality in specialized texts: Selected papers of the 1st CERLIS Conference*, 21–52. Bern: Peter Lang.

Taavitsainen, Irma. 2001b. Middle English recipes: Genre characteristics, text type features and underlying traditions of writing. *Journal of Historical Pragmatics* 2(1): 85–113.

Taavitsainen, Irma. 2004. Genres of secular instruction: A linguistic history of useful entertainment. *Miscelánea: A Journal of English and American Studies* 29: 75–94.

Taavitsainen, Irma, & Pahta, Päivi. 1997. The corpus of *Early English Medical Writing*: Linguistic variation and prescriptive collocation in scholastic style. In Terttu Nevalainen & Leena Kahlas-Tarkka (eds.), *To explain the present: Studies in the changing English language in honour of Matti Rissanen*, 209–25. Helsinki: Société Néophilologique.

Taavitsainen, Irma, Päivi Pahta, Turo Hiltunen, Ville Marttila, Maura Ratia, Carla Suhr, & Jukka Tyrkkö (eds.). 2010. *Early Modern English Medical Texts*, corpus. Amsterdam: Benjamins.

Talbot, C. H. 1967. *Medicine in medieval England*. London: Oldbourne.

Virtanen, Tuija, & Helena Halmari. 2005. In Helena Halmari & Tuija Virtanen (eds.), *Persuasion across genres: A linguistic approach*, 3–24. Philadelphia: Benjamins.

Wear, Andrew. 1998 [1992]. *Health and healing in Early Modern England: Studies in social and intellectual history*. Aldershot: Ashgate.

Wear, Andrew. 2000. *Knowledge and practice in English medicine, 1550–1680*. Port Chester, NY: Cambridge University Press.

CHAPTER 16

Richard III

Fact, Myth, Fiction

Anna Ilona Rajala and Timo Uotinen

On an August afternoon in 1485 near Market Bosworth in Leicestershire, the last significant battle of the Wars of the Roses was won by Henry Tudor (later Henry VII), and Richard III, crowned in July 1483, was slain. The dead king was carried naked on horseback to Leicester and buried in Greyfriars Church. Due to the dissolution of monasteries in the late 1530s and subsequent development of the site, the tomb was lost. In 2012, human remains, showing in situ signs of spinal deformity, were discovered and excavated under a car park where Greyfriars used to stand (see Figure 15 in the Image Gallery). Mitochondrial DNA proved that the remains were indeed Richard's (King et al. 2014). Richard's death marked the end of three centuries of Plantagenet rule, a civil war, and the Middle Ages, and the beginning of the Tudor dynasty, a time of peace and prosperity and the English Renaissance (Schwyzer 2013: 1).

Richard's case is both historically significant and interesting for literary studies because prior to the rediscovery of the remains, both the body and the character of the king were surrounded by myth and political propaganda: Tudor chroniclers sought to discredit Richard as a usurper to reinforce Tudor legitimacy, which lacked strong hereditary grounds. The most well-known depiction of Richard is of course Shakespeare's. Drawing on his contemporary historical sources, Shakespeare portrays Richard as a deformed, limping, villainous hunchback with an arm like a 'blasted sapling withered up' (*Richard III*, 3.4.69).[1]

Richard's posthumous image relied on the Tudors. In their time, the medieval association of deformity with sin and evil still lingered (Comber 2010). A crooked back was considered, as Elizabethan historian Thomas Hill (1571: 179) writes, to 'innuate the wickednesse of conditions: but an

The authors would like to thank the editors of this volume, the editors at Cambridge University Press, and the two anonymous reviewers for their generous comments.

[1] All the Shakespeare quotations are from Greenblatt et al. (2008).

equalitie of the backe, is then a good note'. Richard's crooked outer form reflected his crooked morals and early modern audiences would have recognised Richard's physical deformity and moral depravity 'as a synecdoche for the state' (Charnes 1993: 30). Over time, some suspected that Richard's wickedness and deformity were exaggerations (see e.g. Hay 1754; Legge 1885; Comber 2010; Carson 2013), but without the earthly remains, the deformity could not be proven.

The rediscovery finally answered the question of deformity. Richard had scoliosis (Appleby et al. 2014). No evidence of limping or a withered arm was found. 'So much for Shakespeare's medical credibility' (Modern Healthcare 2014: 36), it was declared. The story of Richard's twistedness was 'the work of Tudor propagandists, especially Shakespeare' [sic] (Meikle 2014). The myth of the defamed king was busted – or was it?

This chapter aims neither to confirm nor deny the accuracy of the scientific, mythical, and fictional depictions of Richard, nor to address his biography, given an abundance of post-excavation research (e.g. Ashdown-Hill 2015; Baldwin 2015; Horspool 2015; Hicks 2019; Skidmore 2018; Lewis 2019). We address the unique cross-genre nexus between historiography, Shakespeare's drama, and modern medical writing to evaluate the received histories of Richard's body – whether mythical, factual, fictitious, or scientific – and to find out what role interpretation and truth play. How is Richard's body described and interpreted within different genres? What kind of implications do interpretation and truth have for different genres that address Richard's body?

Drawing on literary studies, disability studies, health sciences, and the work of Horkheimer and Adorno (2002), we argue that both myth and science are modes of representing Richard that seek to control truth and draw conclusions regarding the uncertain and unknowable, thus relying on interpretation and speculation. The post-excavation science is not opposed to myth and fiction, but a perpetuation of mythology mediated by Richard's mythical and historical baggage. The fictional body of Shakespeare's Richard has 'truth content' (Adorno 1997) because it challenges the disabling and stigmatising attitudes towards bodies that are 'different' by highlighting the disabling attitudes that caused Richard to 'prove a villain' (*Richard III*, 1.1.30). Richard's body bears a socially constructed disability; however, the real bodily deformity also mediates his actions. Thus, for disability studies the case of the 'carpark king' (Buckley et al. 2013) problematises disability as either physical or social; it is both. Regarding literary studies, analysing the cross-genre nexus demonstrates that subjectivity is inseparable from interpretation and reflection regardless of genre, and truth never appears unmediated. Therefore, making subjectivity visible in analyses is not undesirable; it is indispensable.

16.1 How the Myth Came About

During Richard's reign, John Rous (n.d.) wrote that he was a 'mighty prince' beloved of his subjects and an upholder of the law. Rous revised the favourable character descriptions in his *Historia Regum Angliae*, which he had begun in 1480 before Richard's reign, but finished only after Richard's death in 1486. The work, dedicated to Henry VII, mentions points in Richard's favour, but highlights Richard's crude deformities and 'excessively cruel' character (Hanham 1975: 137). He describes Richard as 'small of stature, with a short face and unequal shoulders, the right higher and the left lower' (Hanham 1975: 121).

To justify Tudor reign, contemporary historiography latched onto depictions of Richard as evil, a crooked mind in a crooked body. Polydore Vergil, Henry VII's official chronicler, repeated Rous's depiction almost verbatim:

(1) He was lyttle of stature, deformyd of body, thone showlder being higher than thother, a short and sowre cowntenance, which semyd to savor of mischief, and utter evydently craft and deceyt. (Vergil 1846: 227)

Thomas More, central in forwarding the mythology, wrote in his *History of King Richard III* (written between 1513 and 1524), echoing Rous, that Richard was 'little of stature, ill-featured of limbs, crook-backed, his left shoulder much higher than his right, hard-favoured of visage' (More 2005: 9–10, xxi–xxiii). More's writing is crucial because he fleshed out the witty, evil crook back seen in subsequent works (Myers 1968: 184; Muir 1977: 32; Hammond 1981: 77; Jowett 2000: 16).

Edward Hall used both Vergil and More in his propagandist account of Richard. His *Union of the Noble and Illustre Families of Lancastre and York* of 1548 gives two descriptions: 'he was litle of stature, eivill featured of limnes, croke backed, the left shulder muche higher than the righte, harde favoured of visage' (Bullough 1975: 253). Hall follows More, though adding to Richard's infamy by substituting 'ill-featured' for 'evil-featured'. Hall's other description resembles Vergil's:

(2) As he was small and litle of stature so was he of body greately deformed, the one shoulder higher then the other, his face small but his countenaunce was cruel, and such, that a man at the first

aspect would judge it to savor and smel of malice, fraude, and deceite [. . .]. (Bullough 1975: 300)

Hall degrades Vergil's 'sour countenance' and 'mischief', 'craft and deceit' to 'cruel countenance', linked with 'malice, fraud, and deceit'. Holinshed's *The Chronicles of England, Scotland and Ireland* (1587 enlarged edition) mimics Hall: the Vergil description is nearly verbatim. Holinshed retains More's 'ill featured' but adds a 'rule of physiognomie' pertaining to Richard, 'Distortum vultum sequitur distorsio [sic] morum' [distortion of character follows a distorted countenance] (Holinshed 1808: 362; Jowett 2000: 386).[2]

Two points emerge in the transmission of Richard's description: first, Rous's description of the right shoulder being higher became the left being 'much higher' in More, Hall, and Holinshed – Vergil being non-committal on laterality and severity. Second, the further Richard's death receded into the past, the greater the severity of characterisation. Richard became more evil. In this respect, More is the main perpetrator: he adds the 'crook-back' and shifts the deformity to the left side, making it 'much higher'. Jowett (2000: 32) points out that '*crook* or *crooked* can mean "deviating from rectitude", and the left side of the body, here dominating, was associated with evil'.

Shakespeare's character is inherited, particularly from Rous, Vergil, More, Hall, and Holinshed.[3] While Shakespeare's Richard was undoubtedly influenced by the Tudor agenda (Garber 1987), it also evoked the association of deformity with evil. Shakespeare's misshapen Richard has been interpreted by scholars as 'the primary embodiment of the sinister' (Slotkin 2007: 26) and argued to 'embody' the political turmoil of his times (Charnes 1993: 30).

How did Shakespeare describe Richard? The character appears in three plays: parts 2 and 3 of *Henry VI* and *Richard III* – bodily descriptions appearing in the latter two. In *3 Henry VI*, Queen Margaret calls Richard 'valiant crookback prodigy' (1.4.76). Richard describes his body with physical detail:

(3) Why, love forswore me [. . .]
And, for I should not deal in her soft laws,

[2] Jowett (2000) looks to attribute this passage by Holinshed to More, but the quote could not be found in the corresponding passage in More, at least in the Logan edition (More 2005).

[3] For the seminal study on Shakespeare's sources see Bullough (1975); for a fuller list of historical sources see esp. 222–8).

> She did corrupt frail nature with some bribe,
> To shrink mine arm up like a wither'd shrub;
> To make an envious mountain on my back,
> Where sits deformity to mock my body;
> To shape my legs of an unequal size;
> To disproportion me in every part,
> Like to a chaos, or an unlick'd bear-whelp [...]. (*3 Henry VI* 3.2.153–71)

A few lines later, he refers to his 'misshaped trunk' (3.2.170). In the penultimate scene he repeats the physiognomic rule: 'since the heavens have shaped my body so, | Let hell make crooked my mind to answer it' (5.6.78–9). He also remarks: 'This shoulder was ordained so thick to heave' (5.7.23–4).

Richard never gives an exact description of his deformity in *Richard III*, with one exception in 3.4 (see below). Interestingly, there is an oblique reference to his body when, after unexpectedly succeeding in wooing Anne, Richard says: 'I'll be at charges for a looking-glass | And entertain a score or two of tailors | To study fashions to adorn my body' (1.2.242–4). Margaret makes oblique animal references to Richard's body, alluding to the shape of his crooked back: 'Thou elvish-marked, abortive, rooting hog [...] bottled spider [...] this poisonous bunch-backed toad' (1.3.225, 240, 244). Richard describes his body in the opening soliloquy of the play as 'not shaped for sportive tricks | Nor made to court an amorous looking-glass' (1.1.14–15), 'rudely stamped' (1.1.16), 'curtailed of this fair proportion' (1.1.18), 'cheated of feature' (1.1.19), 'deformed, unfinished' (1.1.20), and 'half made up' (1.1.21).

The one exception in *Richard III* in which he directly describes his body occurs in the scene where the Yorkist stalwart Hastings is arrested due to his hesitance to believe that Richard's arm was 'like a blasted sapling withered up' due to witchcraft (3.4.68–9). This imagery repeats the 'arm like withered shrub' from *3 Henry VI*. Moreover, this is the most direct intrusion of the historical sources regarding bodily description. This scene is already present in Vergil (1846: 180–1), but More (2005: 55–6) is the clearest influence, copied by Hall (Bullough 1975: 264) and Holinshed (1808: 380). More (2005: 55) writes: 'upon his left arm, [...] he showed a wearish [shrivelled], withered arm and small'. Shakespeare never specifies which arm is 'withered', but also adds the horticultural imagery of 'shrub' and 'sapling'. Shakespeare also omits that 'no man was there present but well knew that his arm was ever such since his birth' (Bullough 1975: 264; Holinshed 1808: 380; More 2005: 56).

There is a curious distinction between the two plays. In *3 Henry VI*, Shakespeare's description comes closer to the language of his sources: 'crookback', 'thick shoulder', 'withered arm', 'mountain on my back', 'deformity to mock my body', 'legs of an unequal size', 'misshaped trunk'. *Richard III*, on the other hand, is more abstract: 'not shaped', 'not made to court', 'rudely stamped', 'curtailed of fair proportion', 'cheated of feature', 'deformed, unfinished', 'half made up'. Omitting to mention body parts in *Richard III* links to a kind of creative agency: expressions have an artisanal quality yet an aestheticised abstractedness that lacks bodily specificity. This is mostly Richard's self-description, but the same abstractedness occurs in Margaret's shift from a straightforward 'crookback' to allusive animal imagery. Moreover, a socially reflective aesthetic in *Richard III* is hinted at with 'looking-glass', 'amorous', 'courting', and 'tailors [...] fashions to adorn my body'.

Shakespeare clearly follows the spirit of Tudor tradition especially in *3 Henry VI*, where Richard utters the physiognomic rule of a deformed body inhabiting a deformed mind central to the myth. As Jowett (2000: 11) points out, due to governmental scrutiny of plays, Shakespeare's 'freedom to vary from sanctioned accounts was limited'. However, Shakespeare is clearly doing something different, especially in *Richard III*, which is partially explained in the genre shift from historical to dramatic narrative. Shakespeare makes Richard more diabolically extreme, for example by making him responsible for Clarence's death, which none of the aforementioned historical sources does. Jowett well encapsulates the tension:

> Shakespeare played up to the image of a villainous and deformed Richard. The 'facts' of the play are uglier than those of his sources, but Shakespeare complicates things by making Richard charismatic and attractive in spite of them. (2005: 19)

Shakespeare's imagery is more vivid than the sources, but at the same time less specific in bodily detail. Although Shakespeare's more extreme depiction of Richard can be read subversively (more below), it clearly bears the hallmarks of the Tudor myth, as Myers (1968: 181) clarifies: 'Shakespeare has given immortality to a view of Richard III which was profoundly influenced by the political and emotional needs of Tudor England'.

16.2 The Modern Historical Narrative

The Tudor myth has not gone unchallenged. Myers (1968) provides an overview of Richard's historiography, dividing historians on their pro or anti stance on the 'Tudor Saga' – the main interest being in how historians were influenced by contemporary opinion. This work is influenced by Carr's (1987: 21) seminal work on modern historiography, according to which history consists in 'seeing the past through the eyes of the present and in the light of its problems' and the job for the historian 'is not to record but to evaluate'. Modern historiography puts the historian as the evaluative and interpretive agent at the centre of the process. In contrast, Holderness (2000: 43) remarks that 'history' in the early modern period was influenced by Cicero and meant 'a recovery of the past; a revival of things lost and forgotten; and a renarration of recuperated oblivion'. These ideas 'became a cornerstone of sixteenth century historical thinking, terms that have become for history in our own day intensively problematised: truth, memory, and instruction' (Holderness 2000: 46). The tension between early modern and modern historiography can be seen in how the Tudor period necessitated a skewed view of their near past and how truth, memory, and instruction needed to play along. As interpreters, chroniclers were conditioned by their time to see Richard in this now mythical light.

Goy-Blanquet (2002: 65) maintains that modern historiography satisfies four criteria: secularisation; experimental research; a sense of historical development; and the delimitation of an area of research. Rous, Vergil, More, Hall, and Holinshed could hardly live up to these modern requirements, leading to their being read as more propagandistic historical texts. As the historian Jacob (1961: 645) writes, Richard 'was very far from being the distorted villain of tradition' and undoubtedly there 'was a sound constructive side' to his story. Writing in the Cold War, Myers points out that to those

> who have lived through an epoch of Nazi and Communist double-talk and brainwashing, it seems natural for the untrained mind to think of a Tudor government in terms of equal propagandist efficiency. (1968: 201)

In terms of redrawing history, Logan (More 2005: 11) notes that an x-ray of one of the earliest surviving portraits of Richard revealed tampering: his 'right shoulder has been repainted to suggest deformity, and the eyes narrowed'.

Historiographically, the myth of a deformed, evil Richard has hardly survived intact. The obvious propaganda has been challenged by the fact of Richard being popular among contemporaries in the north of England and Ireland (Jacob 1961: 629; Myers 1968: 190). However, the moralistic view of Richard – the remains of the instructive strain of early modern historiography – is something we should be suspicious of, so as not to insert archaic connections between physical appearance and ethical activity. Physiology does not prescribe psychology. Skidmore (2018: 7), writing post excavation, laments the debate around Richard remaining 'depressingly predictable': his life and reign are defined by the question 'Was he a good or a bad king?' Skidmore reminds us that Richard acted as expected of kings before and after him. Therefore, instead of creating 'a white legend of Richard's personality' – while perpetuating 'a sterile debate' between 'good' and 'bad' – Skidmore (2018: 10) calls for balance and more accurate scholarship. Again, the historian as interpretive agent emerges. However, despite these objections and qualifications, the myth of the mentally and physically deformed Richard, mediated by Shakespeare's historical fiction, still persists.

16.3 The Leicester Carpark Findings

The research team that examined the remains affirmed that Richard had a severe right-sided thoracic scoliosis (with 70–90° Cobb angle), which is a lateral bending of the spine convex to the right, with some axial rotation. The findings were compatible with idiopathic – spontaneous, cause unknown – adolescent scoliosis. The thoracic curve was King-Moe type 3, meaning it was well balanced with cervical and lumbar spine aligned. The team concludes with a description, containing a Shakespearean echo on tailoring:

> The physical disfigurement from Richard's scoliosis was probably slight since he had a well-balanced curve. His trunk would have been short relative to the length of his limbs, and his right shoulder a little higher than the left. However, a good tailor and custom-made armour could have minimised the visual impact of this. A curve of 70–90° would not have caused impaired exercise tolerance from reduced lung capacity, and we identified no evidence that Richard would have walked with an overt limp, because the leg bones are symmetric and well formed [. . .]. (Appleby et al. 2014: 1944)

There is a curious discrepancy between the team's reports. An earlier report by Buckley et al. (2013: 536) suggests that although not all people with scoliosis experience pain, Richard's scoliosis 'may have been progressive and would have put additional strain on the heart and lungs, possibly causing shortness of breath and pain'.

Why the two opposing views? Today, a similar spinal condition with Cobb angle over 50 degrees would indeed be considered progressive from adolescence to adulthood and therefore prompt preventive interventions: intensive rehabilitation, using a back brace, and in some cases surgery (Negrini et al. 2018). The research reports interpreting Richard's remains did not, however, extensively consult clinical research of this fairly common condition. Rather, the interpretive discrepancy between the reports suggests that there is a limit to scientific certainty in drawing conclusions about Richard's body.

The scientific reports and the often sensationalist popular media reporting bear a striking similarity. Kostihova (2016: 2) observes that in the 'public spectacle of excavation' and 'theatre of discovery', both scientific and popular reporting constantly evoked references to Shakespeare, but there was also conflation between the remains and what the remains could reveal about Richard's psychology, his intentions, and his preferences. Connecting Richard's medical condition and psychology – 'as if one might finally uncover Richard's "real" nature by scrutinizing the truths of his "real" body', as Hobgood (2014: 24) poignantly put it – unwittingly confirms the persisting putative causal link between bodily impairment and psychology. Furthermore, as Kostihova (2016: 3) elaborates, the scientific reports did not succeed 'in steering clear of the voyeuristic sensationalism of scrutinizing Richard's deformed body', which the media further bolstered. Such media reporting declared Shakespeare as a propagandist who 'ensured Richard has been seen as hunchbacked for centuries' (Meikle 2014). In a *Daily Mail* article, Phil Stone, chair of the Richard III society, proclaims that Richard's scoliosis confirms the Shakespearean description of a 'bunch-backed toad' as a 'complete fabrication – yet more proof that, while the plays are splendid dramas, they are also most certainly fiction not fact' (Hope & Zolfagharifard 2014). The scientific evidence, in turn, helped the king once 'stripped by the victors' to be 'reclothed in his true identity' (Mantel 2013). Both scientific and media reporting seemed preoccupied with Shakespeare's falsity, not with what modern medical science is able to tell us about Richard's condition without unwittingly evoking the physiognomic rule. The evidence was neither reported nor received with the 'neutrality' or 'objectivity' expected of science.

16.4 Enlightenment Reverts to Myth: The Material Aspect

We suggest that the scientific facts do not stand against myth and fiction, but rather transgress the boundary of medical writing and perpetuate Richard's mythology. To understand this argument, Horkheimer and Adorno's (2002: xviii) thesis that 'myth is already enlightenment, and enlightenment reverts to mythology' proves helpful. Enlightenment, they write, is 'the advance of thought [that] has always aimed at liberating human beings from fear and installing them as masters' (Horkheimer & Adorno 2002: 1). The historical period of Enlightenment and the rise of modern science sought to 'dispel myths, to overthrow fantasy with knowledge' (Horkheimer & Adorno 2002: 1). Quantifications and classifications of science were to explain and control nature, replacing myth. The twist to their argument, on which ours is based, is that myth was an early rationalisation of nature – it sought to control and explain it, and liberate us from the fear of external nature – and not dissimilar to the mode of Enlightenment thinking, and therefore 'myth is already enlightenment' (Horkheimer & Adorno 2002: xviii). In turn, Enlightenment thinking, the all-permeating standard of calculability and utility of instrumentalised scientific knowledge, has become a new mythology: thus 'enlightenment reverts to mythology' (Horkheimer & Adorno 2002: xviii).

Horkheimer and Adorno (2002) suggest a continuum from myth to science rather than science simply dispelling myth or standing against it. Indeed, in Richard's case historiography, myth, fiction, and even modern science are all rationalisations that seek to control truth and draw conclusions regarding the uncertain and unknowable; but they are also inherently interpretive. Truth, here, does not belong to either myth or science, but is found somewhere in between their blurred boundaries. Drawing conclusions about limping, royal tailors, or lung capacity without observing and examining 'the patient' is at best educated guesswork and at worst guesswork communicated as truth with the authority of objective scientific research. Interpretation and speculation are necessarily at play in the scientific reporting – necessary because examining bones confirms little about Richard's psychology or his animated body, although revealing certain lifestyle, structural, and postural information.

Let us consider a few examples. Appleby et al. (2014) concluded that Richard did not have one leg shorter than the other and therefore probably did not limp. However, unequal leg length is not the only cause of limping. People with adolescent scoliosis may show an asymmetry of gait, a sideways sway caused by a difference in the stance-phase duration or a slight muscle imbalance on one side (Bruyneel et al. 2009; Kuo et al. 2011; Syczewska et al. 2012; Yang et al. 2013; Haber & Sacco 2015) that can appear to the clinically untrained eye as limping. Moreover, there might not have been an 'envious mountain' on his back, but scoliosis does cause a unilateral protrusion of the ribcage when bending forward – a common test used to examine scoliosis – and sometimes the protrusion is visible when standing up or lying down. There are also countless physiological and cultural factors that affect the animated body, from metabolism to cultural expectations and habitus. Differences in motor skills – balance, agility, coordination, speed, power, and reaction time, which often depend not only on learning and skills but also on the nervous system – and differences in muscle strength, muscle balance and flexibility, joint range of motion, and different qualities of connecting tissues, also affect how the body moves. There are so many factors that an accurate retrospective functional analysis is simply impossible. Although bones tell us a lot, they tell us little about the animated body; remains and a living body are very different things.

Any speculation, the above included, about Richard's 'past living body' makes, shapes, and disciplines it to fit our modern understanding of scoliosis: it sees 'the past through the eyes of the present' (Carr 1987: 21) because that is all it can do. The truth, here, is not about whether Richard had a limp. It is about the scientific discourse – albeit bearing facts that dispelled some rumours – operating between science, fiction, and myth and thus perpetuating Richard's mythology in its own way. There is a continuum from historiography, myth, and fiction to the post-excavation science forming the modern mythology of Richard.

16.5 Ability and Shakespeare: The Social Aspect

To complete Horkheimer and Adorno's (2002) chiasmic argument, we argue that Richard's fictional body in Shakespeare's plays has 'truth content' (Adorno 1997), thus 'myth was already enlightenment'. To elaborate this, we turn to Shakespearean disability studies (e.g. Mitchell & Snyder 2000; Williams 2009, 2013; Comber 2010; Wood 2013; Hobgood 2014; Wilson 2017, 2018; Gottlieb 2018; Love 2019).

Applying disability studies to Shakespeare might seem anachronistic, because in Shakespeare 'disability' is not employed in the modern sense of preexisting or acquired impairment. The modern sense of disability started to emerge only in the eighteenth and nineteenth centuries (Davis 2002: 3; Metzler 2006: 6). To be 'disabled' in Shakespeare means to 'experience a physical, moral, or economic slowdown', clarifying disability 'as a temporary state conferred upon one by another's – or by one's own – actions or prejudice' (Iyengar 2015: 9). The terminology of 'disability', therefore, raises the question of how we talk about disability in Shakespeare (Wilson 2017). Our use of the terminology of disability is not intended to make claims about early modern language, but rather about our contemporary understanding of disability – acknowledging ourselves as part of the myth-perpetuating discourse described so far, with necessary elements of anachronism in reading Shakespeare through twentieth-century critical theory and disability studies. We suggest that a degree of 'deliberate anachronism' (Williams 2009) functions as a useful vehicle to convey social criticism. As Hobgood and Wood (2013: 190) have suggested, early modern disability studies methodology need not be fixed to historicism, but rather 'develops from a flexible array of historicist and presentist methodologies and textual- and performance-related concerns'. We follow this suggestion because, we aim to show, Shakespeare has relevance to the critical understanding of disability in modern society, not merely in early modern England, and therefore restricting interpretation to the early modern period would restrict the power of interpretation Shakespeare's Richard holds.

Richard's deformity has been analysed from opposing perspectives on a social/metaphorical–material spectrum. Hobgood (2014: 24) argues that throughout *Richard III* Shakespeare's 'intense pathologizing of Richard's physical health through medical discourse' engages an early modern medical model of disability: Richard's disabled body is not merely metaphorical but material. Williams (2009) reads Richard more metaphorically as compensating for the negative associations of his bodily form by employing rhetorical power and performative ability: Richard foregrounds his deformity to advance his political power. Similarly, Comber (2010: 183) argues that people are always affected and disabled by their societies and constructs that convey the meaning of 'difference': people are 'never *just* physically impaired'. For Comber (2010: 183), Richard is 'disabled by an amalgamation of the religious, political, social and dramatic contexts and prejudices of society'. The interplay between material and social/metaphoric echoes the disability scholar Tom Shakespeare (2006), who argues that the social model of disability – the claim that disability does not reside in the body but in the social and physical environment – is not sufficient to account for the experiences of disabled people. Although the social model presents important criticism of the medical model that sees impairments as problems that can be fixed or cured (Eyler 2016: 4), the bodily impairment is not insignificant for disability: it is 'always an interaction between individual and structural factors' (Shakespeare 2006: 55). Shakespeare's Richard, his deformity (impairment), and his disability (stigmatisation) are similarly a sum of different factors.

Indeed, Richard's evil deeds are as much the product of attitudes towards his nature as they are of his nature. Richard is shunned for what his body signifies. He decides to play the part because there is no alternative; not because of some link forged by nature, but because it is expected of him:

(4) And therefore, since I cannot prove a lover,
To entertain these fair well-spoken days,
I am determined to prove a villain
And hate the idle pleasures of these days. (*Richard III* 1.1.28–31)

The material and social/metaphorical aspects of Richard's body can be read as social criticism. As Wilson (2017: n.p.) argues, encountering disability in Shakespeare kindles philosophical and social questions about the 'place of those who are different from the norm'. Shakespeare's Richard bears important 'truth content' that refers to socially critical knowledge – that is not straightforwardly communicable nor irrational – about the modern conditions of life that resides in the experience of an artwork (Adorno 1997). The truth content of Richard is possibly more significant compared to the 'scientifically accurate' Richard, because the play can offer a fruitful medium for challenging disablement, normativity, and normalisation. As Heller (2002: 371) argues, we can recognise ourselves in Shakespeare's 'revelatory truth': 'We are revealed to ourselves'. Holderness (2000: 49) has also argued that '[i]n the historical plays themselves we can find examples of drama both claiming a truth-function, and admitting its own insubstantiality'. Thus, Richard makes an interesting point of contemplation – with critically deliberate anachronism – for disability studies. Richard's socially constructed disability and real bodily deformity mutually mediate his actions, but also critically foreground the disabling and stigmatising attitudes towards bodies that are 'different'.

An important distinction between capacity and disability is in order. In both the historical and fictional body of Richard, his physical deformity does not make him incapable. Hammond (1981: 76) remarks that in historical research, Richard 'was generally conceded to be a brave and effective soldier'. Even Tudor historiographers acknowledge this. At Bosworth, Hall describes how Richard 'overthrew' and 'slew' significant enemies and as

(5) kynge Richardes men were driven backe and fledde, and he him selfe manfully fyghtynge in the mydell of his enemies was slayne and brought to his death as he worthily had deserved. (Bullough 1975: 297)

Moreover, in Vergil's account, Richard could have fled but decided against it:

(6) his corage also hault and fearce, which faylyd him not in the very death, which, whan his men forsooke him, he rather yealded to take

with the swoord, than by fowle flyght to prolong his lyfe, uncertane what death perchance soon after by sicknes or other vyolence to suffer. (Vergil 1846: 227)

Furthermore, Richard's abilities as military leader garnered praise from More:

(7) None evil captain was he in the war, as to which his disposition was more meetly than for peace. Sundry victories had he, and sometimes overthrows, but never in default as for his own person, either of hardiness or politic order. (More 2005: 10)

Similar military prowess can be seen in Shakespeare's drama. In his final battle, Richard – while seeking a horse to continue the battle – wonders: 'I think there be six Richmonds in the field. | Five have I slain today, instead of him' (*Richard III* 5.7.11–12). Furthermore, besides the many battles of *3 Henry VI*, Shakespeare makes the curious decision to insert Richard into the first battle of St Albans depicted in parts 2 and 3 of *Henry VI* – the historical Richard was under three years old and in France. Not only did Shakespeare have him participate but, as Heller (2002: 231) sees it, makes him the hero of the battle by having him thrice save the earl of Salisbury (*2 Henry VI* 5.5.12–24) and brandish the head of the duke of Somerset to the praise of his father, Richard of York: 'Richard hath best deserved of all my sons' (*3 Henry VI* 1.1.18).

Shakespeare's *Richard III* can be read subversively. The shift of genre from historical chronicle to art form (Shakespeare even titles it a 'tragedy') also shifts interpretive framework. Jowett (2000: 21) points out that 'the play is perhaps now more relevant as a study of history as representation, of the politics of historical narrative'. Holderness instructively deconstructs Richard's character through the phrase 'determined to prove a villain', arguing that it captures the

> paradoxical nature of Richard's self-definition, which turns precisely on the relation between historical causation (the modern sense of 'determined', here of course derived from the early modern legal sense of 'limited', 'set by cause') and voluntaristic 'self-fashioning', personal resolution, the freedom to determine one's own destiny. (Holderness 2000: 82)

This is how Shakespeare's extreme depiction can be seen as the Tudor myth externally imposed on the character, but at the same time expressing a sense of free will. Holderness continues:

> the decision to 'prove a villain' is as much a gesture of self-casting, the choice of a character, as it is a resigned submission to historical

> determinism; and an indication that Richard, the historical character, represented via the dramatic role, is presented as self-consciously aware of his own actorly status: he is an actor within the medium of a historical narrative, since he is conscious that his 'character' can be enacted only by the presence of such an actor in concrete theatrical realisation. (2000: 85)

This is in line with the abstract quality of the vocabulary Shakespeare employs to describe Richard compared to *3 Henry VI*. The lack of clear and distinct bodily descriptors (as discussed above) suggests this abstract, artisanal, metatheatrical quality in Richard's opening soliloquy: he is a malleable creature to be moulded or stamped to perform the function he determines. Moreover, commenting on Richard's performed manipulation of events and his exchange on history and fame with his nephew Edward V, Holderness (2000: 99) speaks to the power Shakespeare's use of the Tudor myth[4] wields: 'The substance of history' does not lie in 'physical remains and documentary characters, but rather in myth and legend, oral tradition and story'.

The cross-genre reading of Richard's body teaches us that the 'deformed' and 'disabled' body has political power: Richard's body was used both against him and by him to political ends. Richard is perhaps the most able character in Shakespeare and his body is central: it signifies the deeds that drive both his success and his downfall. Reports of the historical Richard's battle skills affirm his physical prowess. Even Rous, the original maligner of the king, writes that

> he bore himself like a noble soldier and despite his little body and feeble strength, honourably defended himself to his last breath, shouting again and again that he was betrayed, and crying 'Treason! Treason! Treason!' (Hanham 1975: 123)

Evidence of his military prowess – both historical and osteoarchaeological (Kendall 2002; Buckley et al. 2013) – have been seen as evidence of a non-disabled body. Herein lies a problem. We simply do not know the extent to which Richard was impaired by the scoliosis or disabled by the social norms of his time. There is a degree of paternalism, which is opposed within disability studies and disability rights movements, in retrospectively labelling Richard. When disability is considered negative and undesirable, in addition to the stigmatising presumption that disability and psychology are causally connected, then the discourse of Richard reverts to the 'depressingly predictable' writing that Skidmore (2018: 7) has rightly criticised.

[4] Heller (2002: 100) rightly points out that '[t]he stage is essentially historical. Thus, history is the *medium* of the Shakespearean history plays, tragedies, and certain romances and comedies'.

16.6 Conclusion

Richard III mythology has gained a new afterlife in the scientific post-excavation discourse, which constantly evoked myth and fiction. It seems that Myers's analysis on the interaction between Shakespeare and Ricardian tradition still holds true:

> Shakespeare's spell ensures the immortality of the hostile Tudor tradition; it probably also ensures that someone will always be kindly disposed towards the last Plantagenet king. (Myers 1968: 202)

In the mythology, consisting of historical, mythical, fictional, and factual elements, truth is not reliant on empirical verification nor myth reliant on historical fabrications. Truth transgresses the boundaries of genre, as does interpretation. In the case of Richard III, medical facts cannot escape mythology, and fiction offers a fruitful medium for understanding society through reading Richard's body as socially disabled but physically – and politically – capable. The interpreter's subjectivity and reflection are inseparable from the text and discourse produced, and truth never appears unmediated: there are always subjects, traditions, myths, methodologies, ideologies at play. Rather than being undesirable, subjectivity is inevitable. Therefore, it should be made visible to increase the rigour – even objectivity – of analyses across genres.

REFERENCES

Adorno, Theodor W. 1997. *Aesthetic theory*. Robert Hullot-Kentor (trans.). London: Continuum.

Appleby, Jo, Piers D. Mitchell, Claire Robinson, Alison Brough, Guy Rutty, Russell A. Harris, David Thompson, & Bruno Morgan. 2014. The scoliosis of Richard III, last Plantagenet king of England: Diagnosis and clinical significance. *The Lancet* 383(9932): 1944.

Ashdown-Hill, John. 2015. *The mythology of Richard III*. Stroud: Amberley Publishing.

Baldwin, David. 2015. *Richard III*, rev. ed. Stroud: Amberley Publishing.

Bruyneel, Anne-Violette, Pascale Chavet, Gérard Bollini, Paul Allard, Eric Berton, & Serge Mesure. 2009. Dynamical asymmetries in idiopathic scoliosis during forward and lateral initiation step. *European Spine Journal* 18(2): 188–95.

Buckley, Richard, Mathew Morris, Jo Appleby, Turi King, Deirdre O'Sullivan, & Lin Foxhall. 2013. 'The king in the car park': New light on the death and burial of Richard III in the Grey Friars Church, Leicester, in 1485. *Antiquity* 87(336): 519–38.

Bullough, Geoffrey (ed.). 1975. *Narrative and dramatic sources of Shakespeare*, vol. III. London: Routledge & Kegan Paul.

Carr, E. H. 1987. *What is history?* 2nd ed. Harmondsworth: Penguin.

Carson, Annette. 2013. *Richard III: The maligned king*, updated ed. Stroud: History Press.

Charnes, Linda. 1993. *Notorious identity: Materializing the subject in Shakespeare*. Cambridge, MA: Harvard University Press.

Comber, Abigail Elizabeth. 2010. A medieval king 'disabled' by an early modern construct. In Joshua R. Eyler (ed.), *Disability in the Middle Ages: Reconsiderations and reverberations*, 183–96. Abingdon: Routledge.

Davis, Lennard J. 2002. *Bending over backwards: Disability, dismodernism, and other difficult positions*. New York: New York University Press.

Eyler, Joshua R. 2016. Introduction: Breaking boundaries, building bridges. In Joshua R. Eyler (ed.), *Disability in the Middle Ages: Reconsiderations and reverberations*, 1–10. Abingdon: Routledge.

Garber, Marjorie. 1987. *Shakespeare's ghost writers: Literature as uncanny causality*. New York; London: Routledge.

Gottlieb, Christine M. 2018. 'Unaccomodated man': Dismodernism and disability justice in *King Lear*. *Disability Studies Quarterly* 38(4). https://dsq-sds.org/article/view/6079/5133 (accessed 15 June 2020).

Goy-Blanquet, Dominique. 2002. Elizabethan historiography and Shakespeare's sources. In Michael Hattaway (ed.), *The Cambridge companion to Shakespeare's history plays*, 57–70. Cambridge: Cambridge University Press.

Greenblatt, Stephen, Walter Cohen, Jean E. Howard, & Katherine Eisaman Maus. 2008. *The Norton Shakespeare: Essential plays, the sonnets*. 2nd ed. New York: W. W. Norton.

Haber, Cassandra Kay, & Mark Sacco. 2015. Scoliosis: Lower limb asymmetries during the gait cycle. *Archives of Physiotherapy* 5(1): 4.

Hammond, Anthony. 1981. Introduction. In Anthony Hammond (ed.), William Shakespeare, *King Richard III*. London: Methuen.

Hanham, Alison. 1975. *Richard III and his early historians, 1483–1535*. Oxford: Clarendon Press.

Hay, William. 1754. *Deformity: An essay*. London: R. & J. Dodsley.

Heller, Agnes. 2002. *The time is out of joint: Shakespeare as philosopher of history*. Oxford: Rowman & Littlefield.

Hicks, Michael. 2019. *Richard III: The self-made king*. New Haven, CT: Yale University Press.

Hill, Thomas. 1571. *The contemplation of mankinde contayning a singuler discourse after the art of phisiognomie*. London: Henry Denham for William Seres.

Hobgood, Allison P. 2014. Teeth before eyes impairment and invisibility in Shakespeare's Richard III. In Sujata Iyengar (ed.), *Disability, health, and happiness in the Shakespearean body*, 3–40. New York: Routledge.

Hobgood, Allison P., & David Houston Wood. 2013. *Recovering disability in early modern England*. Columbus: Ohio State University Press.

Holderness, Graham. 2000. *Shakespeare: The histories*. Basingstoke: Macmillan.

Holinshed, Raphael. 1808. *Holinshed's chronicles of England, Scotland and Ireland.* London: for J. Johnson; F. C. and J. Rivington; T. Payne; Wilkie and Robinson; Longman, Hurst, Rees, and Orme; Cadell and Davies; and J. Mawman.

Hope, Jenny, & Ellie Zolfagharifard. 2014. Richard III wasn't a hunchback: Scans reveal monarch's spinal curvature could have been concealed. *Daily Mail* 30 May. www.dailymail.co.uk/sciencetech/article-2643056/Richard-III-wasnt-hunchback-did-scoliosis-scans-reveal.html (accessed 15 June 2020).

Horkheimer, Max, & Theodor W. Adorno. 2002. *Dialectic of Enlightenment: Philosophical fragments.* Edmund Jephcott (trans.). Stanford: Stanford University Press.

Horspool, David. 2015. *Richard III: A ruler and his reputation.* London: Bloomsbury.

Iyengar, Sujata. 2015. Introduction: Shakespeare's 'discourse of disability'. In Sujata Iyengar (ed.), *Disability, health, and happiness in the Shakespearean body*, 1–20. New York: Routledge.

Jacob, E. F. 1961. *The Oxford history of England: The fifteenth century 1399–1485.* Oxford: Clarendon Press.

Jowett, John. 2000. Introduction. In John Jowett (ed.), William Shakespeare, *Richard III*, 1–132. Oxford: Oxford University Press.

Kendall, Paul Murray. 2002. *Richard III.* New York: W. W. Norton.

King, Turi E., Gloria Gonzalez Fortes, Patricia Balaresque, Mark Thomas, David Balding, Pierpaolo Maisano Delser, Rita Neumann, Walther Parson, Michael Knapp, Susan Walsh, Laure Tonasso, John Holt, Manfred Kayser, Jo Appleby, Peter Forster, David Ekserdijian, Michael Hofreiter, & Kevin Schürer. 2014. Identification of the remains of King Richard III. *Nature Communications* 5(1): 5631.

Kostihova, Marcela. 2016. Digging for perfection: Discourse of deformity in Richard III's excavation. *Palgrave Communications* 2(1). www.nature.com/articles/palcomms201646 (accessed 15 June 2020).

Kuo, Fang-Chuan, Chang-Zern Hong, Chung-Liang Lai, & Shih-Hsin Tan. 2011. Postural control strategies related to anticipatory perturbation and quick perturbation in adolescent idiopathic scoliosis. *Spine* 36(10): 810–16.

Legge, Alfred Owen. 1885. *The unpopular king: The life and times of Richard III. In two volumes.* London: Ward & Downey.

Lewis, Matthew. 2019. *Richard III: Facts and fictions.* Barnsley: Pen and Sword History.

Love, Genevieve. 2019. *Early modern theatre and the figure of disability.* London: Bloomsbury.

Mantel, Hilary. 2013. Royal bodies. *London Review of Books* 35(4). www.lrb.co.uk/the-paper/v35/n04/hilary-mantel/royal-bodies (accessed 15 June 2020).

Meikle, James. 2014. Richard III was no 'bunch-backed toad', research suggests. *The Guardian* 30 May. www.theguardian.com/uk-news/2014/may/30/richard-iii-no-bunch-backed-toad-hunchback-research-lancet (accessed 15 June 2020).

Metzler, Irina. 2006. *Disability in medieval Europe: Thinking about physical impairment during the High Middle Ages, c. 1100–1400*. New York: Routledge.

Mitchell, David T., & Sharon L. Snyder. 2000. *Narrative prosthesis: Disability and the dependencies of discourse*. Ann Arbor: University of Michigan Press.

Modern Healthcare. 2014. Correcting the twisted facts on Richard III. *Modern Healthcare* 44(23): 36.

More, Thomas. 2005. *The history of King Richard the Third: A reading edition*. George M. Logan (ed.). Bloomington: Indiana University Press.

Muir, Kenneth. 1977. *The sources of Shakespeare's plays*. London: Methuen.

Myers, A. R. 1968. Richard III and historical tradition. *History* 53(178): 181–202.

Negrini, Stefano, Sabrina Donzelli, Angelo Gabriele Aulisa, Dariusz Czaprowski, Sanja Schreiber, Jean Claude de Mauroy, Helmut Diers, et al. 2018. 2016 SOSORT guidelines: Orthopaedic and rehabilitation treatment of idiopathic scoliosis during growth. *Scoliosis and Spinal Disorders* 13(1): 3.

Rous, John. (n.d.). The Rous Roll, c. 1483–1484. *British Library Digitised Manuscripts*. www.bl.uk/manuscripts/FullDisplay.aspx?ref=Add_MS_48976 (accessed 15 June 2020).

Schwyzer, Philip. 2013. *Shakespeare and the remains of Richard III*. Oxford: Oxford University Press.

Shakespeare, Tom. 2006. *Disability rights and wrongs*. Abingdon: Routledge.

Skidmore, Chris. 2018. *Richard III: England's most controversial king*. New York: St. Martin's Press.

Slotkin, Joel Elliot. 2007. Honeyed toads: Sinister aesthetics in Shakespeare's 'Richard III'. *Journal for Early Modern Cultural Studies* 7: 5–32.

Syczewska, Malgorzata, Krzysztof Graff, Malgorzata Kalinowska, Ewa Szczerbik, & Janusz Domaniecki. 2012. Influence of the structural deformity of the spine on the gait pathology in scoliotic patients. *Gait & Posture* 35(2): 209–13.

Vergil, Polydore. 1846. *Polydore Vergil's English history*. London: Camden Society.

Williams, Katherine Schaap. 2009. Enabling Richard: The rhetoric of disability in Richard III. *Disability Studies Quarterly* 29(4). https://dsq-sds.org/article/view/997/1181 (accessed 26 April 2022).

Williams, Katherine Schaap. 2013. Performing disability and theorizing deformity. *English Studies: Shakespeare and Theory: Special Issue II* 94(7): 757–72.

Wilson, Jeffrey R. 2017. The trouble with disability in Shakespeare studies. *Disability Studies Quarterly* 37(2). https://dsq-sds.org/article/view/5430/0 (accessed 15 June 2020).

Wilson, Jeffrey R. 2018. 'Savage and deformed': Stigma as drama in *The Tempest*. *Medieval and Renaissance Drama in England* 31: 146–77.

Wood, David Houston. 2013. New directions: 'Some tardy cripple': Timing disability in *Richard III*. In Annaliese Connolly (ed.), *Richard III: A Critical Reader*, 129–57. London: Bloomsbury.

Yang, Jae Hyuk, Seung-Woo Suh, Paul S. Sung, & Woo-Hyung Park. 2013. Asymmetrical gait in adolescents with idiopathic scoliosis. *European Spine Journal* 22(11): 2407–13.

CHAPTER 17

Images and Paratexts

Peter Murray Jones

This book, *Genre in English Medical Writing, 1500–1820*, is adorned with thirty-five figures. Many of these figures are tables or graphs condensing the evidence and arguments of a particular author into forms that can be appreciated better through visualisation. The authors of chapters employing this presentational kind of figure have used their own computer software to generate them. They have no problems other than those involved in designing the book – how best to fit such figures into the layout of the chapter and the pages in which they are found. Other kinds of figure in this book are not presentational in this way but are quite different. These are images chosen by the author, and they reproduce pages in manuscripts or printed books of the early modern era. The author may refer to these images in the text of the chapter as evidence in pursuit of an argument, or choose them as emblems of the kind of things discussed (and so not essential to the argument). Illustrations that do necessary work for the argument of the chapter are found in the chapters by Peter Jones (Chapter 2), Alpo Honkapohja (Chapter 5), and Maura Ratia (Chapter 13). In the last two cases the argument focuses on the ways in which the same or similar textual matter is represented very differently in scribal handiwork, layout, or typography at different dates. The third kind of emblematic figure is there to engage the interest of the reader, giving material form (manuscript or printed) to the genre under discussion in the chapter. This applies to the figures in the Image Gallery, where Figure 2 is an emblem of London in time of plague, Figure 3 an author portrait, and Figure 6 a satire on man-midwifery, all from early modern printed books. The images supplied for these kinds of illustrative figure must first be obtained from professional imaging services or directly from libraries. In extraordinary times of lockdown, as we saw in the Preface to the Image Gallery, there may be difficulties in getting images or permissions.

All this should prompt us to think about features of books and manuscripts in the early modern era, particularly those features that are paratextual rather than textual, and that can be thought of not as unique to a particular book, but as belonging to image populations existing in time, and thus subject to considerations of changes in availability or occasional disruption. One major general change of this kind was the development of print media alongside manuscripts from the late fifteenth century onwards, and the consequent mutual influencing of these media (to say nothing of the emergence of woodcut and engraved images, see Jones 2020). Manuscripts were models for the design of printed books, and features of printed books were copied by scribes. While the text of the late sixteenth-century Wellcome MS 674 (Figure 9 in the Image Gallery) is quite probably copied from a manuscript version of John Mirfield's regimen of health, the layout of the text in MS 674 is influenced by that of the printed editions of this text by William Caxton and Wynkyn de Worde, as remarked by Lori Jones (Chapter 3). In a different case, early modern handwritten medical recipe books often contained recipes copied out from printed books, but they tended to retain the page design characteristic of earlier manuscripts. This was adaptable enough to allow for centred recipe titles and divisions between recipes drawn on the page, as well as to allow recipes to be added or crossed out (see Figure 14.2). Some designs like the luxury Stockholm parchment roll (see [Arderne] 2014 and Chapter 2 this volume) or pages with coloured marginal illustrations alongside (Figure 7 in the Image Gallery) were never likely to be copied in printed books because of the technical difficulties involved.

Any inventory of images and diagrams used in early modern medical books and manuscripts would have to include an extraordinary range of different kinds, from scholastic branching figures showing how to differentiate in diagnosing illness, to schemata demonstrating the relationship of the macrocosmic universe to the microcosmic human body, to anatomical displays of the interior of the body, to wheels of urine jars showing twenty colours, to patterns of surgical instruments, and many others. They vary in function from the didactic to the practical, and were directed to families and households as well as to medical professionals and university teachers. They were drawn by hand, or designed to be executed in woodcut and engraving, crude or sophisticated. But they were not equally accessible to all.

Scarcity and abundance of resources played their part in determining the form of early modern paratexts. Certain kinds of manuscript were produced for elite patrons and required enormous investments of precious materials and skilled labour. While these investments were most often made in late medieval times for personal religious works like books of hours, or for secular literature targeted at court entertainment (chronicles, romances, and the like), they sometimes were made in medical writings too. A spectacular example is the illuminated page from the beginning of John of Burgundy's plague treatise found in Cambridge, Fitzwilliam MS 261, made for Lady Margaret Beaufort, mother to King Henry VII (Figure 12 in the Image Gallery). On a fine parchment leaf the decorated and inhabited border around the text block, and the initial T within that border, are illuminated with gold and a full palette of colours. The emblems of the Beaufort family are depicted along with roses and other flowers, as well as insects. The script of the text is elegantly written in a fine bookhand by a professional scribe, with added rubrication and decorated paraph marks. This is a layout fit for a queen. No other manuscript of John of Burgundy's text was produced to this standard.

Of course, the early modern era was the great age of epidemic disease in England and Europe too. This accounts for the continuing popularity of John of Burgundy's plague treatise, in print and manuscript versions. In England, plague treatises like that of John of Burgundy were closely bound to the chronology of plague itself – new outbreaks persuaded printers and publishers to pursue new market opportunities. This kind of republication was essentially conservative, insofar as it was cheaper to reuse previous texts and layouts than to commission new ones. The same conservatism is found in the plague orders first produced in print in England in 1579, and reiterated in times of plague epidemics thereafter, though the reasons were more political than commercial. These orders instructed the justices of the peace in every area to appoint searchers to identify those sick of plague, to isolate them in their houses, to burn the clothes and bedding of the sick, and to raise taxes to pay for these policies. Publication of such orders was repeated in times of plague, with little variation in content or format. The kind of public messaging involved became familiar in England and elsewhere in 2020–2021 (albeit through the medium of TV), as viewers watched updates of COVID-19 rules for lockdown on a weekly basis. The framework of such public announcements, with distanced podia for speakers, PowerPoint presentations, and a cast of increasingly familiar scientific experts, is similarly repetitive by design. We are meant to recognise such official channels as informed by expertise and pronounced with authority.

In this volume, Maura Ratia (Chapter 12) investigates innovative uses of print layout, typefaces, and images in English plague publications of the seventeenth century. Bills of mortality were published in London between 1603 and 1666 in broadsheet form (see Table 12.1 for details). This meant that the various kinds of information on the sheet, from burial statistics to explanations of disease, remedies, and prayers, could all be read off from this one large bill. A bill could be purchased for private reading, but also could be studied in a tavern or coffeehouse (from the mid-century), or even displayed on a wall in a public space. At its simplest such a bill could include two columns of text, in one of which numbers of burials could be presented with the use of curly brackets, with three decorative patterned strips made with the use of a roll giving the design coherence and display value (Figure 12.1). In 1665 a strikingly simple mourning cross grabbed the viewer's attention at top centre, and the burial numbers across a number of plague years were fitted into a table of eight columns (Figure 12.4). In the following year the cross was replaced by a picture of a London skyline (an angel appearing in clouds above) with an open field below, in which a cart drags coffins, kneeling figures pray, and a skeleton brandishes an arrow (of plague) and an hourglass. On either side of the bill are decorative strips with emblems of skeletons, skulls, crossed bones, shovels, and winding sheets (Figure 12.5). As well as these attention-grabbing pictorial devices and decorations, the plague bills use varieties and sizes of type, together with variegated ornaments, to enhance visual impact.

Early English Books Online (EEBO) has created a population of digital images of printed pages extending from the first Caxtons to what was published in 1700, so enabling modern researchers to measure continuities and changes in text and layout across the early modern period. (*Eighteenth Century Collections Online*, ECCO, extends this capacity to a further century.) So far as analysis of layout is concerned, *Verbal and visual communication in early English texts* (Peikola et al. 2017) has shown what can be done, and some of the contributors to that work are represented again in this book (Ratia, Chapter 12; Suhr, Chapter 13; McConchie, Chapter 8). Title pages have proved to be remarkably fruitful in terms of tracing changes in layout over the long term, with the early emphasis on visual effects giving way to increasing reliance on textual labels in the seventeenth century. Plague treatises from 1603 to 1666 were used as a case study by Ratia (Chapter 12) and Suhr (Chapter 13) to demonstrate this transition, which occurred somewhat later than in the case of specialised medical treatises. Broadsheet bills of mortality, as we see in the current book, evolved separately from plague treatises and other medical texts.

Some telling additional evidence for changes in title pages can be found in this new study. The title page of Hieronymus Brunschwig, *Buch der Cirurgia* (1518) (Figure 10 in the Image Gallery) consists of a Low

German statement of the book's title at the top, with a woodcut version of the wound man image beneath. This wound man image had been current in manuscript illustrations for more than a century before Brunschwig's print publication. It would have been instantly recognisable to barbers or surgeons who had been exposed to manuscript or print productions as part of their apprenticeship.[1] The evolution from pictorial towards a predominance of textual labels in the title page is taken a stage further in the advertising pamphlet for *Elixir salutis* of 1675 (Figure 14 in the Image Gallery). This title page packs in a wealth of information about the nature of the product, its history, and a promise to provide names of witnesses to its efficacy within, its mode of operation, suitability to all kinds of people, and its power against noxious humours. A separate compartment gives the name and character of its promoter and salesman, with a warning against counterfeiters, and finally, in a further compartment, its publication details and date. Various typefaces, sizes of print, and capitals help to differentiate the many textual elements in this lengthy title page.

These comments have focused on the sociocultural contexts in which paratexts were produced over the early modern period, when enforced lockdowns in the face of epidemic disease were a recurring feature of such contexts. We have come to appreciate this phenomenon with peculiar urgency in 2021. Genres of medical writing would not all have reflected this paratextually in quite the same way, as no doubt further research will discover, but many of the images illustrated by figures in this book can be thought of as sharing this contextual predicament ('lockdown' for short).

REFERENCES

[Arderne, John]. 2014. *De Arte Phisicali et de Cirurgia by John Arderne; from a new digital version of the Stockholm roll*, trans. and commented by Torgny Svenberg & Peter Murray Jones. Stockholm: Hagströmer Biblioteket.

Jones, Peter Murray. 2020. Visualization of medicine between script and print, c. 1375–1550. In M. Kupfer, A. S. Cohen, & J. H. Chajes (eds.), *The visualization of knowledge in medieval and early modern Europe*, 341–60. Turnhout: Brepols.

Peikola, Matti, Aleksi Mäkilähde, Hanna Salmi, Mari-Liisa Varila, & Janne Skaffari (eds.). 2017. *Verbal and visual communication in early English texts*. Turnhout: Brepols.

[1] See Jack Hartnell's forthcoming study of the wound man tradition: https://medievalartresearch.com/2021/02/09/online-lecture-wound-man-three-early-modern-afterlives-of-a-medieval-surgical-image-jack-hartnell (accessed 26 April 2022).

Preface to the Image Gallery

Peter Murray Jones

The unusual conditions during the COVID-19 pandemic have thrown 'normal' authorial and publishing practice into sharp relief. Lockdown in its various forms and degrees has suddenly interrupted normal service. Perhaps a print or manuscript can no longer be photographed, or the curator cannot even enter the building where it is kept. Curators on furlough or working from home cannot easily fulfil an author's demands, even if those only involve processing permissions to reproduce images. Questions of image supply and reproduction of images suddenly loom larger for author and publisher than previously anticipated. This is certainly the case for this book. Chapter 2, for instance, explains how a seventeenth-century English surgeon copied his own designs for instruments by hand into an interleaved fifteenth-century manuscript of the work of a medieval surgeon. It has proved impossible to get a photograph of the surgeon Walter Hamond's new instrument designs, although by good luck the fifteenth-century model was available to the author as a TIFF image.

More positively, however, present-day pandemic conditions have undoubtedly accelerated even further the turn to digitisation as a basic research tool, making a wealth of products from the digitisation of manuscripts and printed books available to scholars. Even if these products could not simply be downloaded to the author's computer and then passed on to the publisher as figures in the author's text, they are increasingly supplied for the author's use, usually free of charge under Creative Commons licences. The author can then requisition a reproduction of the image of publishable quality from the service or the library in which the image was found, and such access has allowed for new analytical approaches, including the comparison of materials from geographically very disparate repositorics. Although lockdowns have in some cases disrupted this apparently inexhaustible cornucopia of images, making them sometimes hard to get or even completely inaccessible, it seems likely that in the long term the digitisation of research materials will be further encouraged by current conditions. Research, after all, is as much a cultural as a scientific phenomenon, as will be repeatedly noted in all the papers in this collection.

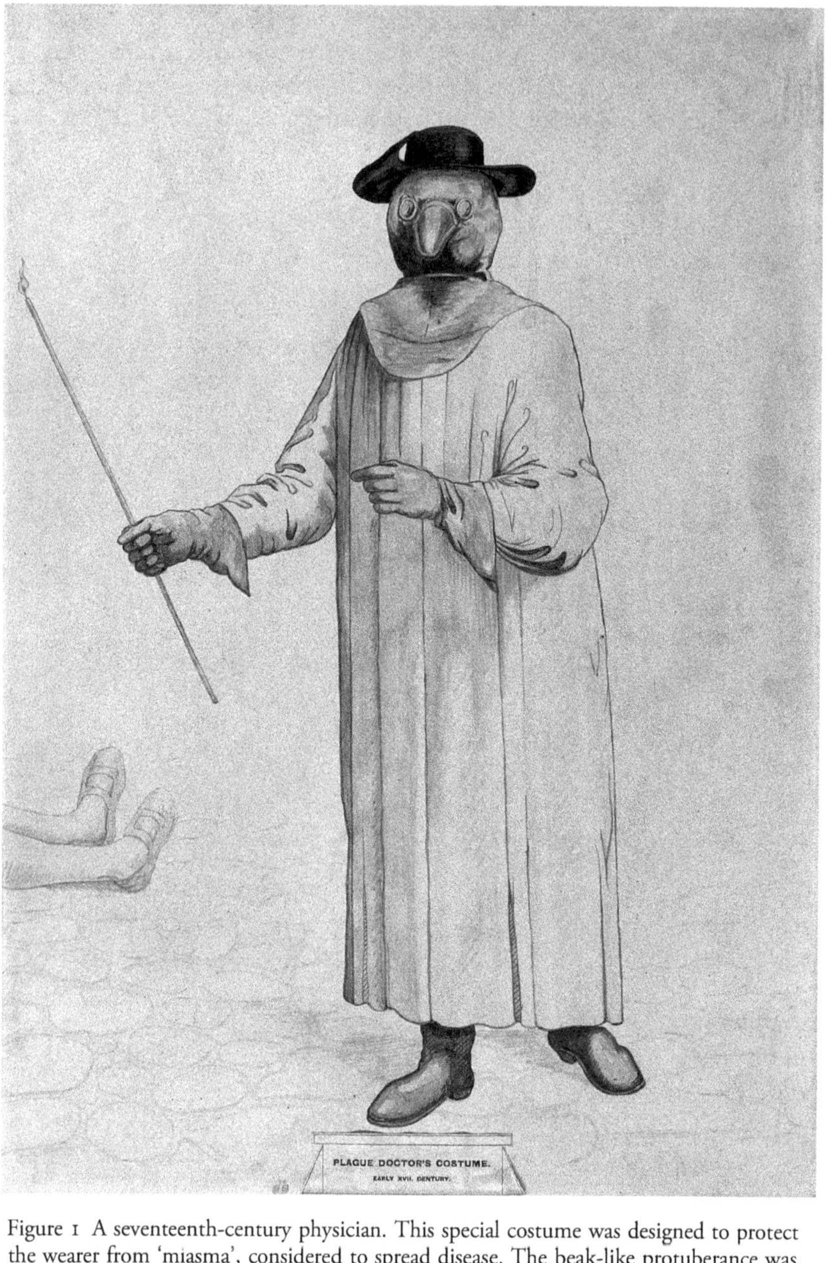

Figure 1 A seventeenth-century physician. This special costume was designed to protect the wearer from 'miasma', considered to spread disease. The beak-like protuberance was filled with aromatic herbs, often lavender. Wellcome Collection. Public domain mark

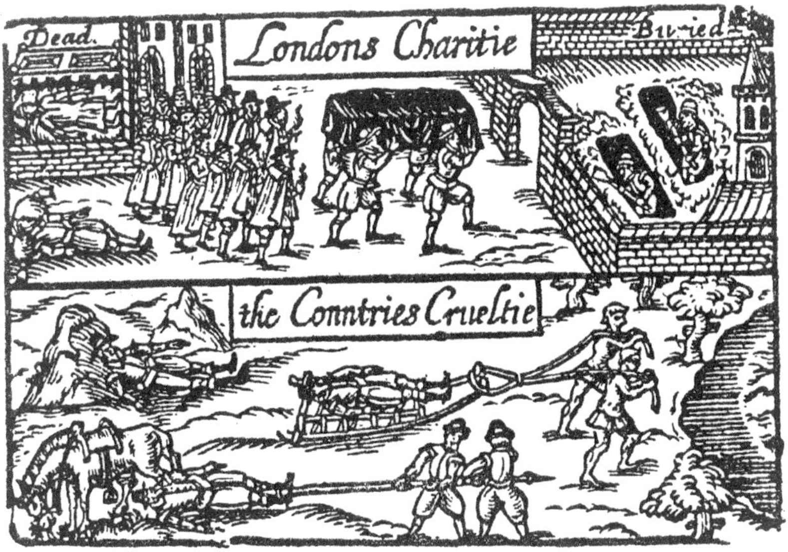

FROM TITLE PAGE OF "LONDONS LAMENTATION," 1641.

Figure 2 A woodcut showing a plague scene: the title page of *Londons Lamentation* (1641), which 'described certaine causes of this affliction and visitation of the plague [. . .] which the Lord hath been pleased to inflict upon us, and withall what meanes must be used to the Lord, to gaine his mercy and favor [. . .].' Wellcome Collection. Image attribution CC BY 4.0

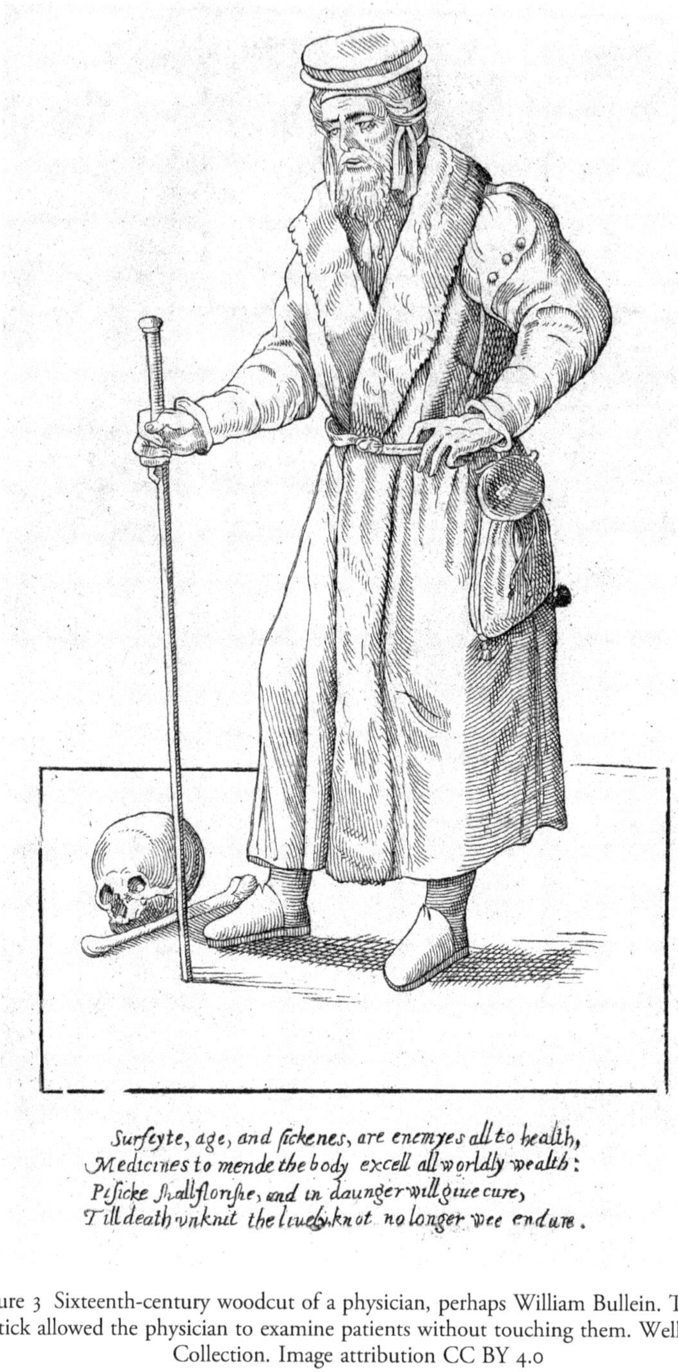
Surfeyte, age, and ſickenes, are enemyes all to health,
Medicines to mende the body excell all worldly wealth:
Piſicke ſhall floriſhe, and in daunger will giue cure,
Till death vnknit the liuely knot no longer wee endure.

Figure 3 Sixteenth-century woodcut of a physician, perhaps William Bullein. The long stick allowed the physician to examine patients without touching them. Wellcome Collection. Image attribution CC BY 4.0

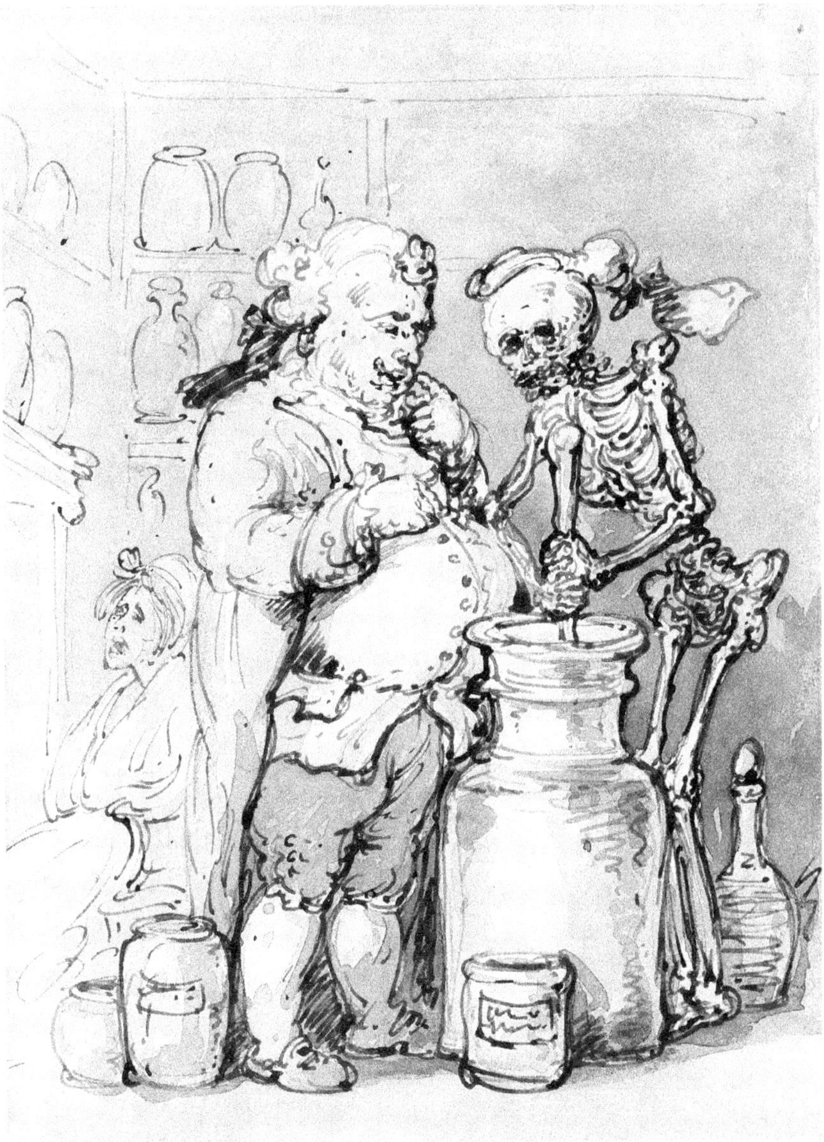

Figure 4 Death as an apothecary's assistant, supervised by its master, making up medicines for a female patient. The watercolour has been ascribed to the well-known caricaturist Thomas Rowlandson (1757–1827), or to one of his followers. Wellcome Collection. Public domain mark

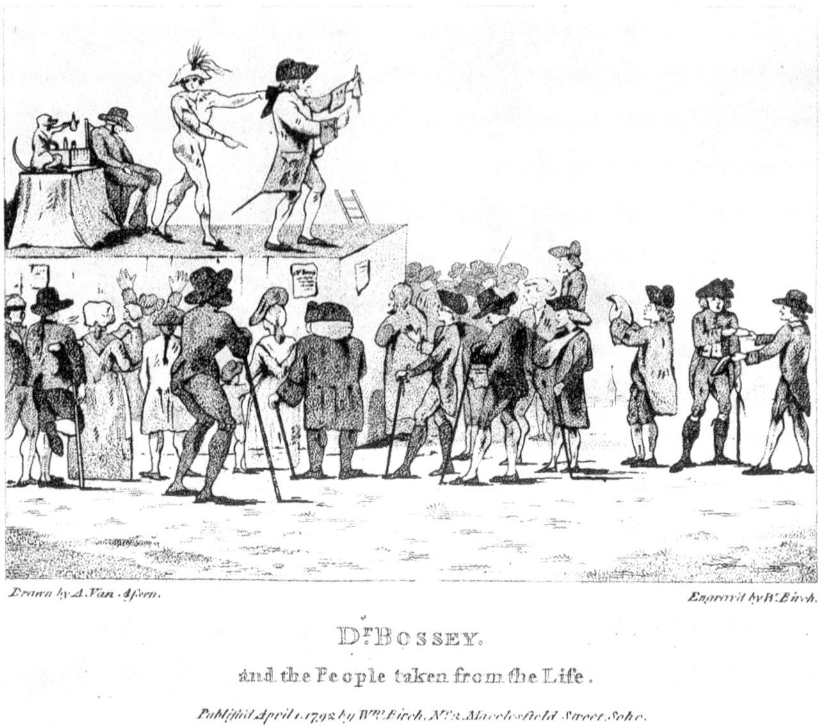

Figure 5 The quack Dr Bossey selling medicines in London in 1792. Behind him are his attendant, who points him out to the crowd, a rather dejected 'patient', and a monkey holding a phial of medicine: an engraving by William Russell Birch. Wellcome Collection. Public domain mark

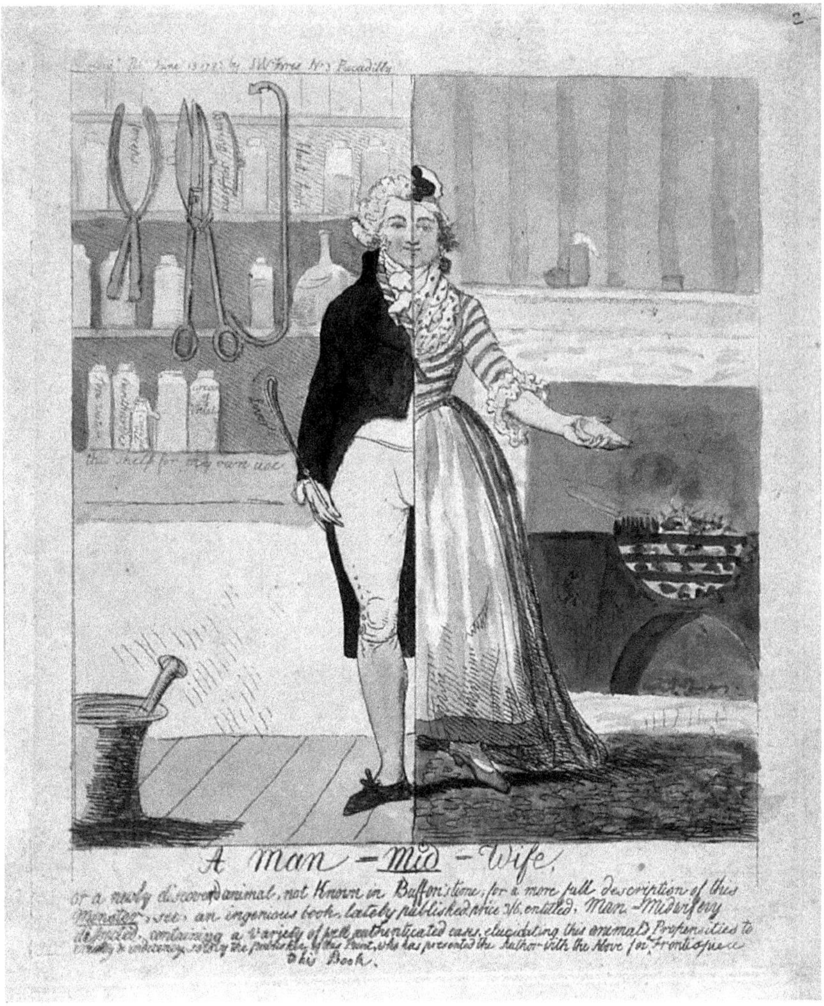

Figure 6 A 'man-midwife' (male obstetrician) represented by a figure divided in half, one half representing a man and the other a woman: a coloured etching from 1793 by the caricaturist Isaac Cruikshank (1764–1811). Wellcome Collection. Public domain mark

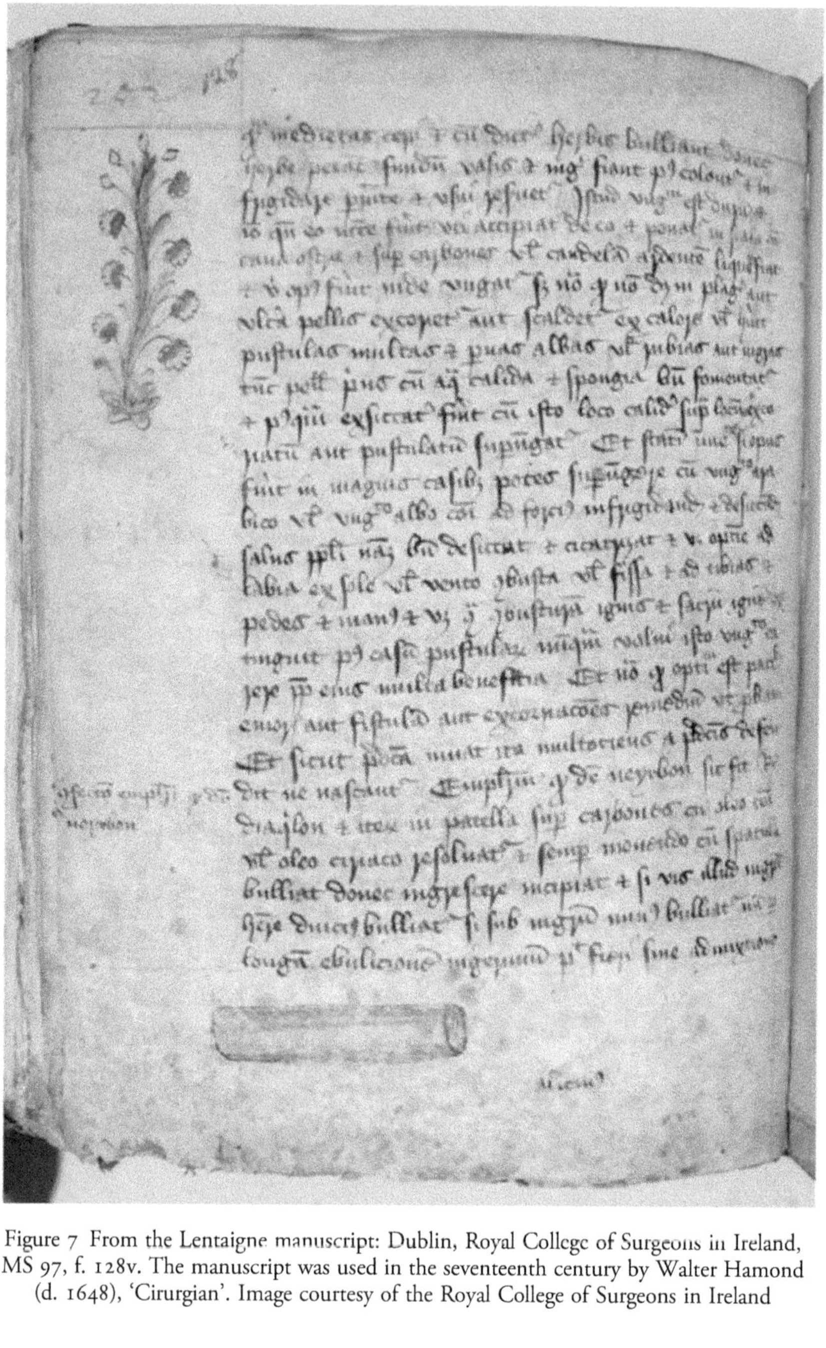

Figure 7 From the Lentaigne manuscript: Dublin, Royal College of Surgeons in Ireland, MS 97, f. 128v. The manuscript was used in the seventeenth century by Walter Hamond (d. 1648), 'Cirurgian'. Image courtesy of the Royal College of Surgeons in Ireland

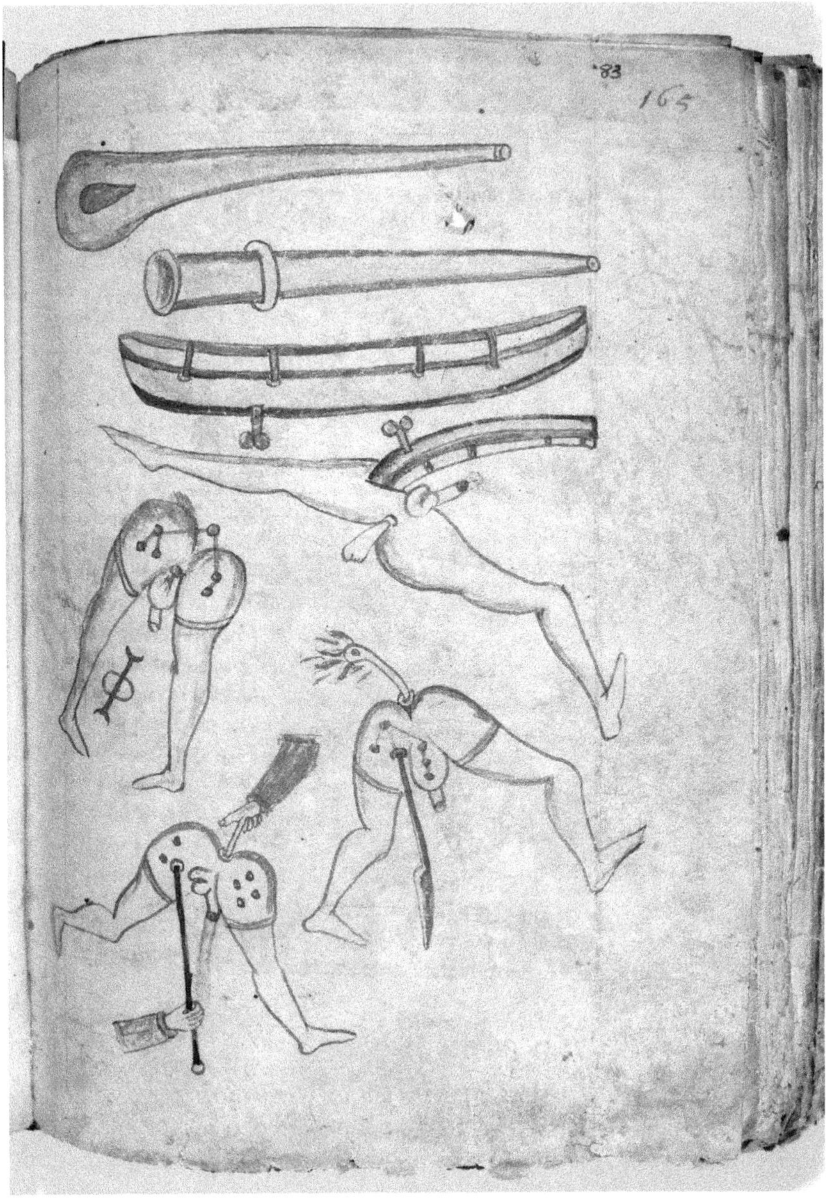

Figure 8 Instruments to be used for the treatment of fistula in ano, drawn by Walter Hamond. The drawings are versions, interestingly modified, of those originally provided for the medieval treatise composed by John Arderne (c.1307–c.1377). From the Lentaigne manuscript, Dublin, Royal College of Surgeons in Ireland, MS 97, f. 83r. Image courtesy of the Royal College of Surgeons in Ireland

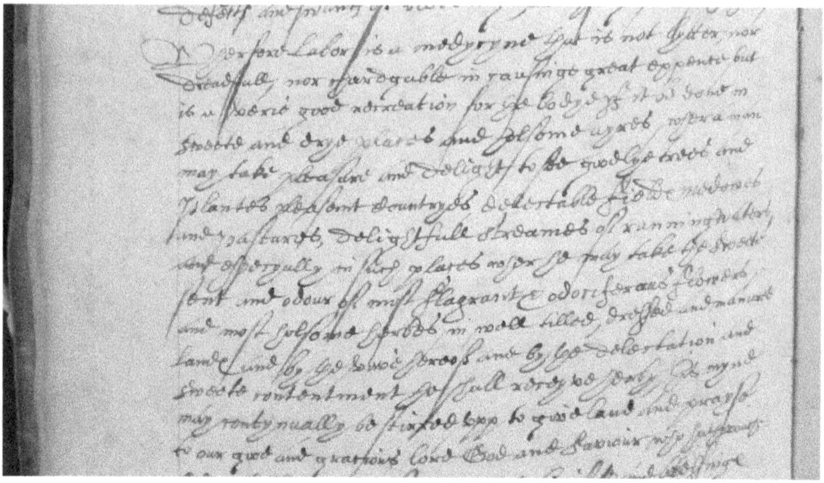

Figure 9 London, Wellcome Collection, MS 674, p. 48: a description of environments suitable for exercise from the *Regiment of Healthe*, a late sixteenth-century version of a treatise first composed by John Mirfield (d. 1407). Author's photo, by permission of the Wellcome Collection

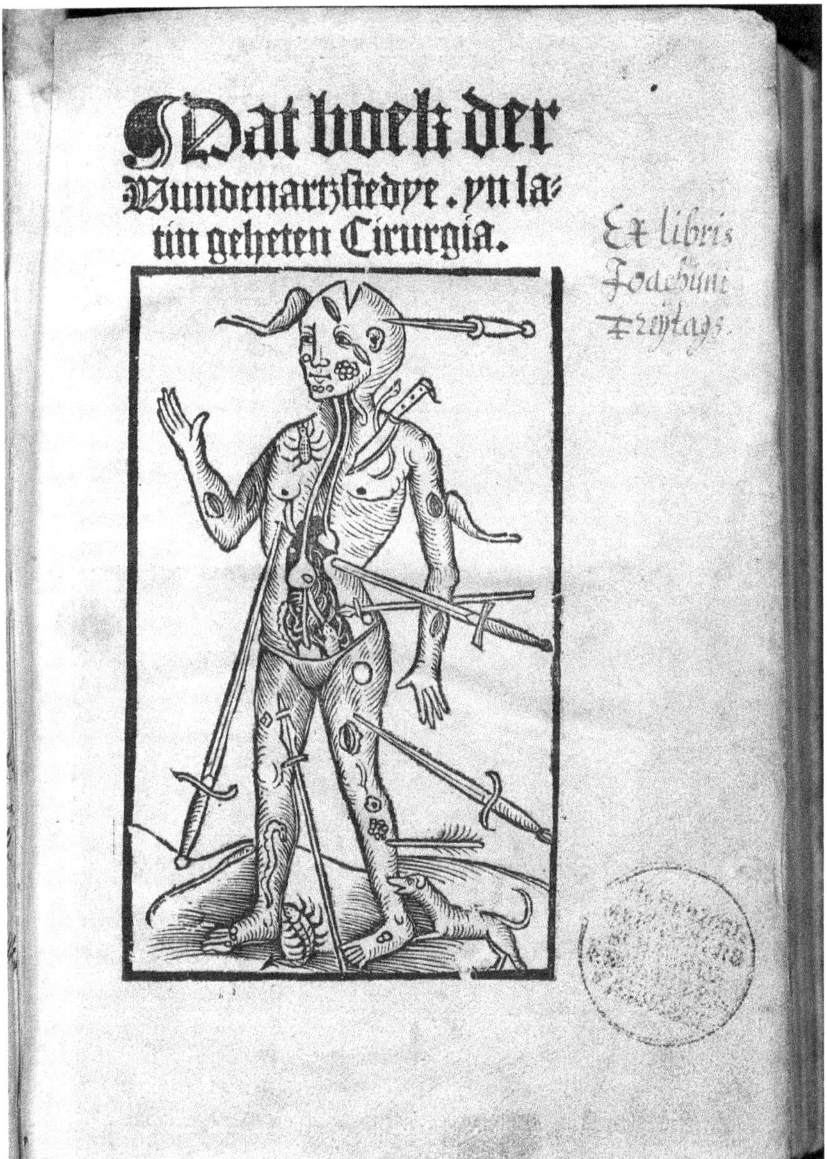

Figure 10 The first page of *Dat Boek der Wundenartzstedye. yn latin geheten Cirurgia* (1518), showing the so-called wound man. Image reproduced by permission of the Landesbibliothek Mecklenburg-Vorpommern Günther Uecker

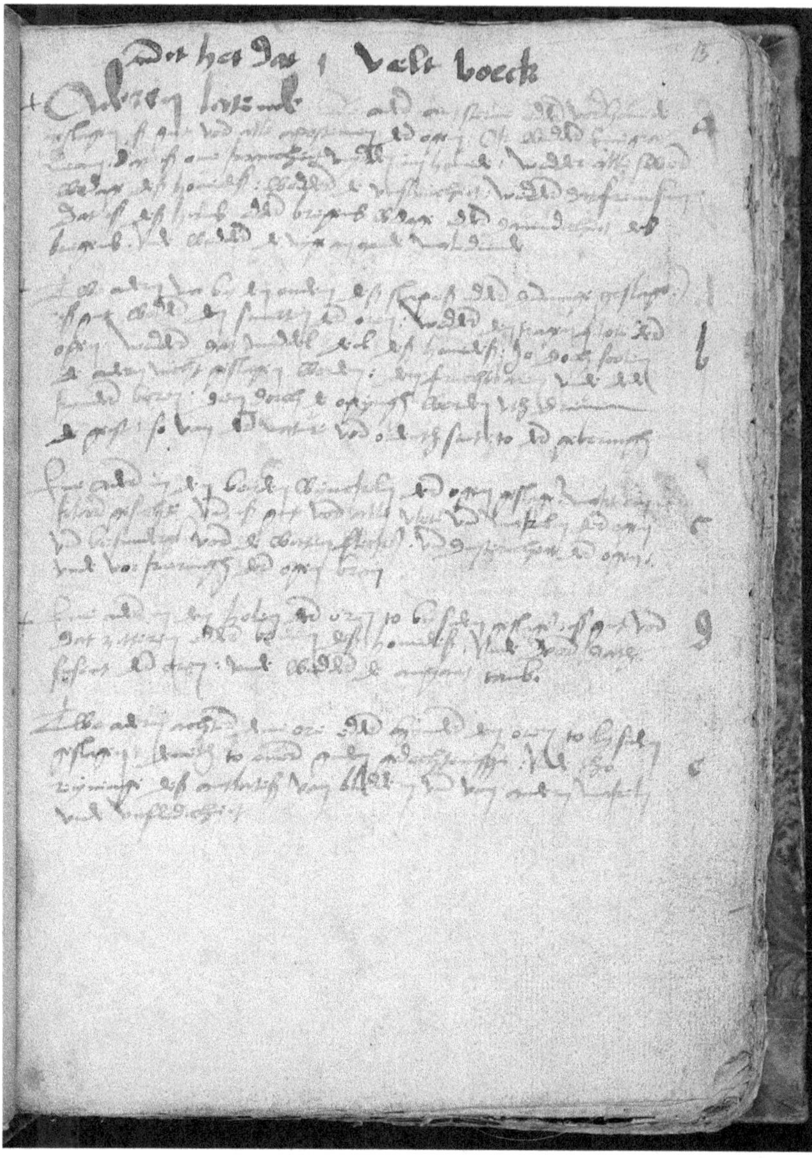

Figure 11 The first page of the fragment of a Low German translation of Hans von Gersdorff's *Feldtbuch der Wundarzney* known as *Dat velt bock*. Image reproduced by permission of the Kongelige Bibliotek, Copenhagen

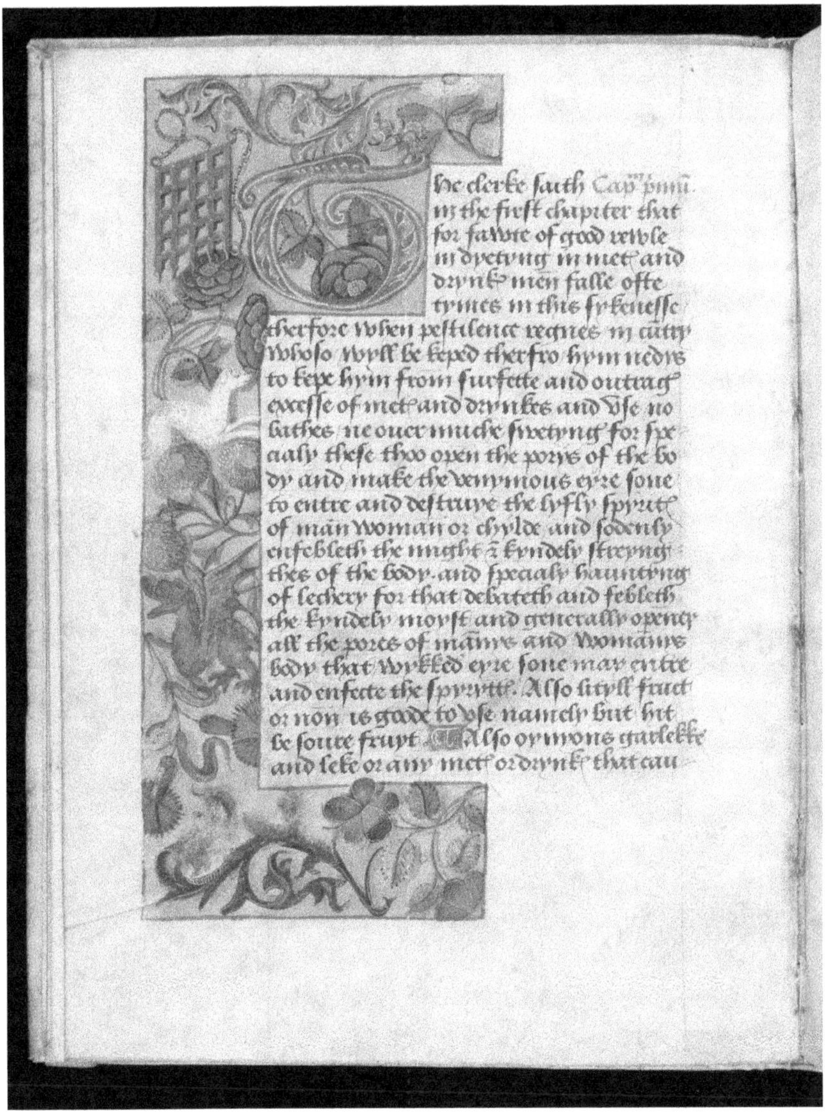

he clerke saith Cap^m primi.
in the first chapiter that
for fawte of good rewle
in dyetyng in mete and
drynke men falle ofte
tymes in this sykenesse
therfore when pestilence regnes in cuntry
whoso wyll be keped therfro hym nedis
to kepe hym from surfette and outrage
excesse of mete and drynkes and use no
bathes ne ouer muche swetyng for spe-
cialy these two open the pores of the bo-
dy and make the venymous eyre sone
to entre and destruye the lyfly spyrit
of man woman or chylde and sodenly
enfebleth the myght & kyndely strengt-
thes of the body. and specialy hauntyng
of lechery for that debateth and febleth
the kyndely moyst and generally openeth
all the pores of mannys and womanys
body that wykked eyre sone may entre
and enfecte the spyrittes. Also litill fruct
or non is goode to use namely but hit
be soure frupt. Also oynons garlekke
and leke or any mete or drynke that cau

Figure 12 A copy of John of Burgundy's plague tract, once owned by Margaret Beaufort (1443–1509), mother of Henry VII. Cambridge Fitzwilliam Museum MS 261, f. 23v. Image reproduced by permission of the Fitzwilliam Museum

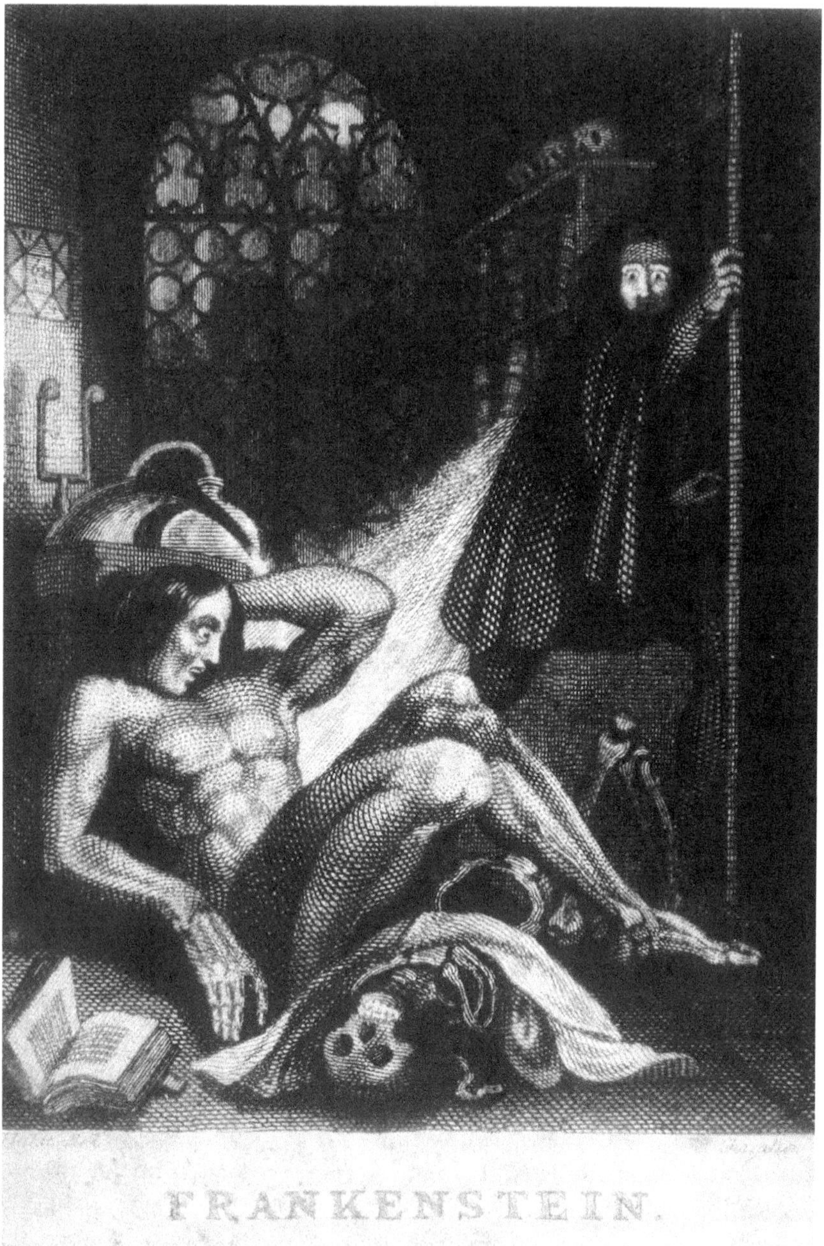

Figure 13 The frontispiece to the second edition (1831) of Mary Shelley's *Frankenstein; or The Modern Prometheus*. Getty Images

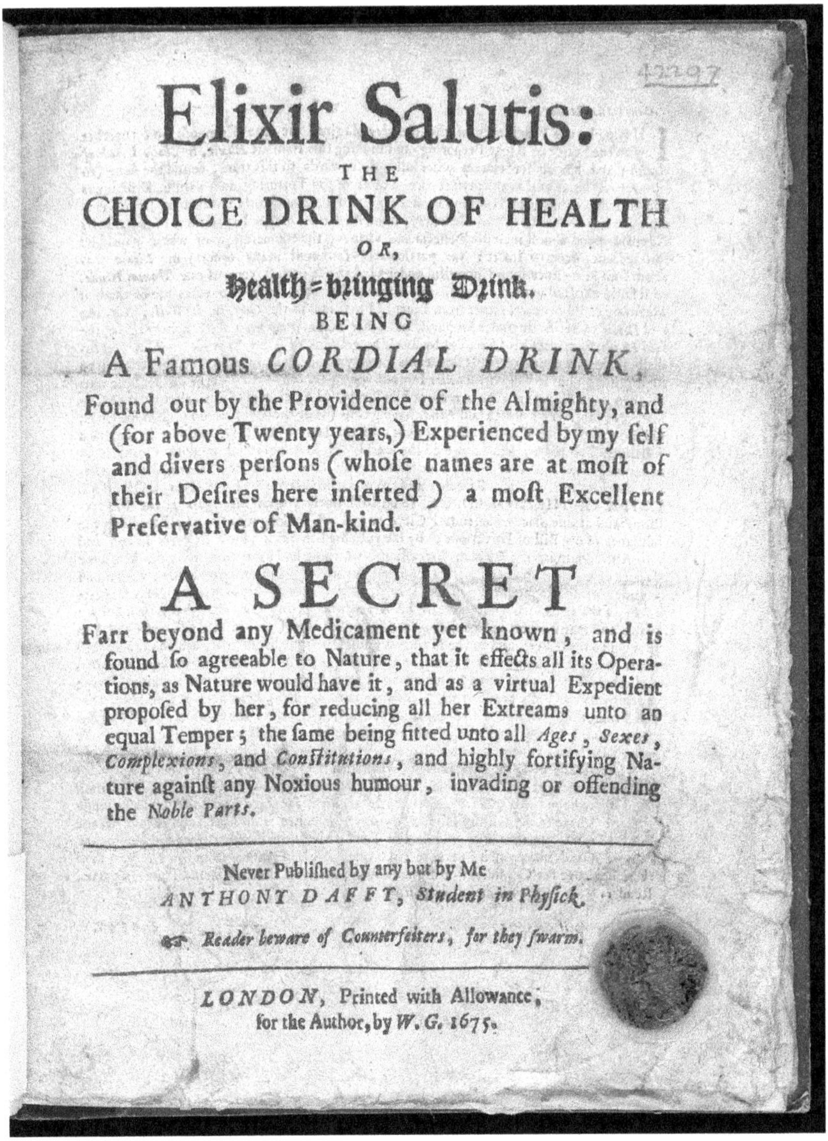

Elixir Salutis:

THE

CHOICE DRINK OF HEALTH

OR,

Health-bringing Drink.

BEING

A Famous *CORDIAL DRINK*,

Found out by the Providence of the Almighty, and (for above Twenty years,) Experienced by my ſelf and divers perſons (whoſe names are at moſt of their Deſires here inſerted) a moſt Excellent Preſervative of Man-kind.

A SECRET

Farr beyond any Medicament yet known, and is found ſo agreeable to Nature, that it effects all its Operations, as Nature would have it, and as a virtual Expedient propoſed by her, for reducing all her Extreams unto an equal Temper; the ſame being fitted unto all *Ages*, *Sexes*, *Complexions*, and *Conſtitutions*, and highly fortifying Nature againſt any Noxious humour, invading or offending the *Noble Parts*.

Never Publiſhed by any but by Me
ANTHONY DAFFT, Student in Phyſick.

☞ *Reader beware of Counterfeiters, for they ſwarm.*

LONDON, Printed with Allowance, for the Author, by *W. G.* 1675.

Figure 14 The title page of Anthony Daffy's pamphlet advertisement (1675) for his proprietary medicine, Elixir Salutis. A manicule at the foot of the page draws attention to a warning against counterfeiters. Wellcome Collection. Public domain mark

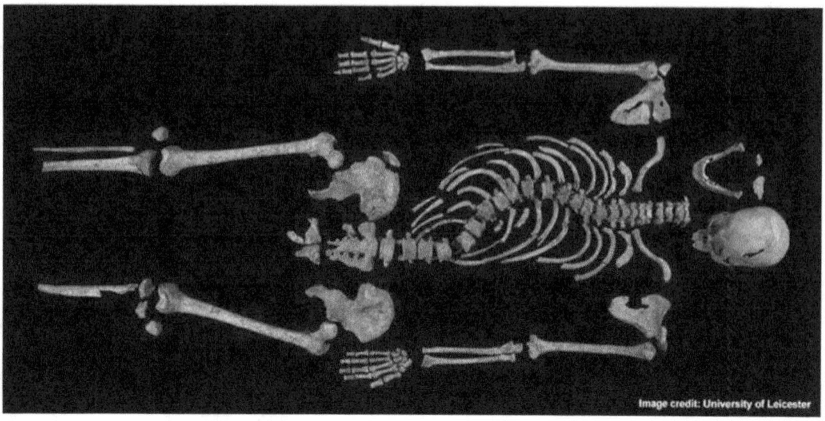

Figure 15 The remains of King Richard III showing scoliosis, or severe curvature of the spine. The wounds to his skull may also be noted, inflicted at the Battle of Bosworth Field (1485). Image courtesy of University of Leicester

Index

For EU product safety concerns, contact us at Calle de José Abascal, 56–1°,
28003 Madrid, Spain or eugpsr@cambridge.org.

www.ingramcontent.com/pod-product-compliance
Lightning Source LLC
LaVergne TN
LVHW011704200926
848484LV00004B/1070
* 9 7 8 1 0 0 9 1 0 0 0 9 0 *